THIS IS BIOETHICS

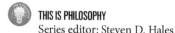

THIS IS PHILOSOPHY
Series editor: Steven D. Hales

Reading philosophy can be like trying to ride a bucking bronco—you hold on for dear life while "transcendental deduction" twists you to one side, "causa sui" throws you to the other, and a 300-word, 300-year-old sentence comes down on you like an iron-shod hoof the size of a dinner plate. *This Is Philosophy* is the riding academy that solves these problems. Each book in the series is written by an expert who knows how to gently guide students into the subject regardless of the reader's ability or previous level of knowledge. Their reader-friendly prose is designed to help students find their way into the fascinating, challenging ideas that compose philosophy without simply sticking the hapless novice on the back of the bronco, as so many texts do. All the books in the series provide ample pedagogical aids, including links to free online primary sources. When students are ready to take the next step in their philosophical education, *This Is Philosophy* is right there with them to help them along the way.

This Is Philosophy: An Introduction
Steven D. Hales

This Is Philosophy of Mind: An Introduction
Pete Mandik

This Is Ethics: An Introduction
Jussi Suikkanen

This Is Political Philosophy: An Introduction
Alex Tuckness and Clark Wolf

This Is Business Ethics: An Introduction
Tobey Scharding

This Is Metaphysics
Kris McDaniel

This Is Bioethics: An Introduction
Ruth F. Chadwick and Udo Schüklenk

This Is Epistemology
Adam Carter and Clayton Littlejohn

Forthcoming:

This Is Philosophy Of Religion
Neil Manson

This Is Philosophy: An Introduction, 2nd edition
Steven D. Hales

This Is Philosophy of Mind: An Introduction, 2nd edition
Pete Mandik

THIS IS
BIOETHICS:
AN INTRODUCTION

RUTH F. CHADWICK

UDO SCHÜKLENK

WILEY Blackwell

Registered Office
John Wiley & Sons, Inc., 111 River Street, Hoboken, NJ 07030, USA

Editorial Office
111 River Street, Hoboken, NJ 07030, USA

For details of our global editorial offices, customer services, and more information about Wiley products visit us at www.wiley.com.

Wiley also publishes its books in a variety of electronic formats and by print-on-demand. Some content that appears in standard print versions of this book may not be available in other formats.

Library of Congress Cataloging-in-Publication Data

Names: Chadwick, Ruth F., author. | Schüklenk, Udo, author.
Title: This is bioethics : an introduction / Ruth F. Chadwick, Udo Schüklenk.
Other titles: This is philosophy (Series)
Description: Hoboken, NJ : Wiley-Blackwell, 2020. | Series: This is philosophy | Includes bibliographical references and index.
Identifiers: LCCN 2020029285 (print) | LCCN 2020029286 (ebook) | ISBN 9781118770740 (paperback) | ISBN 9781118770795 (adobe pdf) | ISBN 9781118770733 (epub)
Subjects: MESH: Bioethical Issues | Bioethics
Classification: LCC R724 (print) | LCC R724 (ebook) | NLM WB 60 | DDC 174.2–dc23
LC record available at https://lccn.loc.gov/2020029285
LC ebook record available at https://lccn.loc.gov/2020029286

Cover design: Wiley

Set in 10.5/13pt Minion Pro by SPi Global, Pondicherry, India
Printed and bound by CPI Group (UK) Ltd, Croydon, CR0 4YY

10 9 8 7 6 5 4 3 2 1

CONTENTS

About the Authors   xi
Preface and Acknowledgments   xiii

1 Introduction to Ethics   **1**
  1.1 Religion and Ethics   6
  1.2 Law and Ethics   9
    1.2.1 Legal and Moral Rights   12
  1.3 Ethical Relativism   13
  1.4 Why be Ethical?   15

2 Ethical Theory   **21**
  2.1 Virtue Ethics   21
  2.2 Feminist Ethics   23
  2.3 Utilitarian Ethics   25
  2.4 Rule-Based Ethics   29
  2.5 'Georgetown Mantra'   30
    2.5.1 Non-Maleficence   31
    2.5.2 Beneficence   31
    2.5.3 Respect for Autonomy   31
    2.5.4 Justice   32
  2.6 Contract Theory   34

3 Basics of Bioethics   **37**
  3.1 History and Scope of Bioethics   37
  3.2 Who Can Claim to be a Bioethicist?   41
  3.3 Organizations and Journals   43
  3.4 Policy Advice   43

3.5	Common Arguments in Bioethics	45
3.6	Playing God	46
3.7	Unnatural and Abnormal	47
3.8	Dignity	48
3.9	Nazi Arguments in Bioethics	51
3.10	Slippery-Slope Arguments	53
3.11	Treating Someone as a Means	55

4   Moral Standing: What Matters **59**

4.1	Moral Standing and Moral Status	59
4.2	Species Membership	60
4.3	Sentientism	62
4.4	Capabilities	64
4.5	Biocentrism	64
4.6	Holism	65
4.7	The Future	66

5   Beginning of Life **69**

5.1	Introduction	69
5.2	Ethical Arguments about Reproductive Rights and Responsibilities	70
5.2.1	Reproductive Autonomy and the Right to Reproduce	70
5.2.2	Consequentialism and Procreative Beneficence	71
5.2.3	'Do No Harm' and the Person-Affecting Restriction	72
5.2.4	The Non-Identity Problem	72
5.2.5	Virtue Ethics	73
5.2.6	Feminist Bioethics	73
5.3	Issues in Assisted Reproduction	74
5.3.1	Genetic Relatedness: How Important Is It?	75
5.3.2	Issues of Selection in Reproduction	77
5.4	Embryos, Fetuses and Abortion	79
5.4.1	Fetuses	80
5.4.2	Judith Jarvis Thomson and the Violinist	81
5.4.3	The 'Future-Like-Ours' Argument	81
5.4.4	The Impairment Argument Against Abortion	82
5.4.5	Women's Character	82
5.4.6	Abortion and Fetal Transplants	83

5.4.7	Savior Siblings	84
5.4.8	Infants and Infanticide	85
5.4.9	Severely Disabled Infants	86
5.4.10	Acts and Omissions	87
5.4.11	Newborn Screening	88

6   Health Care Professional-Patient Relationship   91

6.1	Informed Consent	92
6.2	Paternalism	96
6.3	Deciding for Others	97
	6.3.1 Deciding for Others: Advance Directives	97
	6.3.2 Deciding for Others: Patients Who Never Had Capacity	98
	6.3.3 Deciding for Others: Incapacitated Patients without Advance Directives	99
6.4	Truth Telling	102
6.5	Confidentiality	105
6.6	Conscience Matters	107
6.7	Duty to Treat	110

7   Research Ethics   115

7.1	Elements of Ethical Research	117
7.2	Clinical Research: The Basics	118
7.3	Animal Experiments	120
7.4	Informed Consent	121
7.5	Trial-Related Injuries	122
7.6	Benefits	124
7.7	Benefiting from Evil	125
7.8	Ethical Issues Affecting Clinical Research Involving the Catastrophically Ill	127
7.9	Developing World	130
	7.9.1 Utility of Research Question	130
	7.9.2 Standards of Care	131

8   Genetics   135

8.1	Genetics and Genomics	135
	8.1.1 Introduction – Genetics, Genomics and Bioethics: Is Genetics Special?	135

| | | 8.1.2 | Issues in Clinical Genetics: Genetic Testing and Counseling | 137 |

8.1.2   Issues in Clinical Genetics: Genetic Testing
          and Counseling   137
          8.1.2.1   Non-Directiveness   137
          8.1.2.2   Children   138
          8.1.2.3   Genetic Screening   139
          8.1.2.4   Direct-to-Consumer Testing   139
8.2   Gene Therapy: Somatic and Germline   140
       8.2.1   Is There a Need for Germline Gene Therapy?   142
       8.2.2   Risks and Irreversible Consequences   142
       8.2.3   Future Generations and Lack of Consent   143
       8.2.4   The Iconic Significance of the Germline   143
       8.2.5   Gene Editing   144
8.3   Genomic Research   146
       8.3.1   The Human Genome Project   146
       8.3.2   Biobanks   147
       8.3.3   Feedback of Findings   149
8.4   Personalized Medicine   150
       8.4.1   Human Cloning – Therapeutic Cloning   151
       8.4.2   Reproductive Cloning   153
8.5   Other Issues in Genetics and Genomics   155

9   Enhancement   **159**
9.1   Introduction   159
9.2   Enhancement and Superhumans   159
9.3   The Meaning of Enhancement   161
       9.3.1   Enhancement and Improvement   161
9.4   Alternatives to the 'Improvement' Account   163
       9.4.1   Therapy–Enhancement Distinction   163
       9.4.2   Species-Normal Functioning   164
                9.4.2.1   Quantitative Account of Enhancement   164
       9.4.3   Enhancement: The Umbrella View   165
9.5   Ethical Issues   166
       9.5.1   Is Enhancement Necessary?   166
       9.5.2   Enhancement is Inevitable   167
       9.5.3   A Compromise Position?   168
       9.5.4   Autonomy   169
       9.5.5   The Habermasian Concern   169
9.6   Social Inequalities and Social Justice   170
       9.6.1   Consequences for the Future of Humans   171

9.7   Moral Enhancement   173
9.8   Cognitive Enhancement   176

10   Mental Health   181
10.1   Mental Illness   182
10.2   Diagnosis   184
10.3   Autonomy and Capacity   186
10.4   Least Restrictive Option   187
10.5   Best Interests   188
10.6   Treatment and Detention   189
       10.6.1   Detention for the Good of the Service User   189
       10.6.2   Detention for the Protection of Others   191

11   End of Life   195
11.1   Do You Want to Live Forever?   195
11.2   Terminology   201
11.3   Case for the Decriminalization of Assisted Dying   203
11.4   The Case Against the Decriminalization
       of Assisted Dying   207
       11.4.1   In-Principle Reasons Against
                Assistance in Dying   207
       11.4.2   Slippery-Slope Reasons Against
                Assistance in Dying   208
                11.4.2.1   Pereira v. Downie   210
11.5   Violation of Health Care Professional
       Values and Traditions   213

12   Justice and Health Care   217
12.1   Introduction   217
12.2   Types of Justice   218
       12.2.1   Justice and Discrimination   218
       12.2.2   Justice in Distribution   219
       12.2.3   Procedural Justice   220
       12.2.4   Justice and Exploitation   220
12.3   The Concept of Justice and its Connection
       With Equality   222
       12.3.1   Justice and Equality: Equal Treatment
                and Equal Consideration   222

12.3.2 Justice, 'Deserving', and Personal Responsibility   223
12.3.3 Justice is Giving People What They Need   225
12.4 Theories of Justice   225
12.4.1 Utility and Well-Being   225
12.4.2 Respect for Persons: Rights to Health and Health Care   228
12.4.3 John Rawls and Norman Daniels   229
12.4.4 The Capabilities Approach   231
12.5 Special Cases   232
12.5.1 Personalized Medicine and Justice   233

13 Population Health   **235**
13.1 Global Health Issues   235
13.2 Health Aid Obligations   236
13.2.1 Allocation Priorities   238
13.3 Population Health and Public Health   240
13.4 Communicable Disease Control Challenges   243
13.4.1 Take One: Michael Johnson is Not Culpable   245
13.4.2 Take Two: Michael Johnson is Culpable   245
13.4.3 Take Three: Shared Responsibility   246
13.4.4 Deterrence   246
13.4.5 Private Acts and Social Consequences   247
13.4.6 Novel Coronavirus Pandemic   248
13.4.7 Vaccines   251
13.5 Public Health Promotion   253
13.5.1 Communicable Disease: HIV   254
13.5.2 Non-Communicable Disease: Obesity   256

Bibliography   **261**
Further Reading   **287**
Index   **295**

ABOUT THE AUTHORS

Ruth F. Chadwick is Professor Emerita, Cardiff University and Visiting Professor, University of Leeds. She co-edits the journal *Bioethics* and has served on numerous bodies including the Council of the Human Genome Organisation. She is Fellow of the Academy of Social Sciences, the Hastings Center, New York, the Royal Society of Arts, the Royal Society of Biology and the Learned Society of Wales.

Udo Schüklenk holds the Ontario Research Chair in Bioethics in the Department of Philosophy at Queen's University at Kingston, in Canada. He is a Joint Editor-in-Chief of the journal *Bioethics*. Born in Germany, his academic career has included teaching and research appointments in Australia, South Africa, and the UK.

PREFACE AND ACKNOWLEDGMENTS

Jeff Dean, our then Commissioning Editor at Wiley-Blackwell, suggested to one of us in 2014 to produce a bioethics introductory text. It's always easier to agree to do a thing, then to actually do it, and so it took a 'mere' six years – on and off – to write this volume for you. Marissa Koors, Jeff Dean's successor at Wiley, and Steven D. Hales, our long-suffering series editor for the *This is Philosophy* series at Wiley-Blackwell, showed an unusual degree of patience with us, our book, and our seemingly never-ending delays. There is a German saying along the lines that a good thing takes time. You be the judge on *This is Bioethics*. Last but by no means least, we owe a great deal of gratitude to Nivetha Udayakumar, this book's Production Editor, for a job very well done.

Both of us have spent our academic careers in the field of bioethics, we jointly have been Editors of *Bioethics*, arguably the top philosophical bioethics journal, for more than two decades. Still, as we discovered, it's one thing to successfully author and publish peer reviewed research content, and it's quite another to write content specifically for introductory, and for teaching purposes. We deliberately did not review other bioethics textbooks to decide on what to include or not to include as far as the book's content is concerned. This book reflects what we think a student of bioethics, who takes an introductory course, should – at a minimum – have read and thought about. Quite deliberately we kept the tone informal, aiming to strike a conversational tone. We also quite deliberately avoided technical jargon where that was possible. Some of the external reviewers of an earlier draft of this manuscript had mixed feelings about this. We hope it works for you!

How should you go about reading this book? For one thing, we included plenty of links to sites that we hope won't have disappeared by the time you read this. Check them out if a particular issue catches your interest, and you want to know more. Definitely read Chapters 1–4, in that order, the other chapters can mostly be read independently of each other, even though we have taken care to cross-reference relevant content in other chapters where that was appropriate. We have also added guiding questions at the end of each chapter. We strongly recommend that you take a moment to reflect on these questions. Thinking about defensible answers will assist you in using the concepts and arguments you read about, and so you will gain a better understanding of them and their respective strengths and weaknesses. If you choose to do so, you would likely find yourself in a better position to defend your views on any number of current-day contentious issues, based on sound ethical analysis.

For any bioethics book you hopefully will – you should! – wonder where the authors 'are coming from', what their prior ethical commitments are, and to what extent those commitments influence the content you are reading. Scholars with religious commitments are likely to produce content and arguments that differ from those who are atheists, philosophical utilitarians will differ in their writings from philosophical deontologists, and so on and so forth. We were cognisant of this issue and tried to give views a fair shake, as it were, that we disagree with. We also included references to further reading written by authors whose views we do not necessarily share. Make use of that information, reflect on the arguments given, and form your own considered views.

Ruth F. Chadwick
Udo Schüklenk

1

INTRODUCTION TO ETHICS

Imagine you were running a medical non-governmental organization 1.1
(NGO) established to preserve the lives of poverty-stricken people in
resource poor countries. Your NGO is also usually among the first to provide emergency assistance in case natural emergencies such as tsunamis
strike. However, you did notice that **agencies evaluating your efficiency**[1]
give you a below-average ranking. That is a worry to your fundraising staff,
mostly because you rely on donations and such ratings are said to impact
eventually negatively, on your capacity to raise cash. You investigate what
the problem is, and it turns out that the ratings agency is critical of your
policy of responding mostly in cases of high-impact disasters such as earthquakes, floods or civil wars, because they invariably require a highly
resource intensive intervention. The agency's verdict is that, on the same
capital outlay, you could preserve more lives in developing countries if you
aimed at establishing medium- to long-term health delivery solutions,
including setting up primary health care facilities, beginning vaccination
programs, and other such relatively low-cost means. Chartering private jets
to fly emergency teams in response to disaster also preserves lives deserving
to be rescued, the ratings agency says, but it demonstrably results in a substantially lower number of lives preserved than you could preserve if you
dropped such actions in favor of working toward better health care delivery
infrastructure in the countries you usually serve.

So, if your objective is to preserve lives in developing countries, the rat- 1.2
ings agency might be correct in saying that you only preserve a suboptimal
number of lives. You could do better. Should you change your policy

This Is Bioethics: An Introduction, First Edition. Ruth F. Chadwick and Udo Schüklenk.
© 2021 John Wiley & Sons, Inc. Published 2021 by John Wiley & Sons, Inc.

though? After all, what the ratings agency proposes implies, if you were to act on it, is that those in most dire need, say those living in war-torn countries with minimal health care infrastructure, should be toward the bottom end of your list of priorities, because assisting such people would cost more – per life preserved – to succeed. All other things being equal, more lives could be preserved if the NGO focused on preserving not those most in need but perhaps those whose lives are also threatened but who could be helped with the deployment of fewer resources. Should we only care about the number of lives preserved then, or do other factors matter, too, such as for instance that some people, possibly due to no fault of their own, live in particularly abysmal conditions? Should we factor in the amount of resources required to nurse such people back to a life that would permit them to live independently? Should the age of the to-be-rescued matter? Should it matter whether they have a family dependent on their support? Questions such as these are fundamentally ethical questions. And this chapter is about ethics, it is about right and wrong, good and bad, and how we can go about judging alternative courses of action that might be available to us.

1.3   What are the fundamental purposes of ethics then? Unsurprisingly, one of the purposes of ethics is to *offer us clear action guidance when we are faced with a particular ethical problem*. Of course, action guidance alone is not sufficient, or else an ethicist telling us what we ought to do is not much different to what a preacher or a taxi driver, engineer or medical doctor could tell us. Anyone can admonish us to do this or do that when faced with an ethically challenging situation. All of us almost certainly would have a view on what the NGO chief should be doing. In fact, most of us would probably happily add our two cents worth of opinion when asked what we think the NGO chief should do, policy wise. Thinking about what she ought to do engages with ethics. That takes us to the second objective of ethics. It is to do with the normative justification for the advice given. The preacher's advice would derive its authority from the claim that she knows what a higher authority (say a God) wants us to do. Of course, many people today are **atheists**[2] or **agnostics**[3], and many of those who are not atheists hold a large number of different deities dear to their hearts, all with competing action guidance derived from their respective sources of godly wisdom. For all we know, the taxi driver and engineer might just reply that that is how they feel, or possibly even think, about the problem at hand. Let us leave aside, for a moment, that in ancient Greece there were no taxi drivers or engineers as we understand them today. During those times their approach to ethics would have led to them being labeled as **Sophists**[4], that is a group of philosophers who subscribe to the view that there are no objectively right or wrong answers to ethical questions, and that answers to ethical questions are at best reflective of someone's subjective, strongly held beliefs or feelings. What gave way to the birth of modern ethics were philosophers like **Plato**[5] and his teacher Socrates who both believed that we can actually give right or wrong answers to questions about what is ethically good or bad. We will return to their take on ethics in a moment. How might the medical doctor in our example respond to the ratings agency's ethical challenge? Trying to do better than the Sophists of the world, she could refer to guidance documents issued, for instance by her national **medical association's ethics people**[6], or those issued by the **World Medical Association**[7], a worldwide umbrella organization of national medical associations, or possibly the **World Health Organization**[8]. But what if these organizations have actually omitted to address the problem at hand in their guidance documents? And, even if they haven't, quotes from a document don't constitute an ethical justification. What if the document quoted got it wrong? It turns out, we have good reason to be skeptical about famous historical medical guidance documents such as the **Hippocratic Oath**[9]. Robert M. Veatch explains why the Hippocratic Oath isn't a document medical professionals ought to aspire to. According to Veatch just about everything is wrong about it, from its pledge to questionable Greek deities to a cultish understanding of medicine as a secretive practice to practical guidance that prioritizes individual patient interest always over the greater good of the society (Veatch 2012a, 10–29). To put it in Veatch's own words, 'the Oath is so controversial and so offensive that it can no longer stand alongside religious and secular alternatives. [...] The Hippocratic Oath is unacceptable to any thinking person. It should offend the patient and challenge the health care professional to look elsewhere for moral authority' (Veatch 2012a, 1). Veatch tells us, somewhat reassuringly, that the Oath today is used in so many variations in the world's medical schools that sometimes only fragments of the original document seem to remain (Veatch 2012b).

Be mindful that even if we agreed with the content of the Hippocratic 1.4 Oath or a modern version of it, and even if they actually provided us with guidance for the problem under consideration, we would again have to take it on authority that we should go about the NGO's problem in one particular way and not in another, unless there is an ethical justification provided why we should do what it admonishes us to do. Given that in our scenario almost certainly a lot of people would disagree with whatever it is that is being proposed, policy wise, it is important that we get our justification right. Here is where ethics' second purpose comes in: *In addition to providing us with action guidance, it must also provide us with a reasoned justification for the guidance given.*

1.5   As we will discover, there exist a fair amount of competing ethical theories, some more influential than others, that succeed with varying degrees of success both on the action guidance as well as on the action justification fronts. How should we decide then, which one, or which set of them to adopt for our own purposes? Is it ok to use one set of theories for one type of problem and another set of theories for another type of problem? Couldn't we choose virtue ethics for decision-making at the hospital bedside, but decide to go with utilitarianism for matters of resource allocation decision-making? But why should we do that, as opposed to just the opposite? Could there be a meta-theory telling us which theoretical approach to deploy under what circumstances? Or must we determine which theory is the right one and try to abide by its guidance as best as we can, even if some of that guidance is turning out to be deeply counter-intuitive? Well, these are questions about the nature of ethics; they ask whether there can be a true ethics, whether ethical statements must be of a particular kind, whether they can be objectively true or false, or whether they ultimately boil down to statements expressing our feelings. These and other questions are typically analyzed by meta-ethicists. They don't create ethical theories, rather they create theories *about* ethics. There are also legitimate questions about the extent to which ethical theories truly lend themselves to be 'applied' in some sense or another to problems such as the one mentioned at the beginning of this chapter. We will not engage in this sort of theorizing about ethics in this chapter, with the exception of a few paragraphs on ethical relativism. The reason for this is that the discussions driving meta-ethics are quite technical in nature, and by and large there is no obviously correct solution to many of its controversies. Even in the absence of final answers to many of these questions, however, it is still quite possible to undertake ethical analyses. As we will see throughout this book, some arguments are more plausible than others; certain types of argument, such as for instance slippery-slope based arguments, are almost always flawed, and so on and so forth. However, you can easily read up on meta-ethical theories elsewhere. (McMillan 2018) A wonderful source of superb on-line Open Access content, written usually by the some of the best philosophers around, is the *Stanford Encyclopedia of Philosophy*. Check, for instance its entry on **Theory and Bioethics**[10] (*or* Singer 1991, Part VI: The Nature of Ethics).

Bioethics is specifically concerned with normative issues in the biomedi-   1.6
cal and life sciences. Bioethicists hail these days from many different disciplines, including theology, law, medicine, sociology and many others.
Think of typical problems bioethicists analyze in their research: Should we
permit editing of the human genome? Is it acceptable to use sentient animals in clinical research? Is abortion wrong? Should we decriminalize
assisted dying in some form or shape?

Theologians will be able to tell us what a respective religion would make   1.7
of the problem at hand. Legal experts could tell us what the law currently
says with regard to any of these issues; they might even bravely venture into
an analysis suggesting that the law ought to be changed, if they find it to be
a violation of their country's constitutional values. Health care professionals
should be able to enlighten us with regard to what their professional values
have to contribute to these difficult questions. Sociologists do what sociologists do best, they will ask other people, say taxi drivers, philosophy students,
or a representative sample of a given group of people, what their take is on
these questions. None of these discipline-specific responses is capable of
enlightening us in a moral or ethical sense. The problems flagged earlier can
all be read as asking fundamental ethical questions, namely: Is it ethical to
alter the human genome? Is it moral to use sentient animals for clinical
research purposes? Is abortion immoral? Is the criminalization of assisted
dying ethically defensible? Bioethics relies first and foremost on *ethics* to
sustain reasonable defensible answers to these questions. However, it is not
the type of ethics that many armchair philosophers would recognize as traditional philosophical ethics. There can be no doubt that bioethical reasoning is not as deep or watertight as, for instance, meta-ethical reasoning aims
to be. Rather, with few notable exceptions, it aims to use the normative
frameworks, that we will be looking at, as a rough guide indicative of where,
say a utilitarian analysis would lead us when we consider the morality of
abortion and infanticide. These frameworks are also useful as tools of critical
analysis. They offer us some pretty good guidance and guidance justification
on the types of criteria that we might apply when we go about asking, for
instance whether abortion is a morally good or bad thing. They could even
help us taking a considered ethical stance on markers of fetal development
that are frequently argued over by activists and legislators alike. Say, does the
moment of conception confer moral standing on the developing human? Or,
does the capacity to feel anything matter? Does it matter whether an embryo
would be capable of surviving outside the pregnant woman's womb? These
are the types of questions that ethical theories can indeed shed new light on.

1.8   Before we try to get a quick overview of major ethical theories that exert today a significant influence in bioethics, let us briefly address a few other preliminary issues, namely, that of the place of religion in ethics, the relationship between the law and ethics, the challenge ethical relativism poses particularly in the context of bioethics, and the not completely irrelevant question of why we should bother being ethical to begin with.

1.1 Religion and Ethics

1.9   In the 1850s, the American Medical Association (AMA) was busy developing the content of its Code of Medical Ethics. At the time James L. Phelps, an influential Christian doctor in New York, tried to insert in this code a professional obligation for doctors to preach the truth of the Christian gospel. He referred to 'the paramount duty of the profession to their patients not only as regards their body in disease, but also the higher interests of the immortal soul. And hence, also the just claim of religion, the great anaesthetics of the immortal mind, to be considered an element of medicine or the healing art' (Baker, 2013, 181).

1.10   His fellow doctors at the AMA rejected his approach. They aimed instead for a secular code of medical ethics, and also a secular interpretation of professionalism for its members. Their reasons were entirely pragmatic, as you will notice when you read their rationale: 'the principles promulgated by this code have been assumed as a common ground upon which every member of the Association may stand, without reference to the distinctive principles or doctrines which distinguish the various religious societies existing among the vastly extended and diversified population of our country' (Baker, 2013, 181).

1.11   There are a number of problems with religious approaches to ethics. An obvious one is that many competing religions and claims about God or gods exist. It is in the nature of these claims that they cannot be tested. They rely entirely on belief. Given that we cannot know which of these gods – if any – is the right one, we are better off, in assuming with Plato that even if a God or gods exist, they would also need sound ethical reasons for their ethical judgments. Many people doubt the very idea that a God exists, mostly because of the enduring nature of the terrible evil that persists in the world. This just does not seem to gel well with the idea of an all-knowing, all-powerful and good God of most monotheistic religions. In any case, we do not have to settle the difficult question of whether a God or gods exist, thanks to an ancient Greek philosopher, Plato.

Plato created about 380 years before reportedly the historical Jesus was   1.12
born a now-famous dialogue aimed at addressing various questions to do
with the relationship between God or gods and ethics. The dialogue is
called *Euthyphro*[11] and plays out between Plato's teacher, Socrates and the
said Euthyphro. The story essentially takes place at a plaza in front of a
court house. Euthyphro busily prosecutes no less than his father for man-
slaughter committed on a murderer.

Euthyphro's relatives thoroughly disagree with his actions. When Socrates   1.13
(i.e. Plato's protagonist) questions Euthyphro, he replies, criticizing his relatives, 'Which shows, Socrates, how little they know what the gods think
about piety and impiety.' The dialogue goes on for some time, and during
the course of it Socrates makes among others a crucial point that is salient
to the question of the relationship between religion and ethics: He asks
whether something is good because the God or the gods approve of it, or
does God (or do the gods) approve of it because it is good. This is a crucial
question, because if something is good only because God or the gods
approve of it, ultimately what is good would depend entirely on God's or the
gods' preferences. For all we know God (or the gods) could have approved
of Euthyphro's actions. Slavery might be ok, too. This take implies that the
act in question is neither intrinsically good nor bad, because it is entirely
dependent on what God's or the gods' take is on the issue at hand. It is
doubtful that you consider this answer persuasive. Surely, if God or gods
exist, they need to have some sort of ethical reason for saying that something is morally wrong. Their answer cannot be completely arbitrary.

This leads us to an alternative answer to the question. That answer sug-   1.14
gests that some actions are good or bad as such, and that we are able to
evaluate such acts by means of using the tools of ethical analysis. Or, as
Gordon Graham suggests, 'Plato's arguments in Euthyphro seems [sic!] to
show that ... religion cannot logically serve as a ground for morality'
(Graham 2004, 185–188).

There are other problems, too. Most religious authoritative scriptures,   1.15
such as for instance the **Qur'an**[12] or the **Bible**[13], do not actually provide us
with clear guidance to address most ethical questions that we face during
our lives. Even if, miraculously, all of us would agree tomorrow that one of
these two documents, and not the Hindu's **Bhagavat Gita**[14] is the true God's
source of wisdom, we would discover that it actually would not help us to
solve the ethical problem our NGO-manager faces. We might as well go
back to Plato then and try to figure out ourselves what is right and what is
wrong, what is a good action and what is a bad one.

1.16   To what extent then will religious arguments feature in this book? Not to a great extent. It is true that extensive literature, for instance on the stances of Roman Catholicism, Judaism and Islam on assisted dying, exists. However, these kinds of arguments will not be dealt with in great depth in this book. The main reason for this is that these kinds of arguments are only of relatively uncontroversial moral significance to a subset of people, namely those who subscribe to the views expressed on this issue in the authoritative guidance documents published by these faiths. Obviously, Catholic arguments derived from the Bible only matter to Catholics or other Christians who accept the authoritative status of the Bible. The same holds true for Jewish and Muslim believers and their religious texts. Lisa Sowle Cahill, a professor of Christian Ethics, got it right **when she wrote**[15] (Sowle Cahill 1990):

> Public bioethical discourse (or public policy discourse) is actually a meeting ground of the diverse moral traditions that make up our society. Some of these moral traditions have religious inspiration, but that does not necessarily disqualify them as contributors to the broader discussion. Their contributions will be appropriate and effective to the extent that they can be articulated in terms with a broad if not universal appeal. In other words, faith language that offers a particular tradition's beliefs about God as the sole warrant for moral conclusions will convince only members of that tradition.

1.17   What we are looking for, therefore, are reasons that can best be described as *public reasons*[16]. Public reasons don't rely on us making metaphysical assumptions about gods, afterlives or any number of other beliefs requiring a significant leap of faith, so to speak. Instead they aim to persuade us by way of arguments that reasonably educated people from different cultural and religious backgrounds or other ideological persuasions can accept (Quong 2013). This approach is much in line with thinking going back to the seventeenth century, drawing a clear line between religion and the secular state. The state by necessity must remain neutral with regard to religious affairs, it cannot privilege one religion over another (Locke 1689). That way the citizens' right to hold their own religious beliefs is protected. If the state decided to privilege one religious viewpoint over another, inevitably unjust discrimination of the not-privileged religious point of view would follow. This view is supported by many judgments passed by the highest courts in various countries. For instance, a Canadian Supreme Court judgment notes, 'the State is in no position to be, nor should it become, the arbiter of religious dogma' (Syndicat Northcrest v. Amselem 2004).That makes perfect sense; how could judges possibly adjudicate conflicting views between religious dicta or even within a religion? They are not trained to do so. Accordingly, secular societies remain neutral vis a vis religious points of view, and public discourse relies on public reason based arguments. We will do the same in this book.

Let us turn now to the complex relationship between the law and ethics.   1.18

1.2 Law and Ethics

Although medical lawyers work on bioethical issues, this is not a book   1.19
about law. Nevertheless it is important briefly to consider the relationship between law and ethics and also the difference between legal and moral rights. Bioethics is a field in which reference is frequently made to ground-breaking legal cases (e.g. *Roe v Wade* in the United States), and to relevant legislation such as the Mental Health Act in the United Kingdom. To say of a proposed action 'That would be unlawful' is, however, not a knock-down argument against it.

Although you might hope that the law is always ethical and/or just, real-   1.20
ity quickly proves otherwise. The Nazis had laws discriminating unjustly against a whole range of German citizens at the time. Just think of their 1933 Law for the prevention of Hereditary Diseased Offspring. The Nazis used this law to justify the forcible sterilization of tens of thousands of Germans, even of many who did not suffer from hereditary conditions (Proctor 1988, Chapter 4). Apartheid South Africa had racist laws in place that one would hope will never reoccur on this planet. And before we get too optimistic about the state of laws in democratic societies, the Nazi sterilization laws were at the time widely applauded by eugenicists with direct lines to governments in many democratic countries. In fact, it turned out to be difficult to prosecute certain crimes committed against vulnerable people as war crimes, because similar laws were at the time in effect, for instance in the USA (Proctor 1988, 117).

In the light of these observations, several questions arise: (1) what exactly   1.21
is the difference between ethics and law? (2) Should the law enforce morality? (3) How should individuals, especially health professionals, behave when confronted with a law they believe to be unjust?

1. You may see that ethics and law have certain similarities: they are both social devices to make it possible for people to live together in relative harmony and for society to function. They both offer mechanisms for

dealing with areas of life where interests conflict. Of course, the sanctions that the law has are much more far-reaching than those of ethics, including criminal and civil proceedings, punishments and penalties. The sanctions that ethics has, however, are not negligible. While ethics relies on the power of arguments as far as its action guidance and justification are concerned (as opposed to legislation and precedent in the case of law), the power of persuasion can be considerable. Some have suggested that if there is a strong ethical consensus on a particular matter, say that slavery is bad, what likely would enforce this consensus – if there were no law prohibiting slavery – is societal pressure such as peer pressure. Societal disapprobation can be a very powerful instrument in the absence of legally enshrined norms in a particular matter. Arguably these societal norms can be a force for good as well as a force for bad depending on the circumstances – for example disapproval of voluntary childlessness as 'selfish' may make it difficult for people to choose that. You will surely be able to think of other possibilities.

In addition to sanctions, law and ethics differ in scope. Here is what the American Medical Association has to say on the subject of the difficult relationship between law and ethics: 'Ethical values and legal principles are usually closely related, but ethical obligations typically exceed legal duties.' Although there is clearly some overlap where we regard actions as both morally wrong and rightly prohibited by law, such as violence against the person and theft, morality covers a much wider area of our relationships with each other, with other species, and indeed our responsibilities for our own health. There is a question about how far the law should extend into policing the moral sphere. Think of examples such as drug use, sexuality, and smoking.

2. Should the law, then, be designed to enforce morality? A lot of ink has been spilled in response to this question. The American Medical Association probably got it right: in a good society ethical values and the law should be reasonably closely aligned. There is a potential ambiguity here, however. Some people might think it important that the law is attuned to the social values prevailing at the time (which may be discriminatory as in the examples above), rather than to what can be justified by ethical argument. It is the latter that is relevant in the context of the present discussion. It is important to note, however, that the law can play an important role in changing attitudes. Outlawing discrimination, for example, as well as arguing against it from an ethical point of view, can have an influence in changing attitudes in the longer

term. So legalizing marriage equality may play a part in decreasing anti-gay sentiments, for example.

Is there a criterion to aid us in deciding where the law should not intervene? A liberal legal philosopher, Joel Feinberg, argued some time ago that what he describes as 'harmless immoralities' should not be outlawed (Feinberg 1990). What are harmless immoralities? Basically they are immoralities that affect only the person who, being fully informed and cognizant of the relevant information, voluntarily engages in immoral conduct. This begs the question, of course, whether there can even be such a thing as a 'harmless immorality'. It is worth noting perhaps that there are some kinds of ethical theories, going broadly under the term 'consequentialist theories' that deny that there is such a thing as a 'harmless immorality'. To their mind only harmful conduct can sensibly constitute something immoral. Calling something a 'harmless immorality', on that account, would at best be considered a contradiction in terms.

3. It is always an open question whether the law has got it right on a given issue. This can put people in a difficult situation when they are confronted by a situation where they think the law is wrong. Think of examples of this, such as a doctor who thinks it would be right to prescribe a prohibited substance to bring relief to a patient, or to perform a termination of pregnancy in a society where it is unlawful. Or a doctor being required to participate in a torture program in the context of an oppressive dictatorship. The American Medical Association says:

> In some cases, the law mandates unethical conduct. In general, when physicians believe a law is unjust, they should work to change the law. In exceptional circumstances of unjust laws, ethical responsibilities should supersede legal obligations.
>
> The fact that a physician charged with allegedly legal conduct is acquitted or exonerated in civil or criminal proceedings does not necessarily mean that the physician acted ethically.

As we know, working to change the law can take a long time, and does not help in immediately pressing cases. In some circumstances, it can require significant personal costs. The arguments for such legal change, as well as the arguments concerning choice of action in difficult circumstances, are the proper subject matter of ethics. The fact that an action is unlawful, or legally required, is clearly an important factor, but not the conclusive one, in considering its ethical justifiability.

1.2.1 Legal and Moral Rights

1.23   You will find that in many an ethics debate arguments for or against a particular solution are framed in the language of rights. While the topic of rights is enormous and multidimensional, it is worth pausing at this point to reflect on the difference between legal and moral rights. Let's think of examples. Abortion is an obvious one. Does the (legal) prohibition of abortion by giving (legal) protection to the fetus violate a woman's (moral) right to control her body? Are our (moral) autonomy rights violated in societies where assisted dying remains criminalized? Almost certainly you will be able to add your own examples here.

1.24   Of course, rights exist in law when they are backed by legislation, contract or precedent. Both legal and moral rights may be described as negative or positive. The negative ones are rights not to be interfered with or prevented from doing something, such as expressing publicly an opinion that might offend others.

1.25   While such a negative right may require social resources to protect it, positive rights are generally more expensive in that they require resources. A positive legal right could be your entitlement to access welfare payments in case you become unemployed. Such a legal right only exists in societies where such a right has been established.

1.26   What do these kinds of positive and negative legal rights have in common? One commonality is that the state or some other clearly identifiable institution is going to back them up. The state will enrol you in its welfare program in case you register with the unemployment benefits program on your becoming unemployed. Similarly, in the free speech case: the state will not only not interfere with your offense causing sermon, it might even have to deploy police to protect your legal right to say what you wish to say. *Enforcement then is a crucial feature of legal rights, so is their codification in law.*

1.27   When we turn to moral rights, these are not backed up by law, but by argument. Of course, an argument that someone has a moral right to something may be used to argue for a legal right. A context in which the difference between negative and positive rights becomes very clear is in the context of reproduction. Think of the right not to be involuntarily sterilized (negative right) versus the right to assisted reproduction (positive). These can be regarded as moral rights which may also be backed up by law (but historically have not been in all times and places, as we have seen). Moral rights such as these can be the conclusions of moral argument. For example, an argument that there are moral reasons to give you a certain social good, such as access to assisted reproduction, could conclude by using the language of rights, i.e., say that because of x, y and z, you have a right to it. It could, for instance, be argued on consequentialist grounds that it is good for society as a whole if individuals who cannot reproduce without technological have rights to access such assistance. On the other hand, there are certain moral views that take rights as the starting points, rather than the conclusions of moral argument. On such a view, however, it is negative rights that are typically regarded as starting points and prior to positive ones. For example, if we take as a starting point that humans are by nature autonomous beings, and that interference with an individual's freedom needs to be justified, this might be expressed in terms of individuals having rights, period. It is not that they are given rights in order to promote some social good.

You may also want to look out for arguments which purport to show that other species have rights, and the different ways in which such rights are supported.   1.28

1.3 Ethical Relativism

Ethical relativist[17] arguments take various forms, but those most commonly found in bioethics go along these lines: We should not judge today terrible things that occurred in other cultures and societies many years ago. After all, perhaps what we consider unethical today was considered perfectly above board in another age. And in any case, even if we disagree with the views and practices held at the time, we surely have no ethical proof akin to scientific proof, that what occurred in the past is truly and objectively wrong.   1.29

Bernard Williams famously described this take on ethical relativism as 'vulgar relativism' (Williams 1974–1975). He thinks it is vulgar, because it is obviously flawed. Those who declare that it is normatively wrong to form a normative judgment on the goings-on in a different cultural context and/or time in history would seem to form a normative judgment that, if they are correct, they would not be able to form. They hold the view 'that "right" (can only be coherently understood as meaning) "right for a given society"; that "right for a given society" is to be understood in a functionalist sense; and that (therefore) it is wrong for people in one society to condemn, interfere with, etc., the values of another society' (Williams 1972, 20). In Williams' view this "is clearly inconsistent, since it makes a claim in its third   1.30

proposition, about what is right and wrong in one's dealings with other societies, which uses a nonrelative sense of "right" not allowed for in the first proposition' (Williams 1972, 21).

1.31   In some ways this issue seems also to be a bit of a red herring. The important question is not whether something that occurred in the past was morally good or bad, even though that could have a bearing on, for instance the reparations questions in the context of slavery. Rather the important question is whether *today* when we need to make a normative decision on whether we ought to do a certain thing or omit to do a certain thing, it would be morally right or morally wrong to do so (Williams 1974–1975). What people have done a long time ago realistically cannot assist us in answering that question. Our context today will be very different from the context potentially hundreds of years ago. Our knowledge base is different, our values will have evolved, our resource situation will be different, and so on, and so forth.

1.32   Ethical relativists tend to make two distinct claims: There is widespread disagreement on ethical questions, and this disagreement is not merely a matter of historical distance as ongoing controversies about the morality of abortion, marriage equality for same sex couples and assisted dying demonstrate. This claim is empirically uncontroversial, but the meaning of this disagreement for the possibility of ethics is still subject to controversy. After all, we cannot possibly sustain – without trying – a stance that maintains that it will be always impossible to make moral progress on these issues. The second claim is more far reaching, it suggests that there is no objective, universal and trans-historical truth in an ethical judgment. Rather ethical judgments are a reflection of their times as it were.

1.33   What can be said with regard to these claims? For starters, it might well be true that we have no ethical proof comparable to the kind of proof you would come across in logic or physics. However, consider this: Even in the sciences, scientific paradigms (i.e. scientific truths that have been taken for granted, sometimes for centuries) are replaced radically or evolutionarily by other paradigms. After all, that is the story of science! Scientific truth then seems a more relative matter than most people are willing to concede. However, demonstrably progress is made. Change usually occurs when the old paradigm can be proven faulty and a new paradigm is better able to explain and predict the phenomenon in question. There is arguably no equivalent to this in ethics. However, progress in ethics undoubtedly occurs, too. Today we pretty much agree that slavery is unethical, and we even agree by and large on the reasons for this conclusion. In some ways progress in ethics is not dissimilar to progress that occurs in other Humanities' disciplines. For instance, do we have incontrovertible proof of the causes that ultimately led to Hitler's ascendancy to Chancellor in the dying days of the Republic of Weimar? Historians speak much to the causes, but truth be told, their idea of causation is very different to that of a physicist. And yet, we will still find most historians agreeing on some of the fundamental causes that led to Hitler's coming to power. We encounter similar situations with regard to research conducted by researchers working in other disciplines, such as anthropologists, geographers, and even lawyers, yet the charge that they are unable to prove their conclusions objectively 'right' isn't usually leveled against them. Perhaps progress should be measured taking into account the peculiarities and idiosyncrasies of particular disciplines.

Gordon Graham, a Scottish philosopher and ordained Anglican priest, 1.34 seems to have hit the nail on its head when he writes, 'Provided we accept that our conclusions will in all likelihood fall short of absolute proof or incontrovertible demonstration, the most plausible and intelligent approach to moral questions and disagreements is just to see how far clear and cogent reasoning – assembly of the relevant facts, analysis of the relevant concepts and adherence to the rules of logic – can take us' (Graham 2004, 13). He goes on to say that a point of view that he describes as 'soft objectivism' holds 'that for any moral matter reason may be able to point us to a resolution that (…) is clearer and more cogent than any other and which it would be logically possible but unreasonable to dispute' (14).

1.4 Why be Ethical?

That is an odd question, isn't it? Let us first be clear though about the mean- 1.35 ing of this question! Philosophers have, naturally, argued about that, too. What we are interested in is essentially a question about the authority of morality. Why should someone who subscribes to a particular morality, say utilitarianism, actually act according to what a consistent utilitarian analysis would conclude she ought to do when that is going to result in her losing out in some way, and others, possibly even others in far-away lands, winning? Why act altruistically when an egoistic course of action would result in a much better pay-off for her, others be more or less damned? Truth be told, there is no answer that we have come across that would persuade everyone, i.e. there is no answer following logically from uncontroversial normative premises. In what follows we offer a few possible answers to this question without claiming that they constitute some kind of trump card ending the debate.

1.36   Apparently, knowledge of ethics has only a limited effect on the moral behavior of ethicists themselves. Strangely, professionals who work full-time 'in ethics' **do not in the average appear to be much more ethical**[18] than other people (Schwitzgebel 2015).

1.37   Some philosophers have argued that moral judgments in their own right provide strong **reasons for acting**[19] in a particular way that is guided by those moral judgments. The idea here is that moral properties such as 'right' and 'good' motivate us to act in certain ways and they do so in a manner sufficiently powerful to override other considerations, provided we have a proper understanding of what is morally required of us. Simply put, if we reflected on whether or not we ought to donate to the medical NGO described at the beginning of this chapter and we concluded that it would be the morally right thing to do for us, we are also provided with a motive for actually donating to the NGO.

1.38   In any case, isn't it self-evident that we should act morally? Certainly some philosophers hold that view. With the notable exception of psychopaths most of us do experience bouts of guilt and bad conscience each time we act in a manner that we consider immoral. There might be good evolutionary reasons for this response, too (Katchadourian 2010, 167ff). Most economists will tell you that our actions are driven entirely by self-interest. And yet, if you look a bit around yourself, you can't help but notice that many of us engage in actions that don't seem immediately driven by selfish motives. Tax incentives or no, many of us donate for instance to support charitable causes benefiting people in far-flung corners of the planet, even though there is no demonstrable pay-off to us. Just think of **Life You Can Safe**[20], an initiative by the Australian philosopher Peter Singer. On the initiative's website **he tells a story**[21] of a little girl falling into a pond. Unable to swim, she thrashes about in the water and is about to drown, unless you step in to rescue her. Of course, stepping into the water would wreck your shoes. No doubt most, if not all of us would step into the water to rescue the girl that is struggling for her life, despite the fact that there is no immediate benefit to ourselves, and despite the fact that we would actually incur an inconvenience, possibly even a loss in terms of wrecked clothes. Most of us would do this despite the fact that a legal duty to rescue is not enshrined in the laws of many a country. Singer then goes on to make the point that there is no ethically relevant difference between that girl and another girl that might die a preventable death in a far-away resource poor country because we have not donated the equivalent dollar amount of a pair of wrecked shoes to an initiative aimed at preventing her death. *Life You Can Safe* encourages us to **volunteer**[22] a certain amount of our income to initiatives aimed at preserving such lives.

Consider a completely different example of altruistic behavior. Claire Aitchison, an Australian academic, clearly somewhat disenchanted with the work climate at her Sydney based university, traveled in 2012 to Bali, an Indonesian island. **You might want to read**[23] her account of this visit where she writes of her experiences: 1.39

> Kindness in Bali seems to be a national pastime. I was blown away by the numerous, daily acts of kindness. We were the recipients of so many kindnesses arising from concerns for our welfare, health, enjoyment, comfort and so on; it was almost unnerving. We were invited into people's homes, to ceremonies at the village temple, we were offered food; the list goes on. Each morning and evening someone came to our house to lay out beautifully constructed offerings to protect us, and the home. It seemed extraordinary that this woman would care so much for the welfare of strangers, but by virtue of coming to the village, we were welcomed into their sphere of kindness, it would seem, without question.

According to her account the villagers she met engaged in numerous acts of altruistic kindness. The question we are asking here, is, of course, why should they bother doing this to begin with. It turns out to be the case that to many people living an ethical life means living a life that is meaningful to them. A purely egoistic life involving the accumulation of ever more wealth just doesn't seem to satisfy most of us. To be fair, there are exceptions. Just think of the difference between two billionaires, the late Apple boss Steve Jobs and the investor Warren Buffett. Buffett **aims to donate 99 percent**[24] of his wealth to charitable causes before his death. Steve Jobs, on the other hand, knowing of his impending death, **refused to part with his wealth**[25]. Buffett isn't alone in his quest. To give you just one further example, **Charles Feeney**[26] gave his interest in a major chain of duty free stores to a charitable organization that he founded. His objective was, as he put it, to use his wealth to 'help people.' Since then the charity has disbursed several billion US dollars in a variety of countries. Feeney is proud not to own a house or a car. He travels mostly in economy class and makes a point of wearing a watch not worth more than about 15 US $.   1.40

1.41 Well, be these anecdotal cases as they may, it seems true at least for those who can't find meaning in material wealth alone that living a more ethical life is one possible answer to that all too human yearning for a meaningful life. You might be surprised to learn that many a developed country medical school's professors leave their comfortable resource rich environments behind to volunteer time in resource poor parts of the world. They volunteer their time and expertise under difficult conditions to help others. Peter Singer observes quite sensibly, 'If we are looking for a purpose broader than our own interests, something that will allow us to see our lives as possessing significance beyond the narrow confines of our wealth or even our own pleasurable states of consciousness, one obvious solution is to take up the ethical point of view' (Singer 2011, 293). A good life might only be truly possible for us if we behave morally. Helping strangers could be part of that package.

1.42 Another reason to be ethical appeals ironically to our enlightened self-interest, so perhaps the economists mentioned earlier were not that far off. It has been suggested that we all would be better off if everyone behaved ethically. There is some truth in this, but it also seems to be the case that this claim can only be correct if many or most people behave ethically, otherwise it is quite likely that in an unjust society those behaving ethically would lose out to the unethical people around them. Perhaps that is one explanation for the enduring popularity of contractualist models in ethics. As we shall see in the next chapter, these are models that rely on us voluntarily agreeing to behave in particular, hopefully ethical ways in our interactions with each other. Contractualism with its appeal to our enlightened self-interest relies on reciprocity and on our living up to the promises we make to each other. Much more could – and has been – said by way of answering the question *why be ethical*. If you want to read up on this surprisingly difficult question, you might try Singer (2011, Chapter 12).

1.43 Let us turn now to influential ethical theories that exert significant influence in bioethics. Many books and articles have been published about each of these theories. There is not enough space in this volume to discuss each of these theories at great length. The objective of the subsequent expositions is to flag the main features of these theories as far as they affect reasoning in bioethics; space will also be given to the main criticisms leveled against them. Ideally what you should be able to take away from these expositions is a rough-and-tumble idea of what kinds of issues matter with regard to particular ethical theories. You should be able to make use of these features when you aim to analyze particular ethical issues. Be under no misapprehension: you won't have gained an in-depth understanding of ethical theory at the end of this book. Pay particular attention to the kinds of issues that are relevant for the purposes of these different approaches. You will find that, looking at the same problem, often but not always different features of the same problem matter to those who advance one or another of these theories. Do keep in mind the two primary objectives of ethics: action guidance and action justification. Ask yourself to what extent the following ethical approaches meet those objectives.

Questions

What is your answer to the question of 'why be ethical'? Did you find any of the answers given by ethicists persuasive?

Website Links

1   http://www.charitynavigator.org/
2   http://www.iep.utm.edu/atheism/
3   http:/www.iep.utm.edu/atheism/
4   http:/plato.stanford.edu/entries/sophists/
5   http:/plato.stanford.edu/entries/plato-ethics/
6   https://www.ama-assn.org/delivering-care/ethics/code-medical-ethics-overview
7   https://www.wma.net/what-we-do/education/medical-ethics-manual/
8   http://www.who.int/en/
9   https://www.nlm.nih.gov/hmd/greek/greek_oath.html
10 http://plato.stanford.edu/entries/theory-bioethics/
11 http://classics.mit.edu/Plato/euthyfro.html
12 http://quran.com/
13 http://www.bartleby.com/108/
14 http://www.bhagavad-gita.org/index-english.html/
15 http://www.thefreelibrary.com/Can%2Btheology%2Bhave%2Ba%2Brole%2Bin%2B%22public%22%2Bbioethical%2Bdiscourse%3F-a09330141/
16 http://plato.stanford.edu/entries/public-reason/
17 http://plato.stanford.edu/entries/moral-relativism/
18 http://aeon.co/magazine/philosophy/how-often-do-ethics-professors-call-their-mothers/
19 http://plato.stanford.edu/entries/moral-motivation/

20   http://www.thelifeyoucansave.com/
21   http://www.youtube.com/watch?feature=player_embedded&v=
     onsIdBanynY
22   https://www.thelifeyoucansave.org/
23   http://blogs.lse.ac.uk/impactofsocialsciences/2013/02/20/bali-kindness-
     and-the-neoliberal-enterprise-university/
24   http://www.standard.co.uk/business/warren-buffett-donates-another-178bn-
     in-plan-to-give-away-99-of-wealth-6419853.html/
25   http://dealbook.nytimes.com/2011/08/29/the-mystery-of-steve-jobss-
     public-giving/
26   http://www.atlanticphilanthropies.org/history-and-founder/

2

ETHICAL THEORY

In this chapter, we will give you a rough and tumble overview of major 2.1 ethical theories. They are foundational for much of what follows in terms of the arguments and analyses offered when we look at specific issues in bioethics.

2.1 Virtue Ethics

One of the oldest types of ethical theories can be traced back to an ancient 2.2 Greek philosopher, **Aristotle**[1]. He developed it in his classic **Nicomachean Ethics**[2]. The basic premise driving **Aristotle's account of ethics**[3] is tied to what he considers the highest good in our lives. He identifies that as a flourishing or a good life. There is undoubtedly some truth in this, a good life is surely what we all aspire to, and this good life is not a means to achieve some other objective, rather it is an end in its own right. According to Aristotle a virtuous life is such a flourishing life. But, lest we want to be accused of a question begging account of ethics, what exactly is a virtue? According to Aristotle, a virtue is a kind of character trait or disposition to have feelings resulting in actions that will permit us to live flourishing lives.

What kind of virtuous character traits should a good doctor have? 2.3 Honesty presumably, and integrity perhaps, among others. We can find other such virtues mentioned in the Hippocratic Oath, such as the virtue of maintaining patient confidentiality. This all seems not unreasonable. Surely, we should be able to identify character traits that promote a flourishing, good life and aim to develop those. To be fair, there seems to be more than one possible flourishing, good life possible. Different people will hold different views with regard to what would make their life a flourishing life, but some features hopefully can be agreed upon by well-intentioned, reasonable people, such as for instance living in safe neighborhoods, being in good health, and other basic necessities of life.

2.4   How are we going to decide though whether an agent acted virtuously in a particular tricky situation? Would it be virtuous for a doctor to maintain the confidentiality of the doctor–patient relationship and not disclose a patient's HIV infection to her husband or would the virtuous doctor disclose the HIV infection to protect the husband? It turns out that **virtue ethics**[4] offers space to defend both kinds of actions. The reason for this is that virtue ethics is agent-focused rather than rule- or outcomes-oriented. A virtue ethicist would be concerned about the question of whether or not the doctor possesses a virtuous character, whether or not the doctor had all the relevant information, whether or not the doctor pondered carefully about his or her preferred course of action, and so on and so forth. Whatever the doctor does is right if and only if that is what a person of good character would do. Interestingly, virtue ethics does not require the doctor to take the place of an impartial observer, unlike other ethical theories that we will be looking at in just a moment. On this account it would be quite acceptable for the doctor to prioritize her patient's needs over those of other people who are professionally further removed from the doctor. In fact, the doctor would not necessarily be faulted for prioritizing her friends and relatives over other patients.

2.5   This strategy to explain what makes an action right has been criticized on various counts. The only way to determine whether an action is the right action, is by looking at what a person of virtuous character would do. Evidently, this risks becoming a circular enterprise. Once we have determined that someone is a virtuous person, *whatever* she decided to do would then become a right course of action. But, let's assume that our doctor is a virtuous person, how is she supposed to determine which virtue is the applicable one in this case? Is the applicable virtue the one requiring her to maintain confidentiality, or is it about preventing harm to another patient? It is not a terrible stretch to suggest that a virtuous doctor could go either way here, depending on which set of virtues is strongest. Critics of virtue ethics have expressed doubts about this approach's ability to be action guiding.

2.6   Virtue ethicists respond to this by saying that as far as they are concerned, even if both courses of actions were followed by different virtuous doctors, both actions could be morally acceptable actions. They do away with the idea that ethics requires necessarily that one particular course of action is right, and that all other competing courses of action must be necessarily wrong.

Another assumption made by virtue ethicists has come in for sustained 2.7
criticism, too. Virtue ethics seems to assume that for every particular ethical problem a set of relevant applicable virtues exists, ready to swing into
action in order to guide the virtuous character. John Hardwig has noted
that the same character traits that could be considered virtuous in certain
professional contexts would likely be considered vices in interpersonal relationship contexts. He writes (Hardwig 2000, 19), 'consider, for example,
impartiality and impartial justice, which are a virtue in an employer, but a
vice in a father, mother, or spouse. Thus the dilemma posed by nepotism:
qua employer one should treat all applicants impartially, but qua parent one
is defective if one is not willing to provide special advantages to one's
children.'

Does pointing to what a person of virtuous character would have done 2.8
constitute an ethical justification? Say, if a virtuous doctor withholds from
a terminal cancer patient his diagnosis in order to avoid causing distress to
the dying patient, would reference to the doctor's virtuous character truly
justify the decision in a meaningful way? Justin Oakley suggests that 'most
virtues are not simply a matter of having good motives or good disposi-
tions, but have a practical component which involves seeing to it that one's
action succeeds in bringing about what the virtue dictates' (Oakley 1998,
95). He questions whether the benevolent character traits that motivated
the doctor's decision to deceive her patient is truly benefitting her patient.
Of course, that does not actually settle the justification question, and it
seems question begging. After all, the doctor in our scenario could well
reply to Oakley that he does actually think the course of deception he chose
was the most benevolent available under the circumstances. If the virtue of
benevolence is correctly identified as the relevant virtue, as opposed to the
virtue of honesty, it appears to be the case that Oakley would be unable to
provide us with a virtue ethical argument capable of showing the doctor
wrong.

We will see in Chapter 5 how contemporary virtue ethicists such as 2.9
Rosalind Hursthouse approach the question of the morality of abortion
(Hursthouse 1991).

2.2 Feminist Ethics

As the name suggests, **feminist ethics**[5] takes a distinctly feminist approach 2.10
to ethical issues. To be clear, to be a feminist ethicist you **don't have to be a
woman**[6].

2.11   Early feminist voices included for instance the liberal utilitarian philosopher John Stuart Mill. Feminist ethics was born out of a frustration by many feminist thinkers about the very nature of mainstream ethics, a critique that to a certain extent overlaps with the critical program presented by virtue ethicists. The fundamental concern expressed here is that mainstream Western ethics is male dominated, asks questions that are the result of the unique life experiences of (heterosexual) men and comes up, not surprisingly, with solutions that are a consequence of these men's life experiences. At the risk of oversimplifying this critique, the concern relates to the different spheres in which men and women operated for most of our histories. That is – with few known exceptions – men were in the public domain, they were usually the sole bread-winners, they did politics, they were judges and entrepreneurs while women typically stayed behind at home, supported their husbands' careers and/or looked after family and friends. Think for instance about Aristotle who thought it entirely appropriate for the male citizen to be his slaves', wife's and children's supreme overlord. It cannot surprise then that his approach to ethics prioritizes male experiences over those of women, slaves and children. The lived experiences of women typically do not feature in such approaches to ethics. If you have any doubt about the misogynist state of affairs with regard to leading philosophical male thinkers in most mainstream philosophical traditions, you might want to spend a bit more time reading up on what common views were of the female sex. To give you a fairly representative voice, let us quote the influential eighteenth century German philosopher Georg Wilhelm Friedrich Hegel who claimed that 'the difference between men and women is like that between animals and plants' (Clement 2013, 1927).

2.12   Carol Gilligan wrote a very influential book that continues to impact significantly on what can best be described as an 'ethic of care' (Gilligan 1982; critical Kuhse 1997). Gilligan criticizes a Kant-inspired moral psychologist, Lawrence Kohlberg. Kohlberg proposed a model of human moral development that fits right into the male ethics narrative mentioned already: universality, impartiality and principles feature prominently. Gilligan, on the other hand, proposes instead a female-experiences inspired ethic that values relationships and the partiality that goes with them. Some critics questioned whether an ethic that is born out of women's subordinate status over centuries is necessarily something worth supporting. Even if that wasn't a problem, does feminist ethics actually meet our action-guidance and action-justification criteria? Perhaps it is not too dissimilar to virtue ethics. While there is good reason to listen to its criticism of what historically was considered Western ethics, it is less clear that it provides us with a reasonably clear roadmap to ethical action and justification for action guidance. No doubt though, the concerns that motivate feminist ethics, and perhaps even more so feminist bioethics, are well worth keeping in mind when we look at specific bioethical problems.

Margaret Little outlines why **feminist bioethics**[7] is important to the 2.13 bioethical enterprise: 'First, it can reveal androcentric reasoning present in analyses of substantive bioethical issues – reasoning that can bias not only which policies are adopted, but what gets counted as an important question or persuasive argument. Second, it can help bioethicists to rethink the very conceptual tools used in bioethics – specifically, helping to identify where assumptions about gender have distorted the concepts commonly invoked in moral theory and, in doing so, clearing the way for the development of what might best be called "feminist-inspired" moral theory' (Little 1996). Feminist bioethicists have contributed influential works on a whole range of subjects ranging from reproductive health issues (Mackenzie 1992) to disability studies (Scully 2008), end-of-life decision- making and resource-allocation justice (Sherwin 1992) among others.

2.3 Utilitarian Ethics

Unlike both virtue ethics and feminist ethics, **utilitarian**[8] ethics is decid- 2.14 edly universalist and **impartialist**[9] in its approach to ethical problem solving. You will recall that both virtue ethics as well as feminist ethics make a point of valuing partiality toward loved ones, one's community and so on and so forth. In stark contrast, utilitarians expect you to take the position of an impartial observer. The universalizability aspect requires of us to treat the interests, needs and preferences of others that are comparable to our own in the same way that we expect our interests, needs and preferences to be treated. There is not one rule for me and another rule for others. Also, all other things being equal, distance is unimportant. The interest of someone at the other end of the world to breath good quality air is as important as my own interest in breathing good quality air.

Utilitarianism belongs to a group of approaches to ethics that typically 2.15 are referred to as consequentialist. As the name suggests, consequences or outcomes are pretty much all that matters to utilitarians. While not all consequentialist ethical theories are maximizing in their respective outlooks, utilitarianism is. Utilitarians hold, essentially, that we ought to maximize the greatest good for the greatest number of people or other beings that have the capacity to live better or worse lives. This nineteenth century ethical theory is, in addition to being impartialist, also aggregative, maximizing, and agent-neutral in its response to ethical issues. It derives its name from radical English social reformers who described themselves as utilitarians. Utilitarians usually support welfarist policies. The rightness of an action becomes here a function of goodness. Once we have determined what it is that is good – or bad – utilitarians admonish us to maximize that good (outcome) – or to minimize the bad. The right action is always the action that maximizes the good optimally. This separates utilitarian bioethicists from deontological theorists who hold that we should abide by particular rules because that is the right thing to do, even if such actions do not maximize the good (Kant 1785 [1959]).

2.16   Broadly speaking, two influential varieties of utilitarianism exist: act- and **rule-utilitarianism**[10]. **Act-utilitarians**[11] ask us to determine for every course of action we are contemplating whether or not it would maximize the good. Only the course of action that maximizes the good in a given situation is the morally right course of action. Doing this could lead to outcomes that many would consider unacceptable. If we agreed, for instance, that we ought to aim for the maximization of particular health outcomes, say quality-adjusted life years (see Chapter 12), an act-utilitarian doctor in an intensive care unit might well demand that an elderly patient is removed from a scarce intensive care bed to make space for a younger patient with equal likelihood of successful care. All other things being equal this would lead to a maximization of quality adjusted life years and so result in a perfect utilization of scarce health care resources. Many people would consider it unethical to physically remove a patient who is still alive, and who would still benefit from clinical care, from intensive care in order to make room for a younger patient who is competing for the same resource. The act-utilitarians, defending the removal of the elderly patient, might respond to this by saying that all they are aiming for is to make the best out of a bad situation, and that the bad situation is not of their own making.

2.17   Rule-utilitarianism was proposed by **John Stuart Mill**[12] as an alternative to **Jeremy Bentham's**[13] act-utilitarianism. He wrote, 'The moral rules which forbid mankind to hurt one another (in which we must never forget to include wrongful interference with each other's freedom) are more vital to human well-being than any maxims, however important, which only point out the best mode of managing some departments of human affairs' (1871

[1910], 55). Mill aims to achieve the maximization objective by avoiding the criticism leveled against act-utilitarianism. The idea here is, basically, that we ought to develop rules that cover many different situations and that are known to maximize the good. We then follow these rules without testing in each and every circumstance whether a particular course of action would truly maximize the good. Such a strategy would lend itself to policy making, but clearly on utilitarian logic it could not be considered superior to act-utilitarianism unless it guaranteed that the application of the rule would maximize the good in all individual cases. Some have suggested that rule-utilitarianism would eventually have to collapse into act-utilitarianism if it was serious about the maximization objective. As J.J.C. Smart pointed out, 'an adequate rule-utilitarianism would not only be extensionally equivalent to the act-utilitarian principle (…) but would in fact consist of one rule only, the act-utilitarian one: "maximize probable benefit"' (1973, 11–12).

Preference utilitarianism is an influential variety of modern-day utilitari- 2.18 anism. The preference utilitarian aim is to maximize the satisfaction of the preferences or interests of all those affected by an action. It is partly based on the acknowledgment that not everything we do is based on the utilitarian twin-objectives of reducing pain and suffering and maximizing happiness. As John Harsanyi puts it, 'preference utilitarianism is the only form of utilitarianism consistent with the important philosophical principle of preference autonomy. By this I mean the principle that, in deciding what is good and what is bad for a given individual, the ultimate criterion can only be his own wants and his own preferences' (Harsanyi 1977, 645). Preference utilitarians hold that individuals are likely the best judges of whatever it is that is in their best interest. The rightness of a proposed course of action then is determined by how much it contributes toward maximizing the satisfaction of autonomous individuals' preferences, desires or interests. An important condition here is that not all of an individual's preferences matter, because satisfying any random preferences or desires an individual utters would likely not result in optimal utility. Rather we should aim to maximize the satisfaction of individual preferences and desires that are reflective of a person's true preferences, that is 'preferences he *would* have if he had all the relevant factual information, always reasoned with the greatest personal care, and were in a state of mind most conducive to rational choice' (Harsanyi 1977, 646).

Critics query whether it actually is possible to engage in the utilitarian 2.19 calculus, they doubt whether we have the means to quantify pain and suffering or happiness and well-being in a meaningful way. They also question whether we can truly balance someone's suffering sensibly against someone else's benefits. Concerns have also been raised about utilitarianism's capacity to allocate resource fairly. Think, for instance, about the example in our introductory chapter: a medical NGO's goal is to alleviate ill-health related suffering in the resource poor world. Considering overwhelming need and limited resources, it wants to be super-efficient. Its decisions on where to deploy its resources are determined by getting the biggest bang for our donors' bucks as its CEO never tires of stressing when she talks to donors, staff and anyone else willing to listen. In the context of health care, generating good quality life years is typically seen to be the primary outcome health care resources must produce. Our NGO is faced with a practical dilemma: Some of the most vulnerable impoverished patients it *could* reach are in locations more troubled than those of other equally impoverished patients it *could* also reach. If the NGO decided to aim for the former group it would end up generating fewer such quality life years than it could generate if it instead decided to provide assistance to the latter group. It simply would require more resources per quality adjusted life-year generated to succeed with regard to the former group than it would be with regard to the latter group of patients with otherwise equal needs. All other things being equal utilitarians would have to support those people that it can reach more easily. In other words, the most vulnerable would be least likely to get the life-preserving assistance they so desperately need (Lowry 2009).

2.20   Does this ethic meet our two action guidance and action justification criteria? As we shall see in various chapters throughout this book, it does provide us with clear action guidance, if we have the relevant data available to us. It also provides us with a moral justification for why particular courses of action ought to be followed. Among modern-day Anglo-Saxon utilitarians wielding significant influence in bioethics are those in public health Angus Dawson (2005), and Robert Goodin (1989), in the context of animal rights Lori Gruen (2011), and in end-of-life issues Helga Kuhse (1987, 1997). Peter Singer is perhaps the most high-profile of contemporary utilitarian bioethicists (1995). We will come across views expressed by these utilitarians on a range of issues across this book. Jonathan Baron has advocated utilitarianism as the best theory for practical bioethics and defended its usefulness for a whole range of bioethical questions, including end-of-life issues, drug research and development, resource allocation justice and a host of other topics (Baron 2006).

2.4 Rule-Based Ethics

Rule-based ethics is seen by many as the direct opposite of consequence- 2.21
based ethics. It holds that something other than consequences or utility
determines the rightness or wrongness of an action. That 'other' are absolute rights and absolute wrongs, moral rules that are modeled on the rule of
law. They are categorical, that is they are absolutely binding. Rule-based
ethics has risen to great prominence with influential works written by a
German **enlightenment**[14] philosopher, **Immanuel Kant**[15]. Like utilitarianism his work is universalist and impartialist in its outlook. Kant thought
that our ethical decision-making should be driven by pure reason alone. He
did not provide us with much material guidance regarding the substance of
ethics, rather he was concerned about the form ethics should take, and he
was concerned with the question of what it is that makes an action an ethical action. According to this rule-based ethic, what is it that makes an action
a good action? Kant thought that it is our motivation. We have to act from
the right motive, and that right motive is always that we act according to an
ethical rule because it is the right thing to do so. That is, we don't abide by
an ethical rule because it would help others, but because we want to abide
by said rule for its own sake, we abide by it because we recognize its respect
commanding nature. Philosopher John Hardwig is not the only one skeptical of Kant inspired ethics. He wrote, (Hardwig 2000, 9) 'Although it's been
10 years, I can still see the student, hands on her hips, as she brought my
beautiful lecture on Kant's ethics to a grinding halt: "Is Kant saying," she
demanded, "that if I sleep with my boyfriend, I should sleep with him out of
a sense of duty?" My response: "And when you're through, you should tell
him that you would have done the same for anyone in his situation." What
could I say.' He then goes on to lament that impartialist ethical theories are
something of a no-go area when you are looking for an ethics of personal
relationships. Hardwig isn't entirely correct here, Kant would have answered
the student's question in the affirmative only if the couple had been in a
legal marriage. The student probably would not have considered that
response much more plausible.

Kant wasn't particularly fond of our emotions and intuitions as the basis 2.22
of our moral actions. He recognized that some of these intuitions and
emotions could well result in our doing what is ethically required of us, say
by our supporting the poor. However, he warns that just as well they could
lead us astray, because they are not a result of our reason in analytical
action. There certainly is some truth in this. Think for instance about

Leon R. Kass, an influential bioethicist in the United States. Kass argued that certain views held in bioethics are clearly wrong, because they are repugnant. He argued, among others, that utilitarianism, human cloning and particular ways of eating ice cream were clearly wrong because they were repugnant. He wrote, 'There is something deeply repugnant and fundamentally transgressive about such [destructive embryo experimentation] a utilitarian treatment of prospective human life' (Kass 1997, 26).

2.23   Kass' treatise on the *Wisdom of Repugnance* earned the scorn of many a bioethicist, not least because his line of reasoning arguably leads to arbitrary conclusions about what is right and what is wrong, based on who you ask about their feelings on a particular matter. To be fair to Kass, he advanced other arguments against human cloning that we will be looking at in Chapter 8. Still, strongly felt repugnance is indicative of a sound moral intuition to him.

2.24   Where would reason-based ethics take us in terms of the formal structure of ethics? Kant insists it would take us to something he called the Categorical Imperative. There are slightly differing formulations of the Categorical Imperative, and not unexpectedly they have led to much scholarship generated by philosophers. That notwithstanding, the basic arguments underlying the Categorical Imperative are these: whatever moral rules we identify must be rules that are categorical, that is they are absolute, and they must be binding on us and everyone like us. Accordingly, these rules must be universal rules that we would be happy for all humans to follow them. Like utilitarians rule-based philosophers think that we must not create rules just for ourselves.

2.25   Rule-based ethics has been very influential in bioethics as well as political philosophy generally. Many an admonition in codes of medical ethics is rule-based as opposed to consequentialist in nature. The idea that patient confidentiality must never be breached is an example of this; so is the idea that a doctor must never assist a patient who wishes to end her life. Among influential current day Kantian philosophers writing on bioethical issues are **Frances Kamm**[16] (e.g. 1992, 1994 and 1996) and **Onora O'Neill**[17] (e.g. 2002). We will hear more about their views throughout this book. Kantian philosophers also **contributed**[18] to US President George W. Bush's **Council on Bioethics**[19] deliberations.

2.5 'Georgetown Mantra'

2.26   The Georgetown Mantra isn't actually a mantra endorsed by Georgetown University, a Jesuit college in Washington DC. It's a nickname describing arguably the most influential biomedical ethics textbook's four-principles' approach to bioethical problem solving. It is often referred to as the 'Georgetown Mantra' because of its leading proponents' close affiliation with Georgetown University. Tom Beauchamp and James Childress are the authors of *Principles of Biomedical Ethics*; they developed this approach in successive editions of their popular textbook (2012). These authors do not claim to have developed a fully-fledged ethical theory. However, they insist that four *prima facie* principles they have identified are widely recognized as sensible principles, even across cultures, and that they are compatible with various ethical theories. The Mantra combines consequentialist and deontological approaches to bioethics decision-making. Essentially Beauchamp and Childress believe that four overarching principles suffice to address virtually every ethical problem that we are likely to encounter in bioethics.

The principles they propose are: non-maleficence, beneficence, respect   2.27
for autonomy and justice. Let us have a closer look at each of these principles and at how they interact with – and sometimes against – each other in
order to get a better handle on the Georgetown Mantra. Keep in mind that
these principles are considered *prima facie* by Beauchamp and Childress,
that is – with good reason – every one of them can be overridden by competing stronger demands.

2.5.1 Non-Maleficence

You might have heard of the often-cited 'first rule' when it comes to health   2.28
care practice: *Primum non nocere* – First do no harm. Non-maleficence
means little other than that. This principle is more strongly associated with
Kantian thinking.

2.5.2 Beneficence

Beneficence requires health care professionals do to what is best by their   2.29
patients. As we shall see, this can give rise to justifiable paternalistic actions
by health care professionals. This principle is more strongly associated with
consequentialist thinking.

2.5.3 Respect for Autonomy

This seemingly uncontroversial principle stipulates that the choices under-   2.30
taken by competent, well-informed patients should or even must be
respected. In many jurisdictions this is reflected in law. In Canada, for
instance, it would be illegal for a doctor to ignore a competent patient's

refusal of treatment, even if respecting those wishes would ultimately result in harm to the patient. Note that there is an in-built conflict here between the first two principles and this principle.

2.5.4 Justice

2.31   The last principle is primarily concerned with fairness in the allocation of scarce resources, that is **distributive justice**[20]. This obviously is an important principle given the resource constraints faced by most health care systems. Initially we can reduce the idea of justice to a formal principle often ascribed to Aristotle: 'Equals must be treated equally, and unequals must be treated unequally' (Beauchamp 2019, 268). While uncontroversial, this formal principle doesn't realistically help us when we are faced with distributive justice questions. We need to complement the formal principle with a material principle of justice, in other words, we need to move beyond the formal structure, and add substance to the principle. Once we do that though we are faced with a plethora of competing ideas about what justice entails, ranging from traditional communist, utilitarian to libertarian ideals as well as more recent ones such as those introduced by defenders of what is called the capabilities approach.

2.32   Justice then seems to be a thing that is very much in the eyes of the beholder, subject to the vagaries of one's personal ideological convictions. A Marxist will hold a quite different view on resource allocation justice then a libertarian or a utilitarian (Takala 2001, 73). Finnish philosopher Tuija Takala quite nicely illustrates the problems with this principle by means of describing the political arguments political parties in Finland had during an election campaign:

> In the spring of 1999, there was again in Finland the time for parliamentary elections. During the campaigns it became obvious that there was an overwhelming consensus among the rival parties that justice is important and that we should aim for a more just society. The only small difference between the parties was in the understanding of what justice is and what measures should be taken that justice would prevail. The right wing thought that by lowering the taxation of property and high salaries we would be able to do this. Meanwhile, the suggested solution from the left wing was to lower the taxation of the lower income groups and reaffirm the welfare rights, such as free education, free healthcare, and reasonable unemployment benefits. The political middle, representing the interests of agricultural Finland, reckoned that above all the government should fund the

farmers. Same word, but different interpretations of what justly belongs to whom. Is it to everyone according to their need? An egalitarian principle to be found in Marxist thought as well. Or should we follow the libertarian idea of everyone owning their natural properties in good and in bad. If you happen to be faster, better, and smarter than the rest, you should have the benefits.

And equally, if you get a raw deal in the natural lottery, it is your own problem. Should we in principle guarantee that everyone has equal opportunities, or should we go further and give fair equal opportunities for all? Within the sphere of bioethics, these questions arise especially in an age of scarcity. If we cannot help all patients, by which criteria are we able to say that X is to be treated whereas Y is to be left on his own?

Political philosophy has struggled throughout its history with the question of what justice is. How can it suddenly become a non-question in bioethics?

Similar arguments can be advanced with regard to each of the other prin- 2.33 ciples. It is doubtful that there is actually an uncontroversial cross-cultural consensus on the relevance and meaning of these principles, as Beauchamp and Childress claim there is. Coming to their aid, one of their colleagues at Georgetown University, philosopher Robert M. Veatch, has offered an eloquent defense of the idea that such a 'common morality' exists among all humans (Veatch 2003).

A further critical point is worth noting: the absence of a hierarchy among 2.34 the principles has the potential to leave, for instance, patients subjected to more or less arbitrary and unpredictable decisions by health care professionals, simply because health care professionals could always pick the principle most suited to support their already formed intuitive response to a particular ethical problem. Say, a doctor is willing to respect the patient's do-not-resuscitate advance directive, hence the autonomy principle will be deployed. Another doctor, facing the same situation, might have decided to override the patient's choice, hence the principle of beneficence could be deployed in order to justify a paternalistic course of action. In the absence of an overarching ethical theory that arbitrates conflicts between principles, decisions with regard to what ought to be done might be somewhat arbitrary. If, on the other hand, an overarching theory of this kind was utilized – something not supported by Beauchamp and Childress – it would be unclear why we should not adopt the theory itself and forget about the principles altogether.

However, the Georgetown Mantra has proven to be of enduring staying- 2.35 power in bioethical analyses and debates, hence its inclusion among the concepts this book will make reference to throughout. If nothing else, the principles flag issues that are important to many people and that ought to be considered in ethical analyses.

2.6 Contract Theory

2.36 **Contractarianism**[21] – not to be confused with **contractualism**[22] (Kumar 2013) – is really a theory in political philosophy, but it has a significant impact on many areas of concern to bioethics. Initially it was proposed by philosophers such as Thomas Hobbes and David Gauthier with a view to giving an account of political authority. The basic idea here is that any system of government that the citizens of a given state could agree on would wield legitimate authority. Of course, this very idea of informed, voluntary agreement makes contractarianism also a suitable foundation of an ethical theory.

2.37   John Rawls, a neo-Kantian, offered in his *A Theory of Justice* a contractualist way of using this hypothetical social contract as a means to arrive at particular fundamental ethical or political rules for society. Contractualism has prominently been proposed by philosophers such as Immanuel Kant and T.M. Scanlon. Rawls proposes a two-step strategy: First he asks us to imagine that we wanted to create rules for a society in which we would want to live and that we would be happy to abide by. In order to avoid any bias on our part Rawls asks us to imagine that we are behind what he calls a 'veil of ignorance', that is, that we would have no idea as to whether we would be rich or impoverished, healthy or chronically ill, an ethnic minority member or a member of the predominant ethnic group, male or female, gay or straight, etc. He quite rightly thought that this would eliminate any egoistic biases from the rules that we would likely come up with. This isn't dissimilar to the demands of impartialist and universalist approaches to ethics that we have become acquainted with already. Given that you wouldn't know whether you're rich or poor, so Rawls thought, you would likely aim for a centrist view, for instance providing minimum basic health care to everyone regardless of ability to pay, just to be sure that if you were impoverished you would not end up dying a preventable death due to lack of the financial wherewithal to cover your hospital bills. Equally you would likely not go overboard with the level of health care provision because of the onerous cost implications – after all, many people seem reluctant to pay high taxes for this level of health care. Norman Daniels, a Rawls inspired philosopher, has suggested that what we ought to prioritize is a given ill person's return to what he labeled species typical **normal functioning**[23].

Critics of this kind of theory have noted that the very foundation of con- 2.38 tractualism is deeply problematic. Essentially it offers an exclusive reliance on enlightened self-interest. Critics have questioned whether this could actually function as the normative foundation of a sound ethical theory. Rawls and his followers *assume* that this enlightened self-interest would result in particular practical choices on the policy level. The problem is, simply put, they could be wrong. What if citizens actually chose to gamble all on being wealthy and healthy and so instead opted for no publicly funded provision of health care at all? Would their choice then become any more ethically acceptable just because of how it came about? Equally, if the basis of morality is rational egoism, as this strategy seems to suggest, what would stop dictators from behaving as dictators usually do, as long as they could be reasonably confident that their victims would never end up in a situation where they could take revenge?

This concludes our brief overview of influential ethical theories and 2.39 approaches that have a significant impact on bioethical reasoning. Let us have a closer look now at bioethics itself.

Questions

Now that you have read brief snapshots of major ethical theories, do any of them appeal to you? Do any of them reflect your own thinking, values, or intuitions? Why do you reject the theories that you do reject?

Website Links

1   http://plato.stanford.edu/entries/aristotle/
2   http://books.google.ca/books?id=9SIUAAAAYAAJ
3   http://plato.stanford.edu/entries/aristotle-ethics/
4   http://plato.stanford.edu/entries/ethics-virtue/
5   http://plato.stanford.edu/entries/feminism-ethics/
6   http://malefeminists.com/
7   http://plato.stanford.edu/entries/feminist-bioethics/
8   http://plato.stanford.edu/entries/utilitarianism-history/
9   http://plato.stanford.edu/entries/impartiality/
10 http://plato.stanford.edu/entries/consequentialism-rule/
11 http://runrchic1.hubpages.com/hub/Act-Utilitarianism-versus-Rule-Utilitarianism/

12   http://plato.stanford.edu/entries/mill/
13   http://www.iep.utm.edu/bentham/
14   http://plato.stanford.edu/entries/enlightenment/
15   http://plato.stanford.edu/entries/kant-moral/
16   http://www.fas.harvard.edu/~phildept/kamm.html/
17   http://www.parliament.uk/biographies/lords/baroness-o%27neill-of-
     bengarve/2441/
18   https://bioethicsarchive.georgetown.edu/pcbe/reports/human_dignity/
     chapter13.html
19   http://bioethics.georgetown.edu/pcbe/
20   http://plato.stanford.edu/entries/justice-distributive/
21   http://plato.stanford.edu/entries/contractarianism/
22   http://plato.stanford.edu/entries/contractualism/
23   https://plato.stanford.edu/entries/justice-healthcareaccess/

3

BASICS OF BIOETHICS

This chapter provides you with a brief history of bioethics and its scope. We 3.1
will also look at how bioethicists contribute in ethical review committees to
necessary ethics oversight, and in government appointed bioethics commissions to addressing practical policy issues. This matters, because it is at
this intersection of policy and bioethics that academic ethicists sometimes
wield genuine policy influence. Last but not least we will introduce some
commonly used, yet typically flawed arguments, that you will come across
frequently in public debates on matters concerning bioethics or biopolicy.

3.1 History and Scope of Bioethics

No account of the history of bioethics would be complete without mention 3.2
of a biologist, Van Rensselaer Potter, who is typically – and quite
wrongly – credited with coining the term 'bioethics' in 1971 (Jonsen 2014,
332). Potter wrote: 'I propose the term *Bioethics* in order to emphasize the
two most important ingredients in achieving the wisdom that is so desperately needed: biological knowledge and human values' (Potter 1971, 2). **It
turns out**[1] that the author who actually deserves credit for coining the term
is a German Protestant pastor, Fritz Jahr. In 1927 he published an article
called 'Bio-Ethics: A Review of the Ethical Relationships of Humans to
Animals and Plants.' In that article Jahr aimed to establish bioethics as a
discipline as well as a moral principle (Sass 2007). Unlike Potter, Jahr's work
was quickly forgotten during the turbulence of the Second World War. Fast
forward from 1927 to 1987. Helga Kuhse and Peter Singer, the founding

This Is Bioethics: An Introduction, First Edition. Ruth F. Chadwick and Udo Schüklenk.
© 2021 John Wiley & Sons, Inc. Published 2021 by John Wiley & Sons, Inc.

editors of the leading international journal *Bioethics* described their fledgling new enterprise in the first issue of the journal this way:

> *Bioethics* will publish articles on the ethical issues raised by medicine and the biological sciences. … The prefix 'bio' in our title, then, is used in a narrow sense to refer to the biological sciences, and especially, but not exclusively, the medical and health sciences. It is not being used in the wide sense in which we talk of 'the biosphere' to mean all living things, or anything which affects the ecology of our planet. 'Ethics' is at least a well-established term. We understand it to mean the study of what we *ought* to do, and by 'ought' in this context we mean not prudential 'ought' of self-interest, or even group interest, but rather reference to reason or considerations which can be defended from a universal or impartial perspective. (Kuhse and Singer 1987, iv)

3.3   We will follow in this volume the understanding of 'bioethics' that Helga Kuhse and Peter Singer outlined in their journal editorial. For the purposes of this book we understand bioethics as a field of study inquiring into ethical issues arising in the biomedical and health sciences as far as they affect humans.

3.4   It is a legitimate question to ask whether bioethics should also cover ethical issues in our treatment of non-human animals. Some of the most influential **bioethicists**[2] have written about the **moral standing of animals**[3], not least the just quoted Peter Singer himself, and the morality of using sentient animals for medical research purposes as well as the production of food. We will be touching on this issue, albeit briefly, in the next chapter (Chapter 4) as well as in the chapter covering issues in research ethics (Chapter 7). The **morality of animal experimentation**[4] has been debated controversially for many decades. There are also issues at the interface between species, such as xenotransplantation. You might also wonder why we are seemingly unconcerned about our **natural environment**[5]. Isn't the destruction of the Amazon rainforest, for instance, an ethical problem? Well, we are not, strictly speaking, unconcerned, however, what is true is that we will focus in this book on environmental issues only insofar as they affect human health and human well-being. Environmental ethicists have taken on the task of addressing challenging **environmental ethics questions**[6]. We shall by and large stay clear of those in this book. Our main focus in the remaining chapters of this book will be – broadly – on challenging ethical questions that arise frequently at the beginning and end of our lives, questions that arise in the context of clinical research involving human participants, the ability of genetic research findings to dramatically change who we are, as well as ethical challenges posed by population and global health issues.

A lot and very little could be said about the history of bioethics. 3.5 Historically it certainly grew out of **medical ethics**[7]. Traditionally medical ethicists were concerned about normative questions that arise in the health care professional patient relationship. Medical ethics covered many **clinical ethics**[8] issues such as informed consent in the doctor-patient relationship and professionalism in medicine, but also more contentious issues such as the morality of abortion or euthanasia. It is probably fair to say that varying histories of bioethics as an academic and professional discipline could be written, depending on what country you are looking at. For instance, bioethicist cum historian **Robert Baker**[9] has written a superb volume on the history of medical ethics in the United States leading up to what he calls, quite appropriately, the 'bioethics revolution' (Baker 2013). It is well worth a read if you are interested in how medical ethics evolved over the centuries prior to the rise of bioethics. There are fascinating stories to be found, such as that about J. Marion **Sims**[10], the founder of US American gynecology. He shot to fame during his time for the perfection of surgical procedures, but is much more notorious today for achieving this task by undertaking surgery on enslaved African women – without anesthetic or voluntary first person informed consent (Sartin 2004). This might remind you of the kind of ethical relativist questions that we mentioned in Chapter 1, specifically the second type: should J. Marion Sims be judged by the ethical standards of his times or by today's standards? Well, thankfully this is not actually at issue in this instance. Reportedly one of his competitors, Edinburgh based James **Simpson**[11], noted in those same years, 'I took occasion to make an extensive series of experiments ... upon the relative qualities of different metallic threads ... [on] a number of unfortunate pigs, which were always, of course, first indulged with a good dose of **chloroform**[12]' (Sartin 2004, 505). He found it appropriate to use anesthetics even on the animals he used for his experimental surgery, very much unlike his colleague in the United States who thought nothing of abusing enslaved African women during his research. The ethical relativism question doesn't arise then, because Sims' work was already controversial and criticized by colleagues during his times.

A few books about the beginnings of bioethics have been written (Jonsen 3.6 1998; Rothman 1991; Evans 2012). Not unexpectedly these accounts of the birth of bioethics were not written by philosophers but by professionals hailing from other disciplines. Most of these histories are fairly United

States' centric. Whether they are reflective of how bioethics came of age in other countries or cultural contexts is unclear as these histories still need to be written. Having acknowledged this, North-American bioethics and its conceptual frameworks have proven to be very influential the world all over. We will stick in this chapter, for the purpose of sketching a brief history of bioethics, by and large to the United States. It is reasonable to assume – with variations – that similar phenomena led to the birth of bioethics in other relatively resource-rich countries.

3.7   Bioethics as we know it today is in many ways a creation of the 1970s. Robert Baker writes that the political and cultural changes sweeping through the United States from the mid 1960s created the ideological ground for the birth of bioethics (Baker 2013: 275). Well, what exactly happened during those years? A number of things occurred nearly concurrently. Scandals in scientific research rocked the country. **Henry K. Beecher**[13], a Harvard based medical doctor, published in 1966 an article in a top-flight medical journal, the *New England Journal of Medicine*[14], flagging fairly outrageous unethical research practices in some 22 or so medical studies, many of which were funded by United States' government agencies (Beecher 1966). Beecher's article led subsequently to a US government investigation and a whole slew of policies and regulations addressing ethical standards in biomedical research were introduced and eventually implemented. This wasn't a uniquely United States' problem. Two years earlier **Maurice H. Pappworth**[15], an English physician, blew the **whistle**[16] on scandalous research ethics failings in the United Kingdom (Harkness 2001, 366). You will hear more about these episodes in the history of bioethics in Chapter 7.

3.8   Both medical professionals as well as patients saw also the advent of revolutionary medical technologies, such as dialysis machines, ventilators and in-vitro fertilization (IVF). IVF in particular gave rise to a whole host of controversial normative questions about 'new ways of making babies'. Traditionally understood medical ethics was simply ill-equipped to deal with these issues. Meanwhile various groups demanded specific liberties from oppressive medical practices for themselves. The psychiatrist **Thomas Szasz**[17] fought from the 1960s to liberate people from what he considered to be an oppressive psychiatry (Schaler 2004). Gay activists demanded from the American Psychiatric Association that it remove **homosexuality from its list of mental illnesses**[18]. They denied that there ever was a scientific basis for the profession's mental illness designation verdict of homosexuality (Bayer 1981). These activists succeeded in 1973. Equally, women also fought to gain control over their bodies from the medical profession and the law, campaigning to have abortion decriminalized. In 1973 in *Roe v Wade* the United States Supreme Court **decriminalized abortion**[19]. In 1988 the Supreme Court in neighboring Canada, in effect, declared laws limiting access to abortion unconstitutional (**R v. Morgentaler, [1988] 1 S.C.R. 30**[20]).

In a very general sense, trust that the doctor or medical researcher knows   3.9 best, as it were, was replaced with the idea that competent patients are entitled to make their own self-regarding choices and to see those choices respected by health care professionals and clinical researchers. Today, in many jurisdictions, patients are legally entitled to decline even life-preserving medical care, provided they are competent at the time of their decision-making. Patients became more powerful, medical researchers and doctors' generally saw their powers cut.

Since those relatively early days, bioethics has seen a whole range of spe-   3.10 cializations. Researchers in **public health ethics**[21] address questions to do with moral issues arising in the context of health care delivery on population levels. They are concerned about problems as varied as the ethical treatment of multiple-drug **resistant tuberculosis patients**[22], or the ethical challenges posed by the large number of **young people with minor traumatic brain injuries**[23] caused by popular sporting activities. We will be taking a closer look at public health ethics in Chapter 13. At the other extreme is arguably the equally young field of **neuroethics**[24]. It is concerned with the ethical implications of recent advances in neuroscientific research. Should we provide medication to patients with post-traumatic stress disorder that would make them **forget permanently**[25] whatever traumatic events they experienced? Is it ethically acceptable for students to take **memory or attention enhancing drugs**[26]? Neuroethics research overlaps to some extent with concerns driving **transhumanists**[27]. They are hoping that eventually we would be able to 'upgrade' our flawed bodies by technological means, permitting us to be more intelligent, more moral, live much longer, love better, and generally transcend what biological evolution has so far permitted us to be. You will come across these sorts of questions in Chapter 8.

3.2 Who Can Claim to be a Bioethicist?

This is a trickier question than you might think. Unlike medicine or nurs-   3.11 ing, bioethics is not a **profession**[28]. We agree with Bullock and Trombley that 'a profession arises when any trade or occupation transforms itself through the development of formal qualifications based upon education, apprenticeship, and examinations, the emergence of regulatory bodies with powers to admit and discipline members, and some degree of monopoly rights' (1999, 689). There are no statutory boards regulating the affairs of bioethicists. Bioethicists certainly have no monopoly powers like doctors, for instance, when it comes to the right to prescribe medication. When you consider the earlier mentioned events that gave rise to bioethics in the United States, you likely won't be surprised to learn that academics from a number of disciplines were involved in thinking about some of these normative challenges. Among the founders of bioethics were, of course, philosophical ethicists, but there were also, and quite prominently so, Christian ethicists, legal professionals, health care professionals, sociologists, political scientists, even historians. Christian bioethicists obviously have different conceptual modi operandi than secular bioethicists or bioethicists coming from a legal background. It is worth keeping in mind that no single academic discipline 'owns' bioethics. Empirical sociologists have become increasingly active in the field, engaging in both qualitative and quantitative work on bioethical issues, ranging from the rights and wrongs of abortion, reproductive cloning and euthanasia to any number of other issues. When queried they may or may not wish to identify with the label 'bioethicist', but there are ongoing and important debates about the role of empirical evidence in ethical decision-making and about how the disciplines of Sociology and Philosophy can and should work together. Clearly empirical facts about perceptions or attitudes do not determine what is right. Nevertheless, data about what is regarded as acceptable can and do influence what is politically feasible, challenge the universal applicability of certain policies in the light of cultural differences, and for some, challenge the very possibility of universal ethical principles in ethics.

3.12   A lively debate continues among people working in the field about the question of 'who is a bioethicist'. Today specialized programs exist in universities that award doctoral degrees in bioethics. For the purpose of this volume we are looking specifically at how philosophical ethics bears on bioethical questions.

3.13   However, it is worth noting that, as in any evolving field, bioethicists have expanded the scope of their activities. The field continues to grow in leaps and bounds, both with regard to academic subject matters as well as with regard to efforts to professionally accredit the activities of subsets of bioethicists. Extensive efforts are underway to provide accreditations to clinical ethicists, that is ethicists substantially involved in ethics consultations at the (hospital) bedside. The American **Association for Bioethics and Humanities**[29] (ASBH) has taken the lead on this subject matter and produced handbooks on core clinical ethics competencies and related matters.

3.3 Organizations and Journals

More internationally focused organizations such as the **International Association of Bioethics**[30] (IAB) host international networks of scholars with shared research interests. Specialized networks such as the **International Network on Feminist Approaches to Bioethics**[31] (FAB) also exist. The **IAB**[32] and **FAB**[33] have official academic journals publishing high-quality peer reviewed bioethics content with an international flavor.   3.14

As is to be expected in a growing academic discipline, there is a large number of bioethics journals in existence, in English language as well as in any number of other languages. In case you would like to find out more about at least some of the journals in the field, you might find the **journal listings on this website**[34] as good a starting point for your own investigations as any. Looking over the tables of content of current issues gives you a good idea of the kinds of topics that are of concern to bioethicists today.   3.15

3.4 Policy Advice

Among bioethicists there has been a fair amount of debate about their proper role when it comes to public policy issues, especially regarding whether they should focus on elucidating issues or providing answers. Bioethicists more often than not are working on topics with significant public policy import, we mentioned already the morality of abortion, euthanasia, justice in the allocation of scarce resources, governance of emerging technologies, or the issue of ethically defensible triage criteria in COVID19 like pandemics, as well as other policy matters. Some bioethicists hold the view that bioethicists should refrain from providing any kind of public policy advice. The rationale here is typically that in liberal democracies public policy on any subject matter is the result of processes involving democratic consensus finding. Bioethical analysis typically doesn't lend itself to the negotiation of trade-offs between the negotiating parties. Instead bioethical analysis provides critical normative reflection on the issue of concern and then offers a reasoned   3.16

conclusion with regard to what we ought to do (or what we ought not to do). It does this using mostly normative impartialist concepts that will give weight to particular values. Say, a utilitarian analysis will be single-mindedly focused on outcomes and aim to evaluate these outcomes through the lens of its maximization-principle. In liberal democracies legislators are more likely to take consequences as much into consideration as individual rights and any number of other societal values. Bioethicists then are well-placed to reflect on the meaning of such values to the problem at hand, but they are arguably not the right party to draw up policy proposals reflecting a societal consensus on any bioethics subject matter.

3.17   Governments in many countries have set up national bioethics advisory commissions or councils the job of which is to address bioethical issues that are of current policy concern. Their remits vary significantly, some are free to address issues the commission or council members deem important, others respond to government requests to investigate particular issues. In the United States, Japan and Germany, to name but a few, such commissions have existed for many **years**[35]. In the United Kingdom there is no national government-appointed bioethics committee but the **Nuffield Council on Bioethics**[36] fulfils an analogous role. There have also been commissions appointed for particular purposes at different times. In the United States the **members are presidential appointments**[37] and so do probably reflect to some extent the religious or other convictions of the president of the day. The **German Ethics Council**[38] was established by federal legislation.

3.18   Bioethicists also work in advisory or policy making bodies of medical associations and statutory bodies in the health care professions. For instance, the World Medical Association has created its own **medical ethics committee**[39]. Under its guidance the organization has produced a whole host of **ethical guidance documents**[40] as well as **educational resources**[41]. It is worth noting that the guidance documents produced by the World Medical Association typically do not provide ethical justification, rather the ethical guidelines produced by the organization take their authoritative strength from the standing of the organization itself. The World Medical Association has obviously some claim to represent, as an international umbrella organization, the world's doctors.

3.19   CIOMS, the Council for International Organizations of Medical Sciences is the publisher of its infrequently updated *International Ethical Guidelines for Health-related Research Involving Humans*[42] (CIOMS 2016). You will find in this document research ethical guidelines – 25 of them, no less – ranging from traditional content such as informed consent, standards of care in a trial, conflicts of interest, content on particular participant groups such as children and women, to topics including the social value of research, the collection, storage and use of data, or public accountability of research. As with the documents issued by the World Medical Association, most of the CIOMS guidelines also contain no ethical justification. A draw-back of such a publishing strategy is that because it is unclear why particular guidance is issued, it is difficult to determine for a curious reader whether the advice is worth heeding or whether it can safely be ignored. On the other hand, the CIOMS guidelines have become very long and detailed. If the authors of this document had chosen to provide substantive justification for their guidance, they would have produced a document justifiably called an ethics document, but it may have turned out to be unwieldy due to its length.

Increasingly bioethicists are becoming involved in the development of ethical guidance documents that probably come closer to being regulatory or policy documents. A good example of this are the **binding research ethics guidelines**[43] produced by the Canadian federal research funding agencies for health research, the natural sciences and engineering as well as the humanities and social sciences.   3.20

These guidelines are binding regulatory documents for researchers funded by these agencies, not merely expressions of good intentions or an ethics wish-list of a kind.   3.21

You might want to investigate in what roles bioethicists function in your national medical association, research funding agencies and the like.   3.22

In the next section we will introduce some common patterns of argument that you will come across in bioethics and we will demonstrate where, and how they fall short. The kinds of common fallacious arguments that you can find in bioethics are arguments flagged prominently in any number of critical thinking or rhetoric textbooks. This section is not meant to replace these textbooks (e.g. Hunter 2009; Vaughn 2010). Its objective is to red-flag arguments that you should be concerned about when you come across them in bioethics related articles, whether in academic journals or in the news media.   3.23

3.5 Common Arguments in Bioethics

Some arguments are treated as if they were 'knock-down' arguments. So what is a 'knock-down' argument? In simple terms, it is an argument that is regarded as decisive. Nathan Ballantyne has examined definitions of   3.24

knock-down arguments and suggests that they are arguments that ought to bring about agreement, were everyone to understand them, while lacking 'defeaters' for thinking they understand (**Ballantyne 2013**[44]). In other words, they are not aware of good reasons for rejecting the argument. There is a view, however, that there are no knockdown arguments in philosophy – everything is open to question - and thus in bioethics in so far as it is a sub-branch of philosophy, but certain arguments are used *as if* they were knockdown arguments.

3.25   Sometimes this amounts simply to giving a proposed intervention or policy a description, such as 'that would count as eugenics', the implication being that eugenics is something to which no right-thinking person would subscribe (see the section on slippery slopes, below). Alternatively, someone might say 'That would be unlawful'. But in ethics, what is unlawful is not the end of the story as we saw in Chapter 1. What the law should be is the important question.

3.6 Playing God

3.26   The view that one should not 'play God' is commonly expressed in situations where one person or group of people is making decisions about the lives of others (such as whether they should live or die), or using new technologies that go beyond what humans have been able to do before, for example, using gene editing techniques to 'design' future children. When we start to look into exactly what is meant by 'playing God', however, we are forced to ask if there is anything to it more than mere rhetoric. Is it actually an argument at all, let alone a knockdown one? A generous interpretation, which does not dismiss it entirely, is that it is shorthand for different kinds of claims (**Gillon 1999**[45]). In the first type of case, where someone has the power to decide whether another should live or die, it expresses a point about equality, that it is wrong for someone to consider themselves to be sufficiently superior to another to take a decision about the worthwhileness of another's life. This is at least an understandable argument, but it fails to deal with the fact that sometimes decisions about whom to save are inescapable, although it may be claimed that such decisions do not inevitably involve decisions about the *value* of another's life.

3.27   In the second type of case, 'playing God' may be regarded as a warning about the possible adverse consequences of 'going too far'. In this sense it is closest to what are arguably the roots of the 'playing God' argument, the notion of '**hubris**[46]' in Greek mythology. Individuals who displayed hubris, or excessive pride, were liable to severe punishment for putting themselves on a par with the gods and trying to rise above the proper limits of human beings. Arguments about interfering with nature (see below), and opening ourselves and the planet to unforeseeable risks, express similar concerns.

In this sense the 'playing God' argument may reduce to a type of conse-   3.28
quentialist argument, advising us to be aware of dangerous consequences when taking decisions in conditions of uncertainty. There are well established strategies for assessment and management of risks in such circumstances, but the fact that in dealing with new developments there are many 'unknown unknowns' remains for some a matter of considerable concern.

3.7 Unnatural and Abnormal

In public debates about the introduction of new technologies you will fre-   3.29
quently come across arguments of the kind that the use of certain technologies is variously 'unnatural' or 'abnormal', and that that establishes their moral wrongness. Historically we have seen this initially not so much in the context of technologies but in the context of opposition to homosexuality. The view expressed here was that homosexuality is morally objectionable *because* it is seen as unnatural and/or abnormal. But what is meant by unnatural or abnormal? Homosexuality is something that occurs in nature, both human (Crooks and Baur 2014) as well as non-human (Sommer 2006) It is something that does not violate the laws of physics, so it definitely is a natural thing. What proponents of the view that homosexuality is unnatural really mean is that in their view homosexuality violates their *normative* understanding of what human nature should be like. Influential thinkers as varied as the Catholic theologian **Thomas Aquinas**[47] (1225–1274) and enlightenment philosopher **Immanuel Kant**[48] (1724–1804) have tried to deliver rationales in support of such an understanding, with limited success (**Soble 2003**[49]).

Similar problems arise in arguments involving claims of abnormality.   3.30
Normality describes nothing other than a statistical average. And while it is true that homosexuality is not your average expression of sexuality, it's also true that describing that tells us nothing about the morality, or the desirability or otherwise of homosexuality. People driving Rolls Royce motorcars, flying on private jets, or those owning golden Rolex wristwatches are all abnormal, compared to the average person driving a car, flying on a plane,

or owning a watch. None of that tells us anything about the morality of owning luxury cars and watches or flying on a private airplane. The reason for this is that these types of arguments commit a naturalistic fallacy.

3.31   **David Hume**[50], one of the most influential philosophers of the English-speaking world, argued in his *Treatise of Human Nature* (1739–1740) that it is 'altogether inconceivable' (and a logic error) to form or derive value judgments from facts alone. According to this view empirical premises cannot give rise to normative conclusions (Hume, T3.1.1.27). There is a **great entry**[51] in the Stanford Encyclopedia of Philosophy on fallacies. Henry Sidgwick also offers a good discussion of the problems surrounding ethical arguments based on 'God's will', nature and abnormal in his **Methods of Ethics**[52] (Sidgwick 1907, Book 1, Chapter VI, §1– §2). Give these a read if time permits.

3.32   A naturalistic fallacy is committed when we deduce – always falsely – from the way how things are how they ought to be. So, when people say that reproductive human cloning or IVF – i.e. a new way of making babies – is unnatural or abnormal, and therefore wrong, they have committed such a fallacy (Pence 1998). We cannot deduce a *moral ought* or *should* from a description of something that merely *is*. Even if we accepted that these technologies are unnatural – and, arguably we should not even do that – it would not follow that their use is unethical. If we did agree with such a faulty line of reasoning we would quickly find ourselves in a precarious situation where, for consistency's sake, we would have to object to the use of most human invented technologies. Radiation therapy for various cancers, or MRI scans are no more natural by that definition of naturalness.

3.8 Dignity

3.33 A ubiquitous phrase used liberally in many a bioethical analysis and argument is that of human dignity. Unfortunately, while the language of human dignity is universal, there is no consensus on the moral basis or on the precise meaning of human dignity. Religious as well as secular accounts of human dignity exist, and yet, it remains unclear whether it should best be understood as a basic, or primitive, term of moral language or whether it might reasonably be derived from a moral theory of mainstream appeal. The Australian philosopher Robert Goodin thinks that it is impossible to ground human dignity in a moral theory. He suggests that we should accept 'human dignity' as a logical primitive, 'a fundamental axiom in our individualistic ethical system', as he calls it (Goodin 1981, 97). This, of course, does not resolve the problem at hand. Goodin concedes that dignity cannot be derived from an ethical framework, so, instead, he suggests without further justification, that we should accept it as a primitive term of moral language. The problem is, unfortunately, that the meaning of the term is not self-evident to begin with and so we have no reason to accept this invitation.

Among others this was lamented by Adam Schulman, a contributor to an 3.34 anthology on bioethics and human dignity produced by former US President George W. Bush's Council on Bioethics. In his chapter Schulman analyses promising existing normative foundations for the concept of human dignity, and concludes that they all fail. Schulman takes this challenge as a kind of a conceptual call to arms: 'In short, the march of scientific progress that now promises to give us manipulative power over human nature itself ... will eventually compel us to take a stand on the meaning of human dignity, understood as the essential and inviolable core of our *humanity*' (Schulman 2008, 17). Ruth Macklin has taken a different approach. She argues in a much-discussed article in the *British Medical Journal* that 'a close inspection [...] shows that appeals to dignity are either vague restatements of other, more precise, notions or mere slogans that add nothing to an understanding of the topic' (Macklin 2003). In her view, in secular bioethics at least, talk of human dignity merely means respect for personal autonomy.

David A. Hyman agrees, he writes: 3.35

> ... in every generation, philosophers, ethicists, religious figures, politicians, and professional worrywarts have cited human dignity as a reason to restrict innovation or prohibit it outright. Consider a few examples. Galileo was forced to recant his heliocentric views because the Roman Catholic Church had already embraced the Ptolemaic system as more consistent with Biblical revelation and with man's dignity as God's creation. Indoor plumbing, the printing press, skyscrapers, the suburbs, automobiles, television, the Sony Walkman™, and the franchise for women were all met with the objection that they were inconsistent with human dignity. The Industrial Revolution, which laid the foundation for the modern world, was criticized because machines were expected to destroy human dignity.
>
> (Hyman 2003)

In the medical context, human dignity continues to hold a prominent 3.36 place. The World Medical Association's **Declaration of Geneva**[53] demands that doctors treat their patients with 'compassion and respect for human dignity'. Oliver Sensen points out that human dignity, today forms the moral ground of human rights in UN documents. For instance, in the 1948 *Universal Declaration of Human Rights*, human rights are grounded in 'the recognition of the inherent dignity [...] of all members of the human family'. Sensen sees a problem in the UN approach on this issue. He writes:

> [i]n documents like these [UN declarations, covenants] key terms are deliberately kept vague, since one can only secure an agreement among so many parties at the price of a certain ambiguity. If one were to specify the meaning and grounding force of human dignity, it might be at odds with some parties' deeply entrenched opinions and beliefs. In this case the whole project might fail. Accordingly, there is no explicit attempt to clarify or justify human dignity in these documents.
>
> (Sensen 2011)

3.37   Another example of this phenomenon, in the field of bioethics, is the UNESCO **Declaration on Bioethics and Human Rights**[54]. It uses human dignity to ground the substantive policy guidance contained in the Declaration. David Benatar, a South African philosopher, agrees with Sensen's argument on the popularity of vague language in this dignity-centered declaration. He is suspicious that it is being used by the drafters of this document 'to gloss over disagreement', which is achieved by them choosing words 'that are sufficiently vague that each person can interpret them consistently with his or her own views' (Benatar 2005). Unfortunately, just as is the case more generally, there is no consensus among experts on what the moral basis of human dignity is, if any, and what its specific meaning in the health care context should be taken to be.

3.38   In bioethical discourse dignity often means one thing and its opposite. Unsurprisingly, given its vagueness, human dignity is deployed in ethical, political, and even legal contexts in support of diametrically opposing points of view. For instance, both proponents as well as opponents of assisted dying deploy the human dignity trope for their respective ends. The rhetorical tool of human dignity pervades many public policy debates and it is present in many other spheres of social life. Authors often use it to cloak potentially controversial moral considerations in the language of dignity.

3.39   When you come across dignity arguments in bioethics, always investigate whether there is anything substantive to it, or whether it is no more than a pleasant-sounding word deployed to shame you into agreeing with a particular point of view. We are not suggesting here that it is impossible to create a coherent theory of human dignity, but today it is fair to say that there is no consensus on either the moral basis of human dignity, or its meaning, or its scope.

3.9 Nazi Arguments in Bioethics

Nazi arguments are not arguments that Nazis necessarily have defended or 3.40 put forward. Nazi arguments in bioethics, but not just in bioethics, are primarily deployed to end a particular debate or argument. After all, if a point of view is *analogous* to something the Nazis did or propagated, it is highly likely that there is a serious flaw in it. Equally, if a particular course of action would lead us down a *slippery slope* toward something akin to the crimes the Nazis committed, we would also have good reason to not seriously consider that course of action. The utilitarian Peter Singer, an influential secular Jewish philosopher, was accused of promoting points of view that were supposedly both analogous to views propagated by the Nazis, and that would lead societies adopting those views down slippery slopes toward Nazi style atrocities (Schöne-Seifert 1991; Wright 2000).

Walter Wright describes both the argument from analogy as well as the 3.41 slippery slope argument. Singer, as you will discover in greater detail in Chapter 5 on beginning of life issues, holds a number of highly controversial views resulting in him defending as moral the killing of certain severely disabled newborns. Significantly, he used language in this context that was identical to the language used by the Nazis.

In a nutshell Singer holds the view that newborns are not persons, 3.42 because at birth and for a few weeks after they do not have the intellectual capacities to qualify as such. He also thinks that, by virtue of their disability, some newborns will never reach personhood, even in later life. Only persons have a right to life, so newborns would then not have a right to life. Singer the utilitarian aims to maximize the reduction of the overall amount of suffering in the world and to maximize the overall amount of happiness in the world. He argues in his bestselling book *Practical Ethics* that some disabled newborns suffer irreversibly a quality of life that is so miserable 'as not to be worth living, from the internal perspective of a being who will lead that life' (Singer 2011, 162). There he said it, a life not worth living. Singer thinks that parents of such severely disabled newborns should be permitted to make the choice to have their lives terminated. The troubling thing, for Singer, is that in the 1920s two influential German academics, the leading legal scholar Karl Binding and the medical school professor Alfred Hoche published a book in which they argued for the destruction of lives not worth living (Hoch and Binding 1920). They were not Nazis, and they were arguably driven to some extent by compassion. For instance, they insisted that those lives not worth living should only be terminated if, as Wright quotes them, their life ending 'must be experienced as a release, at least by the victim; otherwise allowing it is self-evidently ruled out' (Wright 2000, 180–181).

3.43   The Nazis, of course, had other ideas when it came to euthanasia and the destruction of human lives they did not consider worth living, and their ideas were quite different from those of the German academics, and they were certainly not analogous to Singer's views. The Nazis liked Binding and Hoche's terminology; in fact, 'life not worth living' was used extensively by the Nazis and their propaganda machine. It is fair to say that the Nazis did use pretty much the same vocabulary Singer uses. However, that is where the analogy ends. Their so-called 'euthanasia' program was eventually directed at people who experienced pretty much any kind of mental illness, were homosexuals, drug users, or simply homeless. What occurred was plainly and simply the murder of people who would have considered their lives very much worth living. This then isn't analogous to the case Singer makes in his argument.

3.44   Unsurprisingly perhaps, when Singer was invited by German academics to lecture on this topic, disability rights and other activists protested and succeeded for some time in their efforts aimed at preventing Singer from speaking at German universities. As far as these activists were concerned, Singer propagated views that were analogous to what the Nazis did (Schöne-Seifert 1991). In reality, while Singer's views were and are controversial, as you have seen, the Nazi analogy is flawed. It was deployed on this occasion to end any further debate on Singer's views with regard to the morality of infanticide involving the termination of the lives of certain severely disabled newborns.

3.45   John J. Michalczyk, a medical historian, warns that 'those who invoke the Nazi analogy in a broad or general fashion are pressing the limits of valid analogy simply because the broader the scope of their reference, the harder it becomes to understand exactly what they think the Holocaust was, and thus why it is of moral relevance to the current issue' (Michalczyk 1994).

Others have suggested that if we began taking Singer's views seriously 3.46
and implemented them as a matter of government policy we would inevitably be led down the slippery slope toward a Nazi kind of end result. We will
now turn to slippery slope type arguments in bioethics.

3.10 Slippery-Slope Arguments

Probably the most frequently used rhetorical tool in bioethics debates 3.47
comes in the shape of slippery-slope type arguments. Slippery-slope type
arguments come in various forms, but typically they are claims that something terrible would happen if we did a certain arguably desirable thing. A
good example of this is: 'If we introduce voluntary euthanasia for mentally
competent terminally ill patients soon the mentally disabled will get murdered, just like the Nazis did.' A conservative Canadian newspaper editori-
alized against euthanasia in that country, warning against '**the slippery
slope of assisted dying**[55]'.

Usually slippery-slope type arguments are both emotionally appealing 3.48
and invalid. There are two broad types of slippery-slope arguments that you
quite likely will come across in bioethical arguments. The first type of slippery slope argument is conceptual in nature. It is not as common as the
causal slippery slope type argument in bioethics. Conceptual slippery slope
arguments claim that the criteria that are proposed to govern new legislation or a new policy are sufficiently imprecise as to open the door to abusive
practices. We will come across examples of this kind of slippery-slope argument in Chapter 11 because conceptual slippery slope arguments appear
frequently in discussions about end-of-life issues (**Somerville 2014**[56]). The
same holds true for causal slippery slope arguments (**Somerville 2014**[57]).
Causal slippery slope type arguments typically claim that if a given (possibly sound) policy were introduced, this would invariably trigger a chain of
events leading to actions or outcomes that are unacceptable (Schüklenk
2011, 47–50).

Conceptual slippery-slope arguments are difficult to evaluate as a matter 3.49
of principle. If you were to legislate that only legally competent individuals
suffering from a terminal illness would be allowed to request a medically
assisted death, would that really lead to a slippery slope endangering the
mentally incompetent or people with depression, say, because competence
assessments are not as reliable as mathematical proof? It is difficult to
address this argument, except by noting that we undertake competency

assessments of individuals in a large number of situations on a daily basis. The proposition that we should never implement legislation unless the concepts are as clear as the laws of physics would in effect prevent us from legislating at all.

3.50   Causal slippery slope arguments are much clearer in nature. They stipulate that if you do X, Y will invariably follow. The claim here is, of course, empirical. The inevitability is what typically is in doubt. 'For example, opponents of genetic testing and screening say that there is no way to control the slippery slope from therapeutic uses of these new techniques to eugenic ones' (Schüklenk 2011, 47). There are several problems with these kinds of argument. For starters, we do not know whether the empirical slope that is claimed here does actually exist. Is the inevitability of what is claimed truly inevitable, let alone likely? Given the slippery slope concerns raised would it truly be beyond our capacity to regulate and legislate against such outcomes? Even if there were actions that could be described as eugenic, would they necessarily be unethical? One problem with this line of reasoning is that it often is rhetorical in nature. A label is attached to a particular outcome, typically in a question-begging manner, with the obvious aim being to persuade us to reject both the outcome and the slippery slope event that led to it. This we are supposedly only able to achieve by rejecting a particular proposed policy or action. Last but not least, there is always the possibility that X occurred, and that Y occurred, and that we concur, on reflection, that Y is undesirable, yet Y turns out to be not actual causally related to X. An example for this scenario could be problematic cases in jurisdictions that have decriminalized assisted dying. Say there was a case where a homeless person was euthanized against their wishes. Opponents of assisted dying legislation would need to do more than point to this case to have a sound argument. They would have to show that there is a causal link between the decriminalization of assisted dying and the case in question. Typically causal slippery-slope arguments fail on this count. Correlation is no proof of causation.

3.51   You should be on high alert whenever someone introduces slippery-slope arguments in discussions not only of matters bioethics, but of any issue. Slippery slope arguments can be (logically) valid, but often they are not. Their weakness usually is lies in the lack of *detail*, all they do is to claim that something might happen, on the sketchiest of evidence, or lacking any evidence (Burgess 1993). You will find fine examples of slippery-slope rhetoric in Chapter 8 in our discussion of reproductive human cloning as well as in Chapter 11 dealing with ethical issues at the end of life.

3.11 Treating Someone as a Means

It is not uncommon to find the thought expressed that it is wrong to treat 3.52
someone as a means, with a (possibly brief) reference to Kant. As Onora
O'Neill has pointed out, what goes under the name of Kantian ethics today
sometimes bears little relation to what Kant actually said (O'Neill 1991).
According to Kant's Categorical Imperative, we should never treat humanity, whether in ourselves or in others, as a means only, but always at the
same time as an end in itself.

We cannot avoid treating each other as means; we do this all the time, for 3.53
instance when we take public transport or use delivery services to get a
pizza. The point is that we should not treat people *merely* as means. What is
involved in treating another human being as an end is unsurprisingly a
matter of debate, but involves at least respecting them as an autonomous
being with goals of their own, whom it would be wrong to use in a way
merely to satisfy our own ends. Difficult questions tend to arise in situations where it seems to us as agents that a person is not treating themselves
with proper respect, e.g. by their choice of ways to make a living. If that is
their choice, does it have to be respected in order to treat them as an end?

In bioethics it might be argued that a savior sibling (see Chapter 5) is 3.54
being used as a 'mere' means. Is that right? The sibling may not have had a
life if it were not for the need for a source of tissue. What conditions need
to be satisfied in order for the sibling to be treated as an end in themselves?
This will be discussed further in Chapter 5.

Two other questions arise, at least. The first is the range of application. 3.55
What must be treated as an end, for Kant, is an autonomous being. This
might seem to rule out from the start the possibility of applying the argument to fetuses. But a Kantian-*inspired* ethic might try to make that move.

The other question is what it can mean to treat oneself as an end. Kant 3.56
himself had many examples of duties towards our bodies, which seem
strange to the modern more liberal minded reader, but this demonstrates
that for him, one's body should be treated with proper respect, as it is not
'mine' it is 'me'. This type of consideration may be appealed to in arguments
about prostitution, as well as in discussions about selling parts of the body
for profit.

The important take-away from this is that we must be careful about 3.57
attempts to argue that something is wrong because it involves treating
another human being as a means, without being clear about exactly what is
involved, and whether what is at issue is treating someone as a 'mere' means.

Questions

We have seen in this chapter that particular, faulty types of arguments keep appearing in ethical analyses. Try summarizing in your own words what kinds of arguments these are, how they work, and why they are faulty.

Given what you have read in this chapter, do you think it is possible to use patients who participate in clinical trials not as mere means? Can you think of slippery slope type arguments that you have come across recently? Were they sound or flawed? Provide reasons for your answers.

Website Links

1   http://www.iep.utm.edu/bioethic/#SH2a/
2   http://gemmacelestino.googlepages.com/Singers1973.pdf/
3   http://www.nybooks.com/articles/archives/2003/may/15/animal-liberation-at-30/
4   http://www.mdpi.com/2076-2615/3/1/238/pdf/
5   http://www.iep.utm.edu/envi-eth/
6   http://plato.stanford.edu/entries/ethics-environmental/
7   https://www.wma.net/what-we-do/education/medical-ethics-course/
8   https://depts.washington.edu/bhdept/ethics-medicine/bioethics-tools
9   https://www.union.edu/philosophy/faculty-staff/robert-baker
10   https://www.medscape.com/viewarticle/479892_3
11   https://www.general-anaesthesia.com/images/james-simpson.html
12   http://encyclopedia2.thefreedictionary.com/chloroform/
13   https://en.wikipedia.org/wiki/Henry_K._Beecher
14   https://apps.who.int/iris/bitstream/handle/10665/74765/vol79.no.4.365-372.pdf
15   https://www.newscientist.com/article/mg23731640-800-the-doctor-who-exposed-the-uks-terrible-experiments-on-patients/
16   https://apps.who.int/iris/bitstream/handle/10665/74765/vol79.no.4.365-372.pdf
17   http://www.szasz.com/
18   https://psychnews.psychiatryonline.org/doi/10.1176/appi.pn.2019.10b11
19   http://www.law.cornell.edu/supct/html/historics/USSC_CR_0410_0113_ZS.html/
20   https://www.canlii.org/en/ca/scc/doc/1988/1988canlii90/1988canlii90.html
21   http://plato.stanford.edu/entries/publichealth-ethics/

22 http://www.plosmedicine.org/article/info%3Adoi%2F10.1371%2Fjournal.
    pmed.0040050/

23 http://v1archives.aansneurosurgeon.org/features/sport-related-mtbi-a-public-health-
    ethical-imperative-to-act/

24 http:/www.neuroethicssociety.org/

25 http:/www.wired.co.uk/magazine/archive/2012/04/features/the-forgetting-
    pill/

26 http:/www.newyorker.com/magazine/2009/04/27/brain-gain?current
    Page=all/

27 https://whatistranshumanism.org/

28 https://en.wikipedia.org/wiki/Profession

29 http://www.asbh.org/about/content/asbh-ceca.html/

30 http://bioethics-international.org/index.php?show=networks/

31 http://fabnet.org/

32 http://onlinelibrary.wiley.com/journal/10.1111/(ISSN)1467-8519/

33 http://www.ijfab.org/

34 https://bioethics.georgetown.edu/using-the-library/bioethics-journals/

35 https://apps.who.int/ethics/nationalcommittees/NEC_full_web.pdf

36 https://www.nuffieldbioethics.org/

37 https://bioethicsarchive.georgetown.edu/pcsbi/node/851.html

38 http://www.ethikrat.org/about-us/our-mandate/

39 https://www.wma.net/members-area/standing-documents/wma-procedures-and-
    operating-policies-apr2019/

40 https://www.wma.net/what-we-do/education/medical-ethics-manual/

41 https://www.wma.net/what-we-do/education/medical-ethics-course/

42 http://cioms.ch/ethical-guidelines-2016/WEB-CIOMS-EthicalGuidelines.pdf/

43 https://ethics.gc.ca/eng/policy-politique_tcps2-eptc2_2018.html

44 https://faculty.fordham.edu/nballantyne/public_html/Ballantyne_
    KnockdownArguments_Erk-preprint.pdf

45 https://www.ncbi.nlm.nih.gov/pmc/articles/PMC1297029/

46 https://www.britannica.com/topic/hubris/

47 https://plato.stanford.edu/entries/aquinas

48 https://plato.stanford.edu/entries/kant/

49 https://philpapers.org/archive/SOBKAS/

50 https://plato.stanford.edu/entries/hume/

51 https://plato.stanford.edu/entries/fallacies/

52 https://www.gutenberg.org/ebooks/46743

53 https://www.wma.net/policies-post/wma-declaration-of-geneva/

54 https://en.unesco.org/themes/ethics-science-and-technology/bioethics-and-
    human-rights

55   https://nationalpost.com/opinion/national-post-view-the-slippery-slope-of-assisted-dying/

56   https://www.catholiceducation.org/en/controversy/euthanasia-and-assisted-suicide/euthanasia-s-slippery-slope-can-t-be-prevented.html/

57   https://www.catholiceducation.org/en/controversy/euthanasia-and-assisted-suicide/euthanasia-s-slippery-slope-can-t-be-prevented.html/

4

MORAL STANDING: WHAT MATTERS

This brief chapter is dedicated to the question of moral standing. Moral 4.1
philosophers have long struggled with questions such as these: Why do people
have moral standing and why don't other animals have moral standing? Do
all people have moral standing regardless of their intellectual capacity? Are
there good reasons for ascribing moral standing to non-human animals?
Does species membership matter? But, what about trees or ecosystems? Do
they have moral standing? And what do we mean when we say that someone has 'moral standing'? Why does 'moral standing' matter?

4.1 Moral Standing and Moral Status

Let us start with the easier bits. What do we mean by 'moral standing'? Why 4.2
does it matter who we ascribe 'moral standing' to? You might be able to get
a good indication of the significance of answers to these kinds of questions
by undertaking a search in your favorite on-line search engine, such as for
instance **google scholar or Microsoft Academic**[1]. A lot of people have a lot
of different ideas about the question of who or what has moral standing,
and we will familiarize ourselves with the most influential of those views
in just a moment. What knowledgeable people seem to agree on is what
moral standing is, and also why it matters. Whoever has moral standing is
someone who can be morally wronged by actions undertaken by moral
agents. A moral agent is someone who has the capacity to distinguish
between what is morally right and morally wrong. If you have moral

This Is Bioethics: An Introduction, First Edition. Ruth F. Chadwick and Udo Schüklenk.
© 2021 John Wiley & Sons, Inc. Published 2021 by John Wiley & Sons, Inc.

standing, my actions affecting you can be morally right or morally wrong. Equally, if you have no moral standing, whatever it is that I do or don't do that affects you has no moral implications. Say, if we agreed that a stone has no moral standing, me kicking the stone along the road is morally inconsequential as far as the stone is concerned. So, if you think that non-human animals or people with certain disabilities have no moral standing, your treatment of them, whatever you might choose to do or not to do, would be a morally neutral activity.

4.3   Allen Buchanan has suggested that we should distinguish between 'moral status' and 'moral standing'. To him saying that something has moral standing simply means that it counts morally in its own right. However, the moral status of entities that have moral standing is not necessarily the same. Some entities with moral standing might have a higher or lower moral status than other entities who have moral standing (Buchanan 2009). This seems to align with the moral intuitions that many of us share. We might agree that sentient non-human animals have moral standing, and so we might also agree that they have moral status. That still permits us to disagree vigorously about whether a non-human animal's moral status should be the same as that of a human being with similar intellectual capacities. What seems uncontroversial is that 'moral status admits of degrees' (DeGrazia 2008).

4.2 Species Membership

4.4   There are, in fact, any number of ways to argue in favor of particular approaches to moral standing. If you consider Immanuel Kant's celebration of reason and rationality, it won't surprise you to learn that to him moral standing was subject to being a person belonging to our species. He derived that view from the value he ascribed to our capacity to reason, act on reason and, ultimately, be held accountable for our choices. Invariably an argument ensued about the moral standing of members of our species who are not capable of reasoning, such as for instance some people with mental disabilities, but also babies or elderly people who suffer from dementia. Would their moral standing change depending on their mental capacities?

4.5   Some have argued that we ought to distinguish between moral persons and membership in our species. Traditionally membership in our species was seen to be identical with moral personhood. A person certainly was considered to be someone who at a minimum had a right to life. As you will discover in the next chapter, that view gave rise to bitter arguments over the question of whether or not fetuses are persons in that sense, because by granting fetuses full personhood an argument might be created that they also deserve to be treated as persons or be treated *as if* they were persons. That in turn might make it more difficult, if not impossible, to sustain an argument in favor of letting pregnant women choose whether they carry their pregnancy to term or whether they have an abortion.

The ethical challenge, essentially, is that in a Kantian sense, a lot of people are not persons because they lack permanently or temporarily the dispositional features that are constitutive of personhood, such as a sense of self, future oriented plans, self-reflection, and so on and so forth. Michael Tooley, in a widely discussed article on abortion and infanticide, argues that neither fetuses nor newborns have a right to life, because they are not persons. He calls the 'tendency to use expressions like 'person' and 'human being' interchangeably ... unfortunate' (Tooley 1972, 41). Tooley, like most moral and political philosophers, holds the view that persons uncontroversially have a right to life. Here are the conditions he thinks someone needs to meet in order to be ascribed personhood. He writes: 'An organism possesses a serious right to life only if it possesses the concept of a self as a continuing subject of experiences and other mental states, and believes that it is itself such a continuing entity' (Tooley 1972, 44). So, as far as Tooley is concerned, for something to have a right to life it must have self-consciousness. Of course, not everyone agrees with him. Don Marquis, for instance, has defended the view that even fetuses have a right to life, because aborting them would rob them of a future of value, of a future like ours (Marquis 1989). We will not delve deeper into this line of reasoning here, however, you will discover more about Tooley's views and possible counter arguments in the next chapter. If we were to accept his argument it would follow that not all members of our species have uncontroversially a right to life, let alone fetuses at their different stages of development. Of course, that does not mean that they might not have other dispositional capacities that we ought to take into consideration that would grant them some kind of moral standing, but possibly not a right to life.

Interestingly, animal rights advocates among philosophers have developed ideas similar to Tooley's. Tom Regan, for instance, has argued that at least some non-human animals have moral standing, and moral rights even. He suggests in an influential book on *The Case for Animal Rights*, that animals who meet what he calls his subject-of-a-life criterion, must no

4.6

4.7

longer be treated as mere means to achieve human ends. They, in his view, are bearers of rights. He wrote (Regan 1988, p. 243):

> Individuals are subjects-of-a-life if they have beliefs and desires; perception, memory, and a sense of the future, including their own future; an emotional life together with feelings of pleasure and pain; preference and welfare-interests; the ability to initiate action in pursuit of their desires and goals; a psychophysical identity over time; and an individual welfare in the sense that their experiential life fares well or ill for them, logically independently of their utility for others and logically independently of their being the object of anyone else's interests.

4.8   Regan claims that many higher mammals meet this standard, and, like Tooley, he also notes that not all humans are subjects-of-a-life, so understood. This would imply both that at least some humans do not have moral rights, while some higher mammals at least would have moral rights. As we have seen, an initial suggestion was that all members of our species deserve moral consideration. That, of course, leads us immediately to the question of when membership in our species begins, is it something that occurs at the moment of conception or something that really only begins after birth, or at morally significant points in-between? We will discuss in the next chapter in greater detail the intricacies of this question, because depending on how one answers it one ends up quickly in hot water with regard to reproductive health issues such as abortion. After all, if membership in our species begins at the moment of conception, and that is sufficient for full moral standing, it would follow that abortion is not a morally neutral activity. However, this does not quite mean then that abortion would be always wrong.

4.9   We will look now at various approaches to the question of moral standing by drawing concentric circles including ever more living, and eventually even inanimate things, and looking at the reasons proposed for why they deserve moral consideration.

4.3 Sentientism

4.10 Some influential ethicists such as one of the founders of utilitarianism, Jeremy Bentham (1789), or modern-day utilitarians such as bioethicist Peter Singer (1975), think that the focus on species membership is deeply flawed. Both Bentham as well as Singer argue that using species membership as the relevant moral criterion really is something akin to racism. Singer calls it 'speciesism'. These thinkers point out that the formal principle of justice requires of us to treat equal interests equally. Jeremy Bentham famously noted in 1789 in his book *Introduction to the Principles of Morals and Legislation* (Bentham 1789):

> The day may come, when the rest of the animal creation may acquire those rights which could never have been withholden from them but by the hand of tyranny. The French have already discovered that the blackness of the skin is no reason why a human being should be abandoned without redress to the caprice of the mentor. It may one day come to be recognized that the number of legs, the villosity of the skin, are reasons equally insufficient for abandoning a sensitive being to the same fate. ... What else is it that should trace the insuperable line? Is it the faculty to reason, or perhaps the faculty of discourse? But a full-grown horse or dog is beyond comparison a more rational as well as a more conversable animal, than an infant of a day, or a week or even a month old. The question is not, Can they *reason*?, nor Can they *talk*? But, *Can they suffer*.

It shouldn't surprise that utilitarians, with their focus on the minimization 4.11 of harm and the maximization of happiness, are not supportive of a standard that involves species membership, because it is undoubtedly true that there are many members of our species that have mental capacities throughout their lives or at certain points during their lives that are well comparable to those of other non-human higher mammals. If we do not inflict gratuitous pain on human members of our species that have mental capacities comparable to non-human higher mammals capable of suffering, justice would require of us that we treat them equally to those humans. Utilitarians are also adamant that intelligence or species membership are irrelevant to the question of whether or not it is acceptable to inflict pain and suffering on someone. Rather, they think we should zoom in on the criterion that is actually relevant: the capacity to feel pain and to suffer. They call it sentientism (as opposed to the human-centered anthropocentrism). Basically, everything that is capable of feeling pain and suffering has moral standing and should be ascribed an interest in not feeling pain and in not suffering. The infliction of pain and suffering on a being capable of feeling pain and suffering is not a morally neutral activity according to this standard, regardless of species membership. As we will see in Chapter 7 (Research Ethics) this take on moral standing has important implications for the ethics of experiments involving non-volunteering non-human animals.

4.4 Capabilities

4.12   Martha Nussbaum, an influential philosopher proponent of the **capabilities approach**[2], has been highly critical of both the Kantian as well as the utilitarian view on animal rights (Nussbaum 2006, 1). She thinks that for us to address the question of what we morally owe to other people we need to begin by asking what they are actually capable of doing and capable of being. She argues that we are entitled to a decent level of opportunity in 10 key aspects of our lives; these areas include: life, bodily health, bodily integrity, senses, imagination and thought, emotions, practical reason, affiliation, other species, play, and control over our environment (Nussbaum 2006, 2). Nussbaum then extends this also to the relations between humans and non-human animals. The moral standing of non-human animals is grounded in their needs and abilities (2006, 1). Essentially this is an attempt at extending human flourishing-centered virtue ethics to non-human animals. Nussbaum concludes that 'each form of life is worthy of respect, and it is a problem of justice when a creature does not have the opportunity to unfold its (valuable) power.'

4.5 Biocentrism

4.13   William K. Frankena has proposed a widely used typology of ethical theories that affect who would be considered a moral patient (i.e. an entity that can be morally harmed or that can benefit from particular actions) and/or a moral agent (i.e. an agent that can morally harm or benefit a particular other) (Frankena 1979). He argues that living non-sentient things might be reasonable candidates for the status of moral patient, because they can be harmed or benefitted by actions undertaken by moral agents. Trees could be harmed if someone cuts them off in order to use them for the production of paper, for instance. Of course, Kantians would disagree because trees don't have the dispositional capacity for rationality. Utilitarians might agree that healthy trees are useful for sentient beings to have around, because they generate much needed oxygen. They would disagree that a tree, as such, has moral standing, because the tree is not sentient. Once we ascribe moral standing to non-rational, non-sentient living things, there is potential for ethical conflicts, as we saw earlier with regard to sentient beings and experiments with non-volunteering non-human animals. A possible answer to the concerns raised by utilitarians with regard to sentient non-human animals could be to live life as a vegetarian or even a vegan, but that would cease to be an uncontroversial option if those food sources were also ascribed moral patient status. Similarly, what would that mean for the moral standing, of, say cancer cells busily replicating in our bodies? Would we owe them the right to express themselves freely, until our eventual demise? What about **Zika virus**[3] carrying mosquitos? To be fair to this account, there are plausible answers to these challenges. For instance, vegetarianism could arguably be defended as ethically preferable even if plants were granted moral standing, because the production of meat for food purposes would require a disproportionately larger quantity of plants to feed the livestock first (Pimentel and Pimental 2003). Still, the destruction of plants, say forests, for the sake of human development, would have to be considered not only because of the potential for harmful consequences affecting future generations of people and non-human animals, but also because of their impact on the plants themselves. This approach is often referred to as *biocentric*[4]. Jon Wetlesen has defended this kind of biocentric approach. He proposes 'equal moral status for moral persons and agents, and gradual moral status value for non-persons, depending on their degree of similarity with moral persons' (Wetlesen 1999).

4.6 Holism

The next circle encompasses whole ecosystems, and nature as such. The most influential writer arguing in favor of legal standing for ecosystems such as oceans, valleys, river systems is Christopher D. Stone (1972, 2010). His argument is essentially legal in nature. Stone holds the view that if we assign legal standing to corporations, we have little reason not to grant rights to, for instance ecosystems. It is noteworthy, perhaps, that there is at least one reported precedent where this kind of reasoning has found its way into court rulings. In New Zealand the Waitangi Tribunal granted legal personhood to the Whanganui River, creating thereby the means to appoint legal guardians with the capacity to fight on behalf of the river and everything in it (Vines et al. 2013). 4.14

Bioethicists began to develop an interest in environmental issues a long time ago. Remember what we learned in Chapter 3 about two of the founders of the field, Van Rensselaer Potter and Fritz Jahr. Both were concerned about our relationship with non-human animals as well as plants. 4.15

4.7 The Future

4.16   In recent years, discussions about the moral standing and status of fetuses, non-human animals, plants and ecosystems have been supplemented by other, equally fundamental concerns. They have much to do with new possibilities open to us as a result of human stem cell research as well as research on artificial intelligence. For instance, it is possible, experimentally, to transplant human stem cells into non-human animals, thereby creating chimeras (Streiffer 2005). It may be possible, in the future, to 'upgrade' such non-human animals. What will this mean for their moral status? Will it rise accordingly?

4.17   You might recall **Data**[5], a fictional character in the science fiction series Star Trek. Data is a highly sophisticated android with human-like characteristics. In various episodes of the series he seems to regret his inability to experience emotions, including joy. In the feature film **Star Trek: First Contact**[6] the **Borg Queen**[7] offers Data what he desires. She reconfigures the android so that he also experiences sensations and emotions. This takes us to challenging ethical questions about the moral standing and status of potential future artificial intelligence entities created by us (or, potentially, created by themselves) that might display characteristics and behaviors similar to our own. Data, for instance, has a line **in one of the series episodes**[8] where he says, 'I chose to believe that I was a person, that I had the potential to become more than a collection of circuits and sub-processors.' **The riposte is delivered**[9] by Beverly Crusher, the star ship's doctor, 'Commander Data, the android who sits here at Ops, dreams of being human, never gets the punch line to a joke…'

4.18   So, while he failed as the pre-upgraded Data to relate to humans, everything changed in terms of his moral status and moral standing after that was done. Once he had an 'emotion' chip installed, and a skin graft that permitted him to feel sensation, he really was like us in morally relevant ways. His status, arguably, might have been pegged somewhere above us, due to his superior analytical skills and speed as well as his bodily strength. That perhaps was the Star Trek writers' answer to the question of what constitutes 'consciousness'.

4.19   The troubling thing about post Borg Queen Data is that we still had to take at face value his expressions of anxiety, stress, fear, and so on and so forth. We didn't know how the skin graft, emotion chip and his android hardware interacted. Was that *really* the same as us experiencing anxiety, stress, fear, and so on and so forth?

It is fair to say that at this point in time there are no androids developed   4.20
anywhere near to a level where a Data-like scenario would even occur as a
serious question. However, if we ever reached a stage where creatures like
humanoid **CY**bernetic **L**if**O**rm **N**ode's could become a reality, i.e. where
we would debate the moral standing or status of bioengineered hybrids of
humans and machines, this empirical question would pose very serious
challenges to address. The main reason for this is that we typically take
expressions of pain, suffering, and happiness at face value. We can never
know, ultimately, whether someone who expresses pain, suffering or happiness actually experiences any of these. One of the first things medical students are taught is to believe their patients when they claim that they are in
pain. This is so, because, despite a few gotcha strategies, we have no means
to investigate the veracity of such patient claims. We act on our own experience of those *feelings* and assume that someone who is physiologically close
to us can experience the same. Our existing ethical analyses – unless they
are specieist – rely on the truth of these assumptions.

It's not too far-fetched to grant the truth of such assumptions with regard   4.21
to beings that are in vital respects like us (as biological chimeras would
arguably be), but where would that leave Data?

Part of the challenge will undoubtedly be to answer the question of   4.22
whether human- or sentient-being-like responses to particular stimuli in an
artificial intelligence entity are morally equivalent to the responses given by
beings that are physiologically capable of having such experiences. Robert
Sparrow has argued for a **Turing Triage type test**[10] to assist us in determining whether an artificial intelligence possesses moral standing. He proposes
a 'test for when computers have achieved moral standing by asking when a
computer might take the place of a human being in a moral dilemma, such
as a "triage" situation in which a choice must be made as to which of two
human lives to save. We will know that machines have achieved moral standing comparable to a human when the replacement of one of these people
with an artificial intelligence leaves the character of the dilemma intact.' His
answer to this challenge is that *if* we decide that moral personhood is only a
matter of cognitive skills, it's just a matter of time until artificial intelligence
attains moral standing. If, on the other hand we create an account of personhood that entails being part of a network of others like us with whom we
socially interact (as in the **African philosophy of Ubuntu**)[11], machines
would have some difficulty passing such a test (Sparrow 2004).

The answer to the question of who matters depends on an answer to the   4.23
question of what we value, and on the reasons we provide when asked why

we value a particular thing. You will learn in the next chapters how significant the implications of the initial normative stances are, that we take, for the answers that we give to many controversial questions in bioethics.

Questions

What do you think about the moral status and moral standing of non-humans? How would you go about deciding to whom or to what you have moral obligations? What are your ethical justifications for your answers?

Website Links

1   https://academic.microsoft.com/home/
2   https://plato.stanford.edu/entries/capability-approach/
3   http://www.cdc.gov/zika/
4   https://www.google.com/?ion=1&espv=2&q=biocentric%20 ethics%20definition/
5   https://memory-alpha.fandom.com/wiki/Data
6   https://www.imdb.com/title/tt0117731/
7   https://memory-alpha.fandom.com/wiki/Borg_Queen
8   https://memory-alpha.fandom.com/wiki/Rightful_Heir_(episode)
9   https://memory-alpha.fandom.com/wiki/Remember_Me_(episode)
10   https://gizmodo.com/what-its-like-to-judge-the-turing-test-5921698/
11   https://www.iep.utm.edu/hunhu/

5

BEGINNING OF LIFE

5.1 Introduction

Reproduction plays a central part in the lives of the majority of humans, but 5.1
the ethical issues to which it gives rise are far from resolved. You may have
noticed that in the context of climate change, it is argued that having a child
adds massively to one's carbon footprint, a new version of older debates
about population control. The twentieth century was a time of unprecedented change in reproductive matters, as in other areas of bioethics. The
default framing of reproduction shifted from 'having the children God
gives' to one of reproductive choice. Enormous developments in assisted
reproduction have taken place since the birth of the first 'test-tube' baby,
Louise Brown[1], in 1978. The subject of much ethical debate, it is now both
widely practised and accepted, although arguments continue about both
the type and extent of choices that should be allowable: choosing the sex of
one's offspring, for example, remains a contested topic. We cannot give
detailed attention to the variety of modes of assisted reproduction, a chapter could easily be written on each, but will aim to address the principal
considerations at stake.

Moral issues regarding the fetuses and newborns remain among the most 5.2
difficult and controversial. (There are issues of moral standing to consider,
as discussed in Chapter 4.) We do not seek to resolve them here but to elu-
cidate some of the principal arguments surrounding both old problems and
new developments. Termination of pregnancy, for example, is an issue upon
which people hold strong views on either side, which appear not to be fully

resolvable by argument. While different ethical theories have been applied in this area, many of the ethical debates are affected by disagreement over the status of the fetus.

5.3   We shall begin with ethical considerations typically used in framing the debates, such as arguments about the rights and responsibilities of adults in reproduction, then proceed to issues surrounding the fetus and abortion, ending with matters of infant life and death.

5.2 Ethical Arguments about Reproductive Rights and Responsibilities

5.2.1 Reproductive Autonomy and the Right to Reproduce

5.4 In the twentieth century the right to reproduce was an important ethical argument against interventions such as unwanted sterilization, and the right to found a family was included in the **European Convention on Human Rights**[2]. Like many other rights it has gradually expanded in content, although its boundaries are contested. Whereas it is now widely accepted that individuals should have the right to choose whether to have children, there are ongoing discussions about the *how*, as in the extent of entitlement to reproductive technology. For some, supporting reproductive autonomy is insufficient, as it may be interpreted narrowly to mean reproductive freedom in the sense of access to contraception and avoidance of sterilization. John Robertson introduced the term 'procreative liberty' which includes the right to reproduce without sex, i.e., access to reproductive technologies (Robertson 1983).

5.5   Josephine Johnston and Rachel Zacharias have argued that it is important to pay attention to the contexts in which women's autonomy is exercised. In conditions of wide inequalities and social injustice, many women cannot have real reproductive autonomy if they lack the economic, political and social conditions which facilitate choice. Tackling these factors is a prerequisite for enabling a 'reproductive autonomy worth having' (Johnston and Zacharias 2017).

5.6   From another point of view reproductive autonomy is insufficient in so far as it appears to offer little room for considering the interests of future children: other ethical arguments provide such criteria for consideration. The view that there should be no limits to reproductive autonomy is challenged because of the perceived implications of some reproductive choices for other people, including present and future members of society. Can you think of examples of such implications, in addition to climate change already mentioned above?

5.2.2 Consequentialism and Procreative Beneficence

A consequentialist perspective facilitates consideration of the interests of 5.7 prospective parents, future children and society as a whole. In reproduction it has been common to speak of conflicts of interest between pregnant woman and fetus, most notably in the abortion debate, but in fact the potential conflicts of interest are increasingly complicated.

In the light of technological developments, there is also an issue over 5.8 identification of who the parents are, when we are thinking of giving them consideration. In the past it was clear that, while fatherhood might be open to dispute, the mother was the one who gave birth. Traditional classifications have arguably been thrown into doubt in, for example, surrogacy, in cases of donated gametes, and developments in mitochondrial transfer, where genetic material from three people is involved in creating the resultant child (Dimond 2015). Transgender parents also lead to a questioning of the traditional biological classifications of parents. Does this matter? There is also a further problem about identification of interested parties and issues of moral standing. When one is caring for a pregnant woman, is there only one patient, or two? If one, is it the pregnant woman or the fetus? (Chadwick and Childs 2012). If two, which should take priority when there is a clash of interests?

Although there are grounds for saying that, in the case of other client 5.9 groups, the boundaries of care also extend beyond an individual patient to, for example, partners and children, the question of other parties with interests is particularly pressing in the context of the fetus and indeed the newborn. This is partly because the latter are never in a position to speak for themselves. In their case, we cannot follow the principle of respect for autonomy, because they do not have the capacity for autonomy. Speaking in terms of potential for autonomy that will develop at a later date is also fraught with problems: a potential x does not have the same rights, for example, as an x, whether for 'x' we substitute king, employee or father.

There are not only questions about what prospective parents should be 5.10 free to do. Within the overall framework of consequentialism Julian Savulescu's argument from procreative beneficence (Savulescu 2001) argues that we ought to produce the children with the best possible prospects, e.g.

those who will have the best possible genetic inheritance (whatever that means), with the aim of achieving the best possible consequences overall. In principle this allows not only for the avoidance of disorder but also for enhancement (see Chapter 9).

5.11   Procreative beneficence has been widely criticized (e.g. by Michael Parker 2007). First, there are many uncertainties about how to define the 'best possible' – as Parker points out it is 'underdetermining'. Secondly there are also uncertainties about the conditions of life that will be available to future offspring. Much more is now known about the ways in which the environment affects how genes are expressed. In a world in which populations are displaced through conflict, migrants in particular are subject to widely different environmental conditions.

5.2.3 'Do No Harm' and the Person-Affecting Restriction

5.12   According to what is called the person-affecting restriction the important thing is to avoid doing harm to persons. In reproduction, however, there are challenging questions about who is directly affected by our actions (recall the point about identifying patients, above). On the person-affecting view if there is no person in existence, then there is no one that can be harmed. In that case it is problematic to say a decision or lifestyle choice could be harming some as yet unspecified future person. To reply that an existing fetus can be harmed will raise the question of whether the fetus is a person. If it is agreed that the fetus is not a person, it still might be argued that the fetus is a potential person. On the other hand, as we saw in the previous chapter, moral standing does not necessarily depend on being a person. We can do harm by causing sentient beings to suffer, even if they do not fall into the class of persons.

5.2.4 The Non-Identity Problem

5.13   A further problem in the reproductive context is Derek Parfit's non-identity problem which he discussed in *Reasons and Persons* (Parfit 1984, see also Parfit 2017) and which is said to arise in the following way. Suppose a person is told that if she has a child this year the child will suffer from a disorder, but if she changes her lifestyle and waits till next year she will have a child free from that. It might be argued that it would be right to wait. The problem is that the child born in a year's time, say George, will not be the same child as the one that would be born this year, Alice – the relevant choice is not between harming Alice or not harming Alice, but between having George and having Alice. If the pregnant woman proceeds to have a child this year that child, even if suffering from a disorder, might still be glad that she has been born. Disability rights arguments sometimes suggest, 'If my condition had been edited out, I would not have been born' and this line of thought is put forward as a reason against thinking there is a duty to choose the 'best possible'. Provided that the life brought into being is considered by the subject of that life to be worth living, no wrong has been done.

5.2.5 Virtue Ethics

Within virtue ethics responsibility in relation to reproduction might be 5.14 regarded as a virtue. There may be differences of opinion about the elements of responsible parenting but they are likely to include, for example, self-restraint in pregnancy with regard to alcohol, and concern for the welfare of the future child. What is considered virtuous will look different according to social context, and arguably the more information about reproduction and genetics we have, the more it makes sense to speak of reproductive responsibility (and the more it may require of us).

The important question is how emerging technologies such as gene edit- 5.15 ing and epigenetics (see Chapter 8) might make a difference to what is expected of the virtuous parent. Given the emphasis on practice and character development in virtue ethics, the implications of epigenetic information about the effects of present day behavior on future generations might be that women in particular could be required from an early age to make lifestyle choices that will maximize their chances of having healthy children.

5.2.6 Feminist Bioethics

Feminist bioethics urges us to look at the real context of power relations in 5.16 which decisions are taken. Ideas about relational autonomy have been prominent: the agent exists in relation to others who may be more powerful. From this perspective it is important to have regard to care for the vulnerable, however these are defined, which may include future people as well as the decision-maker herself. It will be important not simply to accept blame or responsibility but to look at the ways in which other powerful people and organizations can affect the well-being of future people. In whose interests might greater burdens be put upon women parents, in particular? This perspective has been quite influential in the abortion debate.

For women, however, the control of their own fertility continues to be an 5.17 issue, more so in some social settings and cultures than in others. There is a demand for efficient contraception, and for access to abortion in situations such as contraceptive failure. This is a central aspect of feeling in control of women's own lives and bodies. For obvious reasons, this is an issue that affects men less, but it does not follow that they have no interests at all in the matter. Not only have there been cases of men seeking to prevent their partners from aborting fetuses, but there is increasing discussion about the ethics of using technology to produce male pregnancies (see, e.g. Sparrow 2008). Increasingly also, it is argued that for reason of parity, if women are free to choose to terminate a pregnancy then men should be free to choose to avoid fatherhood (Brake 2005). There are thus issues of justice at stake in reproduction as well as other ethical considerations (see Chapter 13).

5.3 Issues in Assisted Reproduction

5.18 A central aspect of control of fertility concerns those who face fertility problems. Technologies such as *in vitro* fertilization (IVF) have made it possible for people who were previously unable to have a child, to do so. Issues that have commonly been raised in this context include whether or not infertility should be considered a disease and whether it should be treated at the public expense, how many treatment cycles people should be entitled to, and on what criteria patients should be considered suitable for treatment. How far, in other words, should we go in trying to satisfy demand in a situation of limited resources? Should women be free to freeze their eggs to allow them to delay reproduction, even where not medically indicated – e.g. for reasons of career or the absence of a partner (see Capps et al., 2013)? Should womb transplants be provided at public expense? (Foley 2012; O'Donovan et al. 2019). The latter question demonstrates the difficulties in establishing the boundaries of a right to reproduce, alluded to earlier in the chapter. If we accept that there is such a right, it does not necessarily follow that there is a right to be helped to reproduce by any means and at any cost whatsoever. Without the availability of womb transplants, women with uterine infertility are limited to adoption or surrogacy, but is it clear that the right to reproduce necessarily includes the right *both* to carry a child *and* to have one that is genetically related?

5.19   One of the key issues in assisted reproduction concerns the introduction of third parties, in cases where donation is required, whether this be the donation of sperm, egg, embryo, womb, or the use of a surrogate. While we cannot deal with all these separately, there is an issue that arises in cases of donation and that is the importance of genetic relatedness. In some cases donation happens by accident, for example, when a couple think they are having assistance only to bring their own sperm and egg together, but the wrong embryo is transferred. You will doubtless have your own view on how important it is to have children that are genetically related. Let's turn to look at this.

5.3.1 Genetic Relatedness: How Important Is It?

Enabling adults to have children that are genetically related is sometimes 5.20 described as making it possible for them to have children 'of their own'. It was regarded as very important by the Warnock Report (Warnock 1985), which took the view that the desire for genetically related children cannot be assuaged by adoption possibilities. Not all types of assisted reproduction, however, provide genetic connection for both or even one partner. The debate about womb transplants introduces a new kind of having children 'of one's own' – via the possibility for an individual to carry a fetus. It is the genetic connection, however, that has received the most attention and which we now consider.

As we have already noted, historically the mother was in a position to be 5.21 sure of genetic connection (except in rare cases of baby mix-up after birth) while for men it was much less certain. Putting aside for the moment the possibilities of male and transgender pregnancies, men have traditionally had genetic connection to their children through a relationship with the mother, and could be mistaken about whether their partner's offspring had a genetic connection to them – hence the importance attached to female fidelity. The development of assisted reproduction has in fact facilitated cases of loss of genetic connection for both partners. Although both partners of a couple may contribute their gametes, if an embryo from other people's gametes is transferred to the womb, then neither partner has genetic connection with the offspring, even though the woman partner has given birth. Such cases are particularly likely to come to light when it is clear that the resulting child cannot be related to their supposed parents, e.g., because of signs of different ethnic origin.

Sometimes called genetic affinity rather than genetic connection or 5.22 genetic relatedness, the loss of it might be considered a harm to parents. But what about the child? For genetic affinity is a reciprocal relation, is it not? It is indeed reciprocal but it is not symmetrical. While everyone has a genetic parent, somewhere, not everyone has genetically related offspring. As Marilyn Strathern has commented, we can look at anyone and see a child. We cannot look at anyone and always see a parent (Strathern 1994). Nevertheless, genetic affinity may be important to both parent and child, in different ways. Parents may want to have genetically related offspring and to know who they are, children may want to know their genetic origins. The good of knowing is not, however, and should not be regarded as, an unalloyed good. As we can see from false paternity cases, where people discover that they are not, in fact, genetically related to their partner's offspring, it has to compete with the potential harm to relationships of disclosure of the genetic facts. In the case of children the perceived good of knowing may be grounded in curiosity, entitlements (e.g. to inheritance), a sense of belonging, health issues, or identity. There have been publicized cases of assisted reproduction clinics where one man has provided sperm for multiple pregnancies. A child produced from donated sperm might want to know their genetic parentage in order to avoid marrying, in ignorance, a sibling, for health or identity reasons or both.

5.23   So, what are the arguments for the importance of genetic affinity? Is it sufficient to say that people have desires and wishes for it? There are other arguments to consider. In the case of parents, the good of genetic affinity may perhaps be grounded in a right to reproduce, in so far as it has an aspect of a right to pass on genetic material rather than just having a child to bring up. Alternatively, it might be grounded in legitimate expectations that people may have, of their partners or of providers of reproductive services. The former may have promised faithfulness: the latter may have contracted to transfer embryos produced from the gametes of the commissioning couple, and not an unrelated embryo. In other words, from the perspective of this argument, it is an issue of keeping a promise or abiding by a contract.

5.24   Despite these considerations, in cases of loss of genetic affinity brought about by transfer of the wrong embryo, there are reasons based on public policy for reluctance of courts to grant damages. First, it may be argued that the birth of a child (even from the 'wrong' embryo) must be regarded as a positive good. Second, if commissioning parents seek redress for the birth of a child based on ethnicity, there are concerns about implications of racism. However, a Singapore case in 2017 did recognize the loss of genetic affinity as a compensatable harm (*ACB v. Thomson Medical Pte Ltd*, 2017).

5.25   Was this a move in the right direction? The issues surrounding knowing in relation to genetic affinity, and the harm of its loss, are ones that are the result of the development of reproduction technology itself. At a time when relationships are increasingly more fluid, however, along with the undermining of once fixed categories of race and gender, can the genetic tie retain its importance? Perhaps it should be regarded as a marker for other goods such as belonging? Is our identity rooted in our genetic ancestry rather than in shared history and experience?

The issues surrounding donation may lessen with the development of **in vitro gametogenesis**[3] (Carter-Walshaw 2019), a technique whereby individuals can have gametes made in the laboratory from their own cells. In that case it will no longer be necessary to ask for donated gametes. This will facilitate genetic relatedness and may also make reproduction easier for transgender couples. It may even be possible for an individual to have two gametes made from their own cells. This would be a step even beyond reproductive cloning which we will discuss in Chapter 8. Nevertheless, as long as there is a requirement for assisted reproduction involving embryo transfer, there will always be possibilities of mix-up. 5.26

5.3.2 Issues of Selection in Reproduction

Another issue which remains contentious is to what extent attempts should be made to control the quality of children, either in terms of preferred sex or genetic characteristics. This does not only arise in assisted reproduction but the fact of assisted reproduction opens up additional possibilities of it. This is a different issue from genetic affinity. Decisions about quality may be made at various stages: genetic counselling for potential parents; preimplantation genetic diagnosis and embryo selection; screening of the fetus with the possibility of an offer of termination; and in some cases disabled newborns have been allowed to die (Kuhse and Singer 1985, pp. 1–17). 5.27

One argument against selection is that we should not 'play God' by deciding what sort of people should exist (see Chapter 3). We cannot avoid taking decisions, however: it is argued by some that we influence the characteristics of our children even by our choice of sexual partner: the extent to which this will be consciously directed to producing a particular type of child (by for example women seeking the **sperm of Nobel prizewinners**[4]) will of course vary and it has long been observed that this is fraught with uncertainty, as in the anecdote according to which Isadora **Duncan**[5] wrote to **George Bernard Shaw**[6] asking him to be the father of her child saying, 'A combination of my beauty and your brains would startle the world.' He is said to have replied that things could turn out the other way round. 5.28

5.29   For many people, whether they support the principle of procreative beneficence or not, it is clear that if we have a choice between bringing into the world a child that suffers from a disorder and one that does not, everything else being equal we should choose the latter. So, in selecting an embryo for implantation, it would seem clear that one that is free from disorder should be selected. Problems arise here, however, over how 'disorder' is to be understood. In the case of deafness, for example, there have been strong arguments for the view that deafness should not be regarded as a disorder or disability, and that people should be free to exercise their autonomy to choose to have a deaf child (see, e.g., Chadwick and Levitt 2016). The general point is that, even if there is agreement that it is good to avoid disorder, it cannot be assumed that there is agreement about what constitutes a disorder.

5.30   The 'expressivist' argument suggests that the very process of selection expresses negative attitudes towards those who have a disability (see, e.g., Shakespeare 2006). It may be possible to disentangle different strands of argument, so that the view that it is preferable, other things being equal, to avoid disability where possible, is not taken to imply that persons with disabilities do not or cannot have worthwhile lives. Clearly, disabled people can and do, but it does not follow from this that it is wrong to try to avoid disability. Nonetheless, in the context of a society which is not disability-friendly, the expressivist argument may have some force (Holm 2008).

5.31   There is even less agreement over whether it is permissible to make choices about what characteristics our children should have, beyond the avoidance of disorder. Sex selection is a case in point (Strange 2010; Strange and Chadwick 2010). Although arguments for reproductive autonomy suggest that people should be free to choose the sex of their child, for example to produce a 'balanced' family, critics are concerned about the implications for social values such as equality between the sexes, and pressures on women, especially in societies where there is a preference for children of a particular sex.

5.32   The procreative beneficence argument (Savulescu 2001) is relevant again in this sex-selection context. As we have seen it moves beyond a choice-based argument in its statement that 'couples (or single reproducers) should select the child, of the possible children they could have, who is expected to have the best life, or at least as good a life as the others, based on the relevant, available information' (Savulescu 2001, 41). Some of the concerns about procreative beneficence have been introduced above. The social context in which decisions are taken is highly relevant. In a very sexist society in which it was difficult for girls and women to flourish, it might seem that selection of a boy would be morally required. The long-term implications of the move beyond the binary divide between male and female remain to be seen.

Let's turn now to examine the issue of abortion.   5.33

5.4 Embryos, Fetuses and Abortion

In the continuing debates about abortion in particular, questions arise   5.34
which seem to lack definitive answers. As mentioned already in Chapter 4 there is a difference of opinion, for example, about whether or not embryos and fetuses can be defined as human beings or persons. Some arguments in this debate try to sidestep the issue of personhood and introduce other considerations. We will be looking at such arguments shortly. We do need to address, however, the status issues.

Let's take embryos first. In one sense, they are arguably human beings, in   5.35
that they are alive, and they are uncontroversially part of the human species. Questions of their status come to the fore when there are issues about the fate of frozen ones, for example. But, it is argued by many that we owe respect only to *persons,* and while they may have the potential for personhood they are certainly not actual persons.

On this view, to be a human being is not necessarily to be a person. So,   5.36
when does personhood start? Some argue that being a person is a matter of possessing certain *characteristics,* such as rationality, language or moral capacities. On these criteria, even infants and some adults would not qualify. Others point to a particular *event* which marks the beginning of personhood, such as birth, but it is not clear why movement from one place (inside the womb) to another place (outside) should make such a difference. Rather, it seems to be a continuum, the development into personhood is a process.

What is clear is that there remains considerable disagreement. What Mary   5.37
Warnock said in her **report**[7] on the issues in 1985 remains relevant today:

> Although the questions of when life or personhood begin appear to be questions of fact susceptible of straightforward answers, we hold that the answers to such questions in fact are complex amalgams of factual and moral judgments. Instead of trying to answer these questions directly we have therefore gone straight to the question of *how it is right to treat the human embryo.*
>
> (Warnock 1985, Para. 11.9)

5.38   The question to which Warnock directs us is also, however, a matter of controversy. Let us agree, for the sake of argument, that embryos are both human beings and potential persons. Even if we agree on this, there is disagreement about how they ought to be treated. After all, even if we conceded that an embryo is a potential person, it would not follow that it should be granted the rights of an actual person. The principle of autonomy, as already indicated, does not help us, for we are dealing with beings that have no actualized capacity for autonomy.

5.39   Some argue that the life of the embryo has absolute value from the moment of fertilization and that it is wrong to take its life. Those of a consequentialist outlook, on the other hand, may say that we have to consider what will lead to the best consequences, and that while the life of an embryo might have some value, it does not have absolute value, such that it can override all other considerations. For example, we should consider the value of the embryo's life, and the effect of its existence on others, when considering embryo selection and the fate of 'spare' embryos.

5.4.1 Fetuses

5.40   The status of the fetus is as difficult to resolve as that of the embryo, and for similar reasons. Again, it is not a simple matter of fact, but depends on what value we put on fetal life. However much we know about the facts of fetal development, controversy will continue. In a classic article, 'Abortion and infanticide', Michael Tooley put forward a criterion of personhood based on the requirement of self-consciousness. He argued that the right to life is the right to continue as a subject of experiences and other psychological states. This right presupposes the desire to continue with those states, but fetuses and infants cannot have this desire. Only a thinking self-conscious agent can do so (Tooley 1972).

5.41   For some, the question of personhood settles the issue, but for others it does not. This becomes obvious if we allow, for the sake of argument, that the fetus is a person, or at least a potential person. It depends on what ethical theory we apply: there is a fundamental clash between 'pro-choice' and 'pro-life' standpoints. The law in a given country lays down parameters within which choice can be exercised, but does not settle the ethical debate.

5.42   The view that the morality of abortion depends on the status and/or right to life of the fetus is challenged by much discussed arguments, by Judith Jarvis Thomson, Don Marquis and Perry Hendricks.

5.4.2 *Judith Jarvis Thomson and the Violinist*

Judith Jarvis Thomson published a famous article on abortion that aims to 5.43
demonstrate the shortcomings of the argument against abortion which
turns on the right to life of the fetus (Thomson 1971): it depends on holding
that the right to life of the fetus is stronger than the pregnant woman's right
to bodily integrity. She uses a thought experiment in which someone wakes
up in hospital to find that a famous violinist is attached to her circulatory
system in order to use her kidneys, which he needs to use for nine months,
or he will die. Accepting that the violinist has a right to life, does that right
outweigh the right to bodily integrity of the person whose kidneys he is
using? There are limits to the right to life: the violinist does not have a right
to the use of someone else's body and neither does the fetus, should the
woman decide to withdraw it.

This argument has provoked much discussion and proved very contro- 5.44
versial. It might be argued that it only justifies abortion in the case of rape.
Where a woman has voluntarily taken part in sexual intercourse, does the
analogy break down? Another problematic aspect of the analogy is that the
violinist is a stranger, whereas a fetus is related to the woman in question.
While people may take different views on this – for example – does it make
a difference if the person whose body is being used will die as a result? – what
Thomson has shown is that the 'right to life' argument has to deal with the
conflicting right to bodily integrity and it cannot simply be assumed that it
trumps it.

5.4.3 *The 'Future-Like-Ours' Argument*

Don Marquis has put forward an argument for the wrongness of abortion 5.45
also without relying on whether the fetus is or is not a person. He argues
that abortion is wrong because it denies a fetus a future of value, a 'future-
like-ours' (just as murder denies an adult human being a future of value).
The argument thus depends on a theory of the wrongness of killing
(Marquis 1989).

The loss of one's life is the greatest loss one can suffer because it deprives 5.46
one of all experiences and activities. So, killing is wrong because it inflicts
one of the greatest possible losses. But what about the possibility that there
are cases in which the fetus does not have a future of value? Marquis says
that in most cases abortion does deny the fetus a future of value. There are
difficulties with this account, however, about determining how we judge
that a fetus does or does not have a future of value.

5.4.4 The Impairment Argument Against Abortion

5.47 Perry Hendricks's impairment argument (Hendricks 2019) is based on the premise that it is wrong to impair a fetus by causing it to have fetal alcohol syndrome (FAS), and introduces the impairment principle, which is that if it is immoral to impair an organism to the nth degree, then, other things being equal, it is immoral to impair it to the n+1 degree. The argument proceeds to claim that abortion impairs the fetus more than FAS, because it causes it to cease to exist. Hendricks also claims that this is an argument that does not depend on whether the fetus is a person.

5.48 How good is this argument? One objection is that abortion does not impair the fetus in the same way that FAS does. Blackshaw writes, 'It is unclear that a fetus can be described as impaired if it no longer exists' (Blackshaw 2019). FAS damages an individual's future interests whereas an aborted fetus has no future interests. Another way of criticizing the argument is via the 'other things being equal' clause. Dustin Crummett argues that it does not apply. Other things are not equal: there *is* a significant moral difference between causing FAS and abortion, and that is in terms of burdensomeness. Carrying a fetus is significantly more burdensome than refraining from excessive drinking for that period: while the burdensomeness of carrying a fetus for nine months may justify an abortion, burdensomeness cannot justify causing FAS (Crummett 2020.

5.49 Let's now explore what virtue ethics has to contribute to this debate.

5.4.5 Women's Character

5.50 Rosalind Hursthouse, a virtue ethicist, lays out in an influential article her analysis of the ethical permissibility of abortion. Unsurprisingly women's reasons for wanting to have an abortion feature prominently (Hursthouse 1991). Hursthouse is careful to note that she does not wish to argue whether women are morally entitled to have abortions. Her point is that women might well have a moral, perhaps even a legal right to have abortions, and for good reasons, and yet their exercise of that right in a particular circumstance is morally questionable from a virtue ethical point of view. Recall that central to virtue ethics is the question of whether the decisions flowing from particular character traits contribute to human flourishing. Hursthouse then proceeds to discuss a variety of possible abortion scenarios, trying to show that motives and circumstances matter. She wants us to replace common questions about the moral standing of the fetus, questions of the kind we have discussed just a moment ago, with other questions such as these: 'How do these facts [about fetuses] figure in the practical reasoning, actions and passions, thoughts and reactions, of the virtuous and the non-virtuous? What is the mark of having the right attitude to these facts and what manifests having the wrong attitude to them?' (Hursthouse 1991, 237).

Hursthouse notes that 'abortion for shallow reasons in the later stages [of 5.51 pregnancy] is much more shocking than abortion for the same reasons in the early stages in a way that matches the fact that deep grief over miscarriage in the later stages is more appropriate than it is over miscarriage in the earlier stages' (Hursthouse 1991, 238). A woman who chooses a later stage abortion for reasons of convenience, say because it would interfere with a skiing holiday, would display a non-virtuous character trait on this account, because she would display an attitude toward family and parenting that is not compatible with a flourishing, virtuous life. If, on the other hand a woman was to choose an abortion, say because after having given birth to a number of children already, she is concerned about her future capacity (Hursthouse 1991, 241) to be – in Hursthouse's words – 'a good mother to the ones she has', she might show a virtuous character.

The difference to the impartialist approaches to abortion we discussed 5.52 earlier is that on this virtue ethics account it matters a great deal which character a woman displays when she chooses to have an abortion.

The question about the moral acceptability of abortion takes place both 5.53 at the individual level, concerning particular abortion decisions, and at the social level, concerning what social policy should be. While health care delivery has to take place within the parameters of legislation on such issues, from time to time debate is of course revisited: the UK House of Commons, for example, deliberated sex-selective abortions in 2015. An argument, of a consequentialist sort, for a liberal abortion policy is that a more restrictive one would do more harm overall, because women, if denied legal ones, will continue to seek abortions illegally, not only adding to their distress but also endangering their health. Even in a society in which the law permits access to abortion, provided that certain conditions are met, women still face multiple pressures, including possibly being subject to protests outside abortion clinics (Bradley 2015). This phenomenon is also, of course, a threat to medical personnel as well.

5.4.6 Abortion and Fetal Transplants

An issue that affects the public policy aspect of abortion is that of fetuses as 5.54 a source of transplant material. Fetal transplants for patients have been of interest since the late twentieth century for patients suffering from Parkinson's disease and remain so today, despite increasing interest in embryonic stem cells (**Transeuro**[8] 2015). While an effective and safe treatment for Parkinson's is clearly desirable, the issue is clouded by its link with abortion. Anti-abortionists clearly have a reason for opposing this technique. Problems would arise if people were persuaded or coerced into having abortions *in order to* provide material for transplant. It is not only anti-abortionists, however, who might think that the practice could lead to a larger number of abortions being performed, that it shifts the debate away from women and their needs, and might change how abortion is performed (Vawter et al. 1990). From a consequentialist perspective, however, if an abortion has occurred, and there is certain material in existence that could be used to help another to regain health, it would seem wrong *not* to use it.

5.55   In order to prevent the potential clinical value of the use of fetal tissue influencing decisions about and practice of abortion, it is important that decisions are kept separate: the decision on whether to abort must be made before any discussion of transplantation; and discussion of when and how to abort must be based on concern for the pregnant woman. In the UK guidance on the use of fetal material (the separation principle here described) was set out in 1989 in the Polkinghorne Report (Polkinghorne 1989a, 1989b). Similar considerations were supported by the American Medical Association (American Medical Association 1996) and they remain valid (MRC 2014).

5.4.7 Savior Siblings

5.56 You might want to compare the issue of using tissue from fetuses for transplants with another issue, that of savior siblings. You may recall we flagged this up in Chapter 3. In the fetal tissue case, as stated above, there has been concern over the possibility of the abortion decision being influenced by the need for tissue, which is not in women's interests if they feel under pressure or if the choice of abortion method is made to maximize tissue collection. In the savior sibling case the issues relate to the morality of deciding to have a child, with the possibility of using embryo selection and tissue typing, in order to provide a potential donor of tissue for a sibling (whom we will call Jack).

5.57   One worry is over treating the donor child (let's call her Jill) as a means, but as you will remember, the Kantian approach asks us, not to avoid treating someone as a means, but to avoid treating someone as a 'mere' means. People regularly have children for purposes of their own, e.g. 'to complete a family' (Sheldon and Wilkinson 2004). It can reasonably be argued, even if the parents would not have had Jill had they not needed a donor to save Jack, that this fact alone does not show that they are treating Jill as a mere means. Jill will have a life of her own and may be loved just as much as Jack. What, you may ask, about the issue of consent? The fact that a child has been selected to be a particular tissue type as a potential donor does not eliminate the need for consent, so worries at the extreme about children being created as organ farms are misplaced. As Wilkinson points out, 'as far as the law is concerned, selected savior siblings do and will continue to benefit from the same protections and safeguards as other children, both specifically in relation to organ donation, and generally as regards their welfare' (Wilkinson 2008, 107). The fact that normal consent rules will apply to Jill is further support for the view that she is not being treated as a mere means. This provides an interesting contrast with the fetal tissue case. If an individual were to choose an abortion specifically to provide tissue, there would be no resulting life for the donor. This will only be an issue, on the 'mere means' argument, for those who think that the fetus comes into the category of beings whom it is wrong to treat as mere means.

From a consequentialist point of view things look very different. In the savior sibling case, if the overall outcome is treatment for Jack plus a life worth living for Jill, then the intentions of the parents are irrelevant. The assessment of net benefit to Jill will need to take into account, among other factors, worries that some have about possible psychological harm. Against that, it is possible that psychological benefit will accrue to Jill from knowing that she has saved a life (if that is indeed the outcome). In her book *Saviour Siblings*, Michelle Taylor-Sands argued that in considering the welfare of the child it is a mistake to focus on an individualistic approach to the child's interests which sets those interests in potential conflict with other family members. Rather, a relational approach should be adopted which sets the child within the family and takes into account the interests she shares with other family members (Taylor-Sands 2013). 5.58

You may be able to think of other arguments that may be brought forward in relation to savior siblings. The slippery slope argument, for example, has been brought up in this context (for a discussion of this see Sheldon and Wilkinson 2004). For a brief reply to Michelle Taylor-Sands, including the applicability of the principle of procreative beneficence in this context, see **Wilkinson 2015**[9]. 5.59

5.4.8 Infants and Infanticide

Some people think that an infant has a status that is totally different from that of a fetus. In an obvious sense, it has joined society by becoming a 5.60

visible member of it. Others, however, think that there is no difference in principle between a being that is inside the womb and one that is outside it: it is simply a matter of geography.

5.61   Let us return briefly to an important implication of Michael Tooley's analysis, that we discussed earlier. In his view not only are fetuses not persons, neither are infants. If we agree with this conceptualization of person-hood, not only would it be morally defensible to undertake abortions, but possibly also infanticide, the killing of newborns. Most people intuitively recoil at the idea of infanticide. We consider newborns as vulnerable humans deserving of our protection, and not as non-persons that we might be permitted to kill under certain circumstances.

5.62   Peter Singer thinks that newborns deserve to be granted no higher moral standing than fetuses, due to their dispositional capacities shortly after birth. As he puts it, 'the *intrinsic* wrongness of killing the late fetus and the *intrinsic* wrongness of killing the newborn infant are not markedly differ-ent' (Singer 2011, 154). Jointly with his colleague Helga Kuhse, Singer argued that we should consider permitting infanticide – on parental request – of certainly severely disabled newborns (Kuhse and Singer 1986). Jeff McMahan, an Oxford based philosopher, agrees with Singer and Kuhse that moral consistency requires of those who reject infanticide but support abortion to reconsider their views (McMahan 2013). He notes that many of us consider abortion, even late-stage abortion in, say, the second or third trimesters of the pregnancy, ethically defensible. Many even agree that abortion beyond the point of viability is morally acceptable in case of severe fetal abnormality. McMahan argues that all those who hold such views but reject infanticide are morally inconsistent in their views, because the dispo-sitional capacities of newborns are comparable to those of fetuses past via-bility. Surely, he argues, the location of the termination of the human life does not change the moral standing of the life in question.

5.63   It is difficult to accept, then, that the status of the newborn infant is sig-nificantly different from that of the fetus. This view is supported by the increasingly earlier viability limit.

5.4.9 Severely Disabled Infants

5.64   In the Netherlands the Groningen Protocol, which was drafted in 2004, allowed for euthanasia of severely ill newborns under certain conditions, with parental consent, including where the prognosis is hopeless and there is the prospect of unbearable suffering (Verhagen 2005). The Protocol was accepted as a standard of practice by the Dutch National Association of Paediatricians. It is worth noting at the outset that the Protocol, while it has led to significant international debate, is only very rarely used (Schüklenk 2014).

The clash between consequentialist and other values comes into play 5.65 here starkly. Should we take the view that an infant, however bad the prognosis, has a life that should be protected and prolonged indefinitely? Or should we think about the consequences, for the infant, its family, and society, of the infant's continued existence?

The Groningen Protocol has attracted controversy, not only because of 5.66 the difficulty of assessing quality of life but because active euthanasia in the case of human beings who are not in a position to express a view crosses an important line (Jotkowitz and Glick 2006). The question whether active ending of a life is worse, ethically speaking, than allowing death is ongoing.

In discussing a **case of a neonate with heterotaxy syndrome**[10], which we 5.67 suggest you look at, with a very poor prognosis, Gilbert Meilander, saying 'no to infant euthanasia' (2014) has argued against a perspective which amounts to thinking of ourselves 'not as fellow human beings and fellow suffers with this child but, instead, as people who are fit to exercise a kind of ultimate authority over another' (Meilander 2014, 533). He argues instead that the goal should be to 'affirm life even in the midst of death, and to commit ourselves to helping to shape a death we can live with" (ibid. 534). Against this Udo Schüklenk, surveying the principal ethical arguments typically brought to bear, including the lack of reflective wishes on the part of the infant, argues that termination of life is a prima facie reasonable option when in line with parental choice and when the quality of life of the newborn will remain such that their lives are not worth living in the best judgment of the parents and attending neonatologists (Schüklenk 2014).

5.4.10 Acts and Omissions

The heterotaxy case introduced in the last section also raises the questions 5.68 of acts and omissions. When a decision is taken, for whatever reason (perhaps from compassion), that an infant's life should not be extended, what does this imply? Let us imagine, for example, that parents reject the baby. Historically there have been one or two well-publicized cases, such as the John Pearson case in the UK and the Baby Doe case in the USA (cf. Kuhse and Singer 1985, pp. 1–17).

It is not always the case, of course, that the parents' rejection of the baby 5.69 entails its death, but in some cases it does, where they refuse permission for a life-prolonging intervention. In some cases like this, health care professionals have brought about or hastened the death of the babies in question by not treating them, and sometimes by not even feeding them, thus relying on the principle of acts and omissions, that it is worse to kill than to allow to die. It could be argued, however, that such a death can be more cruel (or, has worse consequences) than a quick and painless death brought about by an injection of a lethal cocktail of drugs.

5.70   One argument against active euthanasia is that it will lead to less respect for life in general. This is a typical slippery-slope type argument. Kuhse and Singer assessed evidence from other societies where infanticide is practiced and concluded that the killing of newborn infants does not necessarily have unwelcome implications for the manner in which other people in society are treated (Kuhse and Singer 1985, pp. 98–117). This is not because infants suddenly turn into persons at a particular point, but it does show that, psychologically speaking, a sharp distinction can be and has been drawn between our responses to infanticide and to the taking of other forms of human life. As already recognized, however, it is not unlikely that technological developments will change the options and the ways in which we think about these issues.

5.4.11 Newborn Screening

5.71   We will end this chapter by noting that caring for newborns is not always concerned with matters of life and death. Newborn screening is not a new issue: the newborn blood spot test is carried out to screen for a number of serious health conditions. This is justified on the grounds of the health and wellbeing of the infant, because it enables appropriate action. Developments in genetic technologies are leading to discussion of the possibilities of genetic profiling of newborns, in the expectation that in the future it will enable personalized medicine (see Chapter 8).

Questions

Do you think it important to assist people to have children 'of their own'? If so, why? If not, why not?

In the light of the arguments in this chapter, to what extent do you think the permissibility of abortion depends on whether the fetus is a person?

Website Links

1 https://www.britannica.com/biography/Louise-Brown
2 http://www.echr.coe.int/
3 https://www.fertilitysmarts.com/definition/1222/in-vitro-gametogenesis-ivg/
4 http://mentalfloss.com/article/12753/sperm-bank-nobel-prize-winners/
5 https://www.biography.com/people/isadora-duncan-9281125#!/
6 https://www.nobelprize.org/nobel_prizes/literature/laureates/1925/shaw-bio.html/
7 https://embryo.asu.edu/pages/report-committee-inquiry-human-fertilisation-and-embryology-1984-mary-warnock-and-committee/
8 http://www.transeuro.org.uk/
9 https://jme.bmj.com/content/medethics/41/12/927.full.pdf
10 http://www.jtcvsonline.org/article/S0022-5223(14)01302-6/fulltext#intraref1030/

6

HEALTH CARE PROFESSIONAL-PATIENT RELATIONSHIP

We will review in this chapter a number of ethical issues in the health care 6.1 professional patient relationship, beginning with informed consent, one of the foundations of this relationship. Next up is the ethics of paternalism in this relationship, the question of who should decide if the patient is incapable of deciding for themselves, and what criteria should guide those proxy decision-makers. Also, what is the doctor's responsibility vis-a-vis truth-telling and confidentiality of patient information? Are doctors obliged to treat patients even if those patients pose a risk to them, for instance because they're infected with a deadly disease? And, what is the morality of doctors refusing to provide professional services to patients on grounds of individual conscience?

Much of what governs the ethics of the health care professional patient 6.2 relationship is driven by clinical ethics. Clinical ethics is best understood as the practice of ethical decision-making in the health care delivery context. Many of the issues we are looking at in this volume have a bearing on clinical ethics. Efforts are currently underway in various jurisdictions to professionalize clinical ethics consultants. The American Society for Bioethics and Humanities, for instance, has produced a **number of guidelines and training manuals**[1] aimed at facilitating that. Clinical or health care ethicists are employed today in many health care systems, government health departments, health insurance companies and hospitals. Clinical ethics committees exist in many hospitals today.

This Is Bioethics: An Introduction, First Edition. Ruth F. Chadwick and Udo Schüklenk.
© 2021 John Wiley & Sons, Inc. Published 2021 by John Wiley & Sons, Inc.

6.1 Informed Consent

6.3 Any discussion of ethical issues in the health care professional patient relationship would be incomplete if it didn't cover informed consent. We mentioned in Chapter 3 the historical shift in the health care professional-patient relationship from 'doctor knows best' to 'patient decides'. Of course, if the decisionally competent patient is the decider, a procedural tool is needed to accomplish this. In health care today that is informed consent. Informed consent is not only relevant in the therapeutic doctor-patient relationship. You will, for instance, read more about the significance of informed consent in the context of medical research in the next chapter.

6.4   Informed consent basically authorizes the health care professional to interfere with the patient's body, after the patient has been informed about the procedure in question, and after the patient has consented to that type of interference. The authorization is given by the patient, or it is denied by the patient. Something else is required to render informed consent truly valid. It must also be uncoerced, or substantially voluntary. Unsurprisingly, the question of what constitutes true informed consent, and what exactly is meant by substantially voluntary has led to much debate, not only among ethicists, but also among lawyers thinking about how to make sense of these concepts for regulatory purposes.

6.5   A good way to get a handle on this is by asking what the moral basis of informed consent is. The moral basis of informed consent arguably lies predominantly in the value we ascribe in modern societies to respecting persons as well as the self-regarding choices they make for themselves. However, it isn't quite about respecting just any kind of choices that decisionally competent patients make. Autonomous decision-making is not the same as giving informed consent. We can make an autonomous decision without being informed. As patients, we might, for instance, make an autonomous choice to let the doctor decide what they think is best for us (Schüklenk 2019).

6.6   However, we have good consequentialist reasons for valuing informed consent (Schachter et al. 2008; Faden et al. 1986). Informed patients are at a lower risk of misinterpreting, say, postoperative pain as an indication that something may have gone wrong. Having had a say in one's clinical care could also lead to being personally more invested in that care and its outcomes, possibly resulting in better compliance in terms of adhering to treatment protocols.

One of the conditions that renders informed consent ethically valid is 6.7 that it is uncoerced. It is meant to reflect a patient's considered, sufficiently informed, voluntary choice.

There has been quite a bit of debate over the question of what constitutes 6.8 sufficient information. An initial patient's response to the question, 'How much information would you like?' could be: 'Give me full information!' Unfortunately, it is not feasible to disclose all possibly relevant information without taking up an indefensible amount of health workers' as well as patients' time. Some have proposed a so-called 'reasonable doctor standard', that's basically the kind of information a doctor would provide a similarly well-educated other doctor with. The problem with that level of information is – obviously – that most of us are not medical doctors, and so we would not be able to make much sense of that sort of information. So we are left with two other options. One is called the 'reasonable patient' standard, and that is the standard that is applicable in most jurisdictions today. The patient should be provided with information that someone like them would find worth knowing if they found themselves in comparable circumstances. The Canadian Medical Protective Association, while advising its members about the legal background that led to this definition, asks its doctor members to 'walk in the shoes of the patient'. The legal case in question is *Reibl v. Hughes*. Here a patient suffered a massive stroke during or shortly 'after an endarterectomy, which paralyzed the right side of his body. The trial judge found no negligence in the performance of the operation, but awarded compensation to the patient based on the allegation that the patient had not given his informed consent to the operation' (**CMPA**[2]). The country's Supreme Court concurred, noting that the patient's doctor didn't put sufficient emphasis on communicating to the patient the stroke risk. The judges of this highest Canadian Court thought that a reasonable patient might not have opted for the surgery had they been provided with the relevant information.

What then does a reasonable patient want to know? Today doctors are 6.9 expected to disclose what other patients would usually consider worth knowing who find themselves in similar circumstances. They then add what they think their patients ought to know, thereby acknowledging that patients might not necessarily cover ground that should be material to their decision-making, due to their lack of clinical expertise. Ideally they would encourage their patients to ask follow-up questions.

Here is a good example[3] of practical legally informed advice on what 6.10 doctors should take into account during the informed consent (or refusal) process. It is excerpted from the website of the **Canadian Medical Protective Association**[4]. Kenneth G. Evans drafted it for the benefit of the association's members (Kenneth G. Evans 2016).

1. Insofar as may be possible, tell the patient the diagnosis. If there is some uncertainty about the diagnosis mention this uncertainty, the reason for it and what is being considered.

2. The physician should disclose to the patient the nature of the proposed treatment, its gravity, any material risks and any special risks relating to the specific treatment in question. Even if a risk is a mere possibility which ordinarily might not be disclosed, if its occurrence carries serious consequences, as for example paralysis or death, it must be regarded as a material risk requiring disclosure.

3. A physician must answer any specific questions posed by the patient as to the risks involved in the proposed treatment. Always the patient must be given the opportunity to ask questions.

4. The patient should be told about the consequences of leaving the ailment untreated. Although there should be no appearance of coercion by unduly frightening patients who refuse treatment, our courts now recognize there is a positive obligation to inform patients about the potential consequences of their refusal.

5. The patient should be told about available alternative forms of treatment and their risks. There is no obligation to discuss what might be clearly regarded as unconventional therapy but patients should know there are other accepted alternatives and why the recommended therapy has been chosen.

6. Physicians must be alert to a patient's individual concerns about the proposed treatment and deal with them. It must be remembered that any particular patient's special circumstances might require disclosure of potential although uncommon hazards of the treatment when ordinarily these might not be seen as material. Courts have made it clear that the duty of disclosure extends to what the physician knows or should know the particular patient deems relevant to a decision whether or not to undergo treatment.

7. Although any particular patient may waive aside all explanations, may have no questions, and may be prepared to submit to the treatment whatever the risks may be without any explanatory discussion, physicians must exercise cautious discretion in accepting such waivers.

8. When, because of emotional factors, the patient may be unable to cope with pre-treatment explanations, the physician may be justified in withholding or generalizing information which otherwise would be required to be given. This so-called "therapeutic privilege" should be exercised with great discretion and only when there are compelling reasons dictated by clinical circumstances.

9. In obtaining consent for cosmetic surgical procedures or for any type of medical or surgical work which might be regarded as less than entirely necessary to the physical health of the patient, physicians must take particular care in explaining fully the risks and anticipated results. As in experimental research situations, courts may impose on physicians a higher standard of disclosure in such circumstances.

10. Encouragement about optimistic prospects for the results of treatment should not allow for the misinterpretation that results are guaranteed.

11. Where a part or all of the treatment is to be delegated, patients have a right to know about this and who will be involved in their care. Consent explanations should include such information.

12. A note by the physician on the record at the time of consent explanations can later serve as important confirmation that a patient was appropriately informed, particularly if the note refers to any special points which may have been raised in the discussion.

You should be able to find similar information for your country.   6.11

Informed consent requires, of course, that a patient is decisionally com-   6.12
petent at the time of decision-making. There has been some discussion about the question of whether there should be such a thing as a risk-related standard of competence. The underlying argument is that we might be competent to decline a particular course of clinical care when the stakes are low while we might not be sufficiently competent to refuse a particular course of clinical care when the stakes are really high, say, when our life might be at stake. So, perhaps we should require of a patient a higher degree of competence when the latter is the case. The justification here is paternalistic. Joel Feinberg, for instance, has argued, 'if a layman disagrees with a physician on a question of medical fact, the layman can safely be presumed wrong (and the state is justified in intervening) to protect him not from his own free and informed choices, but from his factual ignorance' (Feinberg 1986, 128). Feinberg questions an otherwise competent patient's capacity to make an informed choice when they choose a course of action that is

unreasonable. Buchanan and Brock proposed that 'the standard of competence ought to vary in part with the expected harms or benefits to the
patient in accordance with the patient's choice' (Buchanan et al. 1990, 51).
There is an obvious threat to the informed consent process and patient
autonomy here in so far as there is a risk that 'standards of understanding,
reasoning, and so forth will be set arbitrarily and unattainably high by those
who believe that paternalism is justified when perceived risks are great'
(Wicclair 1991).

6.13   We will return to informed consent in the context of research ethics in
the next chapter.

6.2 Paternalism

6.14   Joel Feinberg mentions paternalism as a possible justification for overriding
patient decisions. Paternalism is, as the name suggests, derived from the
Latin word '*pater*', i.e. father. It has today, wrongly so, a bad reputation in
liberal societies. What it refers to is the overriding of someone's choices for
their own benefit, much like a good parent would override a decision their
child may have made. In clinical practice that could involve circumstances
where patients are incompetent to make their own considered choices, for
instance, because they are drunk, in a state of shock, or any number of other
reasons that render them incompetent to make informed, autonomous
choices. This sort of paternalism is relatively easy to ethically justify. A
health care professional acts in a benevolent way by overriding an incompetent patient's choices. They do so, often on the understanding that the
patient, if they were competent, would consent to the proposed procedure.
The Georgetown Mantra's principle of beneficence, as was as the consequentialist ethical frameworks that underlie it, provide sound justifications
for such a course of action. The kind of paternalism applicable here is often
called weak paternalism or soft paternalism. It is uncontroversial in so far
as most jurisdictions permit such actions.

6.15   More problematic, and certainly more controversial, are paternalistic
courses of action that override a competent patient's considered self-regarding choices. Here a competent patient was or perhaps wasn't even informed
by a health care professional about their options and the health care professional's preferred course of action. Overriding the patient's decision under
those circumstances amounts to what is often called strong paternalism. It
is much more difficult, if not impossible to ethically justify, even if such a

course of action would be objectively in a patient's best clinical interest. This has much to do with the importance we ascribe in liberal societies to self-determination and self-governance. Indeed, in most jurisdictions such a course of action might lead to assault charges against the health care professional.

6.3 Deciding for Others

An important issue in clinical ethics involves the need to make decisions on   6.16
behalf of patients who do not have the capacity to make decisions on their
own behalf. There are different categories of patients to whom this applies:
(a) patients who never had legal capacity to make decisions; (b) patients
who had legal capacity but lost it and left no advance directive; as well as (c)
patients who created an advance directive while they had capacity and there
is an argument between care givers and family members about the interpretation of the advance directive.

6.3.1 Deciding for Others: Advance Directives

Advance directives are becoming a more common tool in medical decision-   6.17
making. Do not confuse them with advanced directives; advance directives
(ADs) may be advanced, as in sophisticated, but really their focus is their
future directedness. So, an AD, as the name suggests, is a directive that is
future-oriented. It permits competent patients to make decisions with
regard to what they'd like to see to happen to them when they lose capacity.
ADs typically occur toward the end of patients' lives, they could for instance
affect patients concerned about the effects of dementia, or Alzheimer's disease. Dementia is becoming a fairly frequent condition in the ageing populations of the countries of the global north, but it is worth keeping in mind
that roughly half of all patients living with dementia globally live in middle-
and low-income countries. The **World Health Organization**[5] predicts that
globally the number of dementia patients is bound to double by 2030 and to
triple by 2050 to an estimated 115 million people.

What is the ethical justification for ADs? Unsurprisingly perhaps, they   6.18
are firmly based on respect for competent patient choices. If we have a right
to refuse life-sustaining treatment while we are competent, we should be
able to issue ADs that address a situation where we might not have the
capacity any longer to make such a choice. This is no different from respect

for the choices we make with regard to our estate. There are a number of benefits that can be derived from a regulatory regime that respects ADs. One of them undoubtedly is that patients will be less stressed about losing capacity, because they know that they will be able to retain some degree of control over what will happen to their bodies after they lose capacity. That will be reassuring to many of us. ADs also seem a good safeguard against undue paternalistic actions by doctors or even family members.

6.19   Allen Buchanan has raised a number of concerns against ADs, some of which are remediable, others less so (Buchanan 1988). Among the latter is this: ADs cannot predict future developments in medicine and so they might not be a true reflection of what a patient would have wanted had they known about those developments. He also mentions another, somewhat related concern, namely that in case of a competent patient family members and health care professionals would at least have a chance to reason about possible courses of action with the patient. None of that would be possible in the case of ADs.

6.20   Another ethical argument against ADs has been raised by Rebecca Dresser. She points out that if the moral justification for ADs is to respect the choices of competent individuals with regard to what will happen to their bodies when they have lost decision-making capacity, it seems the moral case for ADs turns indefensible. After all, ADs *only* come into effect when the patient in question has lost psychological continuity. All that is left at that stage is bodily continuity. It is arguable that the person that inhabited and owned that body is no more, so why should that person's wishes with regard to that body matter any longer? (Dresser 1986) Might a consequentialist approach to the problem at hand not be more ethically defensible? Should a decision about the clinical care for such patients not depend entirely on their quality of life and the resources needed to be utilized in order to maintain the patient above a certain threshold level of quality of life?

6.3.2 Deciding for Others: Patients Who Never Had Capacity

6.21   Of course, regardless of what your views are on ADs, they will never resolve all case challenges where patients are unable to express views on their ongoing treatment options. Some patients may not have been able to issue an AD, not due to an omission of their own, but because they never had the capacity to make considered choices about their ongoing care. In this category of patients we would find patients who were born with serious irreversible brain injuries, such as newborns with **anencephaly**[6]. This condition affects about 3 in every 10,000 births, translating into roughly 1200 newborns suffering that condition in the United States alone, each year. Anencephalic newborns lack a part of their brain and skull that results invariably in their death shortly after birth, usually within a few days. Tragic as such cases are, there can be conflicts between what kind of care the biological parents or other legal proxies might consider appropriate clinical care and what doctors consider reasonable under the circumstances. Most hospitals would not provide anything other than palliative care to the newborn as we have no means to change the nature of the underlying clinical problem. There are other severely disabled newborns who arguably have no reasonable likelihood of living a life worth living. This does raise the question whether it could be ethical – from the perspective of the newborn, its parents, as well as from a resource allocation point of view – to actively end the life of the newborn, at least in jurisdictions where that might be a legal possibility. This is a view that has been defended by various authors (Kuhse et al. 1985; Schüklenk 2015). Helga Kuhse and Peter Singer, for instance, argued in a monograph published a few decades ago, that it would be the ethically right thing to do to terminate the lives of such newborns if that was considered the right course of action by their doctors as well as their parents. Infanticide, of course, is illegal in most, if not all jurisdictions. This has much to do with the sanctity-of-life doctrine in medicine that precludes courses of action such as that proposed by Kuhse and Singer. The view held by doctors following that doctrine is that *all* human life, no matters its quality of life, is worth maintaining, or, at a minimum, that we have a moral obligation not to end such lives pro-actively prematurely (Kuhse 1987).

6.3.3 Deciding for Others: Incapacitated Patients without Advance Directives

Another category of patients for whom life and death decisions might need to be made, on their behalf, by others, are patients who are permanently incapacitated, for instance as a result of serious accidents. While typically it is these patients' loved ones who will be charged with the difficult task of deciding for the patient, conflicts may arise between what medical doctors believe is the clinically best course of action, and what those loved ones consider appropriate. These conflicts often surround decisions about the switching-off of life-support machines for patients with irreversible brain damage. An extreme example of this is the case of a Californian teenager,

6.22

Jahi McMath[7]. She underwent surgery for tonsillectomy. The operation was successful, but shortly thereafter McMath suffered serious loss of blood and cardiac arrest. Eventually experts concluded that she was brain dead, there was no blood flow to the brain, no measurable activity on an electro-encephalogram, and she was unable to breathe without the assistance of a mechanical ventilator. After some back and forth in the courts, that is not relevant for our purposes, eventually a coroner declared that McMath was deceased. The parents disagreed with that finding and insisted that McMath receive continuing medical care. The problem is, of course, that it would be a violation of medical codes and health care delivery regulations to 'treat' a dead person, that is to effectively interfere with a corpse. Eventually the family found a religious facility willing to maintain the dead body. Medical ethics experts by and large agreed that the doctors were right in refusing continuing care for what they considered to be a deceased person. After all, a dead person cannot benefit from continuing medical care, and so the deployment of continuing death support would constitute a waste of medical resources.

6.23   This case also raises the question of whether there would be something ethically objectionable about interfering with the body of a deceased person. By definition, a deceased human cannot suffer as a result of whatever clinical manipulation. In this case, maintaining her body would not have benefitted her, but it appears to have benefitted her family members. It is a difficult question indeed whether the family and their private donors should have been permitted to use the dead body in the manner they did in order to satisfy their psychological needs. What would speak in favor of that course of action is arguably that no actual harm was done to the deceased. In consequentialist terms: The deceased was not worse off as a result of the course of action proposed by the family, the family was better off for it, and no public resources were expended, hence resource allocation justice concerns do not feature here.

6.24   The issues are not always this comparably straightforward. Consider the following case involving a Canadian patient **Hassan Rasouli**[8]. Rasouli went to a hospital in Toronto to receive surgery. The objective was to remove what was considered to be a benign brain tumor. Various complications resulted in Mr Rasouli being eventually seriously and irreversibly brain damaged. His doctors eventually declared him to be in a **persistent vegetative state**[9] (Dilling 2007). For a patient to be diagnosed thus they need to meet the following clinical criteria (Multi Task Force 1 1994; Multi Task Force 2 1994):

1. No evidence of awareness of self or environment; no interaction with others.
2. No evidence of sustained, reproducible, purposeful or voluntary behavioral responses to visual, auditory, tactile or noxious stimuli.
3. No evidence of language comprehension or expression.
4. Return of sleep-wake cycles, arousal, even smiling, frowning, yawning.
5. Sufficient hypothalamic and brainstem autonomic functions to survive if given medical or nursing care.
6. Bowel and bladder incontinence.
7. Variably preserved cranial nerve and spinal reflexes.

In the considered professional opinion of Rasouli's doctors it served no   6.25
clinical purpose to continue efforts aimed at keeping their patient alive, given that he would not benefit from medical care. They proposed instead to provide continuing **palliative care**[10] until his foreseeable demise. His family disagreed with that decision and insisted that Rasouli be kept alive, at very significant cost to the tax funded public health care system in Ontario, the Canadian province where the Rasouli family resided. Rasouli had left no AD for the situation that he found himself in.

In conflicts such as this it is not unusual that cases are heard by committees   6.26
such as **Ontario's Consent and Capacity Board**[11], where decisions about the continuation of medical care will be reached based on a list of criteria that primarily focus on the patient's objective best interests. Among others, the Board in Ontario is required to take into consideration criteria such as these:

> (a) The treatment (i) will or is likely to improve substantially the condition of the person to whom it is to be administered, and the person's condition will not or is not likely to improve without the treatment; (ii) or the person's condition will or is likely to deteriorate substantially, or to deteriorate rapidly, without the treatment, and the treatment will or is likely to prevent the deterioration or to reduce substantially its extent or its rate; (b) that the benefit the person is expected to obtain from the treatment outweighs the risk of harm to him or her; (c) that the treatment is the least restrictive and least intrusive treatment that meets the requirements of clauses (a) and (b).

In Rasouli's case it was difficult to see what objective interest could be   6.27
ascribed to this patient who suffered irreversible brain damage and would have been unable to benefit from any kind of medical intervention.

Still, who should in such situations have the final say, the doctors or the   6.28
family members or a third impartial party like the mentioned Consent and

Capacity Board? Given that this case was heard by the province's Consent and Capacity Board, we know how regulators approach the matter in this Canadian province. The rationale behind removing the decision both from family members as well as the attending clinicians is that both might face conflicts of interest that could cloud their respective judgments. A transparent, objective standard against which decisions are evaluated seems a reasonable procedural solution to what are challenging clinical ethical problems.

6.29   Eventually, as it should be in a liberal democracy, the decision made by the members of the Consent and Capacity Court may be appealed in the courts, too.

6.4 Truth Telling

6.30 Even if we occasionally are not entirely truthful, we do know that our friendships, other relationships, even our society cannot function if we cannot trust that the person we are communicating with is honest. Would you lend money to a friend who you know lies about their intention and ability to repay the loan in order to get it from you? You would likely not do so. Truth telling has also a special place in the doctor–patient relationship. Some of the ethical reasons for this are rather obvious. The doctor–patient relationship is fundamentally a trust-based one. The maintenance of trust requires honesty (Hebert et al. 1997). Truth-telling is a necessary condition for patients to consider treatment options and make decisions that align with their authentic values. An autonomous choice is not feasible in the absence of true information about one's state of health and one's options. True patient first person voluntary informed consent is only feasible if the patient has been informed truthfully about the nature of their condition, their treatment options, cost associated with those treatment options, and so on and so forth. Patient autonomy is disrespected by doctors who are not truthful with their patients (Higgs 1985).

6.31   We could leave it at this if there were not situations where doctors have doubts about whether particular patients might not be best served by not being told the truth. You can see that this shapes up to be a kind of paternalistic rationale. Is it possible then that there is, or should be, a special dispensation for doctors that diverges from standard societal norms entailing truth telling? Examples that should give us pause for thought might be situations where the truth would likely distress the patients, for instance in case of catastrophic often-lethal illnesses for which no successful treatments are available, and where truth telling might lead to a deterioration of the patient's health. Or, should psychiatrists tell a suicidal – but competent – patient suffering from treatment resistant depression that they have run out of treatment options? Would the Hippocratic Oath – despite its problems – provide a justification for lying under such circumstances with its *primum non nocere*, first do no harm, principle?

The view that doctors are in such situations justified in breaching trust   6.32
and telling untruths is often referred to as the 'paternalistic prerogative'. As the name suggests, it's the idea that the doctor's beneficence obligations toward their patients can sometimes justify telling outright lies or deceiving their patients, at least in circumstances where the doctor thinks that the patient would likely benefit from a lie or a deception. You can guess what Immanuel Kant would have made of this. He wrote in a short essay entitled *On a Supposed Right to Lie from Altruistic Motives*: 'truthfulness is a duty that must be regarded as the basis of all duties founded on contract, the laws of which would be rendered uncertain and useless if even the least exception to them were admitted. To be truthful (honest) in all declarations is therefore a sacred unconditional command of reason, and not to be limited by any expediency' (Kant, transl Abbott 1909). There is little room here for a beneficence based paternalistic lie or deception on part of the doctor.

Kant, as we have discovered, wasn't a consequentialist, but he may have been   6.33
interested to learn that there are some known good consequences flowing from doctors being consistently truthful, as well as more harmful consequences. As Hebert and colleagues write in the *Canadian Medical Journal*:

> Truth telling increases patient compliance, reduces the morbidity such as pain associated with medical interventions and improves health outcomes. Informed patients are more satisfied with their care and less apt to change physicians than patients who are not well informed. Some studies suggest that truth telling can have negative consequences. For example, the diagnosis of hypertension may result in decreased emotional well-being and more frequent absence from work.
>
> (Higgs, Roger, Op. cit. 227)

Another aspect might be worth mentioning in the context of doctor   6.34
truth-telling, and that is culture. Reportedly in some cultures patients traditionally seem to expect doctors to withhold bad news from them. There it is expected that bad news is shared with the patient's family and the decision

on disclosure is made by designated family members. The same, incidentally, might hold true for some elderly patients who grew up at a time when medical paternalism ruled the day.

6.35   A medical doctor, in a 1927 essay describes in vivid examples from his practice that patients often do not wish to know burdensome truths and that telling the truth sometimes undermines the medical mission, which is to make the patient better (Collins 1927). Here is one such example:

> There are other lies, however, which contribute enormously to the success of the physician's mission of mercy and salvation. There are a great number of instances in support of this but none more convincing than that of a man of fifty who, after twenty-five years of devotion to painting, decided that penury and old age were incompatible for him. Some of his friends had forsaken art for advertising. He followed their lead and in five years he was ready to gather the first ripe fruit of his labor. When he attempted to do so he was so immobilized by pain and rigidity that he had to forgo work. One of those many persons who assume responsibility lightly assured him that if he would put himself in the hands of a certain osteopath he would soon be quite fit. The assurance was without foundation. He then consulted a physician who without examining him proceeded to treat him for what is considered a minor ailment. Within two months his appearance gave such concern to his family that he was persuaded to go to a hospital, where the disease was quickly detected, and he was at once submitted to surgery. When he had recovered from the operation, learning that I was in the country of his adoption, he asked to see me. He had not been able, he said, to get satisfactory information from the surgeon or the physician; all that he could gather from them was that he would have to have supplementary X-ray or radium treatment. What he desired was to get back to his business which was on the verge of success, and he wanted assurance that he could soon do so. He got it. And more than that, he got elaborate explanation of what surgical intervention had accomplished, but not a word of what it had failed to accomplish. A year of activity was vouchsafed him, and during that time he put his business in such shape that its eventual sale provided a modest competency for his family. It was not until the last few weeks that he knew the nature of his malady. Months of apprehension had been spared him by the deception, and he had been the better able to do his work, for he was buoyed by the hope that his health was not beyond recovery. Had he been told the truth, black despair would have been thrown over the world in which he moved, and he would have carried on with corresponding ineffectiveness.

6.36   While consequentialists might consider individual lies morally called for, under such circumstances, in order to avoid greater societal harm, they might find it difficult to draw clear lines for policy purposes.

6.5 Confidentiality

Another issue that is not quite straightforward is that of confidentiality in   6.37
the doctor–patient relationship. This relationship is a trust-based relationship, with the patient assuming that the doctor is a professional who will do
what is in that patient's best interest. In some ways the doctor is a patient
fiduciary. A doctor is only able to deliver on this if patients are sufficiently
trusting that they will disclose relevant health risk behaviors to the health
care professional. Patient trust in the confidentiality of what transpired
during a meeting between doctor and patient is evidently important. This,
of course, is a consequentialist take on confidentiality. There are also other
moral reasons in support of its importance. It has been argued by some
authors that confidentiality is a corollary of respecting a more important
value, namely patient privacy. All of us construct our lives to a large extent
around the private information about ourselves that we share with others.
Children grow up learning to control their information by getting more and
more informational privacy privileges from their parents, until they reach
maturity and have nothing to share with their parents about their private
lives, unless they wish to.

It should come as no surprise that among the World Medical Association's   6.38
Declaration of Geneva's[12] lofty pledges there is also this, 'I WILL RESPECT
the secrets that are confided in me, even after the patient has died' (WMA
2017). This statement is uncontroversially of a deontological nature, there
are no if's or but's, doctors are expected to maintain confidentiality, no
matter what.

Undoubtedly such a promise will contribute a fair bit toward maintain-   6.39
ing trust in the doctor-patient relationship. Patients might well assume that
doctors are duty bound to maintain the confidentiality of their private
health information, much like a **Catholic priest**[13] is duty bound to abide by
the confidentiality promised to the confessor.

The reality, to the surprise of probably quite a few patients, is more   6.40
complicated. Doctors are indeed generally expected to maintain patient
confidences, but there are also clear limits. For instance, if the life or
well-being of another person is threatened by past or future patient conduct, doctors are legally obliged to breach confidentiality as a matter of
law. Here is an example of a tragic case that occurred in the 1960s, on the
campus of the University of California at Berkeley. An international student from India, Prosenjit Poddar mistakenly thought that he was in a
relationship with another student, Tatiana Tarasoff. When she rebuffed

him in no uncertain terms he began stalking her. His mental condition deteriorated rapidly during this period. Poddar sought psychological assistance from the university's counselling services, while Tarasoff was absent from campus. He confided to a psychologist, Dr Moore that he intended to kill Tarasoff. Moore had Poddar admitted to a mental institution because he considered him a serious threat to Tarasoff's life and well-being. However, Poddar was released after a short period in detention because he managed to persuade the professionals there that he was stable. Poddar stopped seeing Dr Moore and stabbed Tarasoff after her return, killing her. This led to a **high-profile court case**[14], it established that doctors do not only have obligations to their patients, but also to those to whom their patients might be threats. The judge writing for the majority in the case included this influential line in the judgment, 'the public policy favoring protection of the confidential character of patient-psychotherapist communications must yield to the extent to which disclosure is essential to avert danger to others. The protective privilege ends where the public peril begins' (**Tarasoff**[15]).

6.41   This argument explaining the Tarasoff verdict is of a consequentialist nature. Ironically, the strongest argument against a duty to disclose confidential private patient information happens to be also of a consequentialist nature. The judge writing the minority opinion in the California Supreme Court case argued (quoting from an article in a law journal), 'the very practice of psychiatry depends upon the reputation in the community that the psychiatrist will not tell.' This is a fairly powerful counter argument to the stance taken by the majority opinion in the Tarasoff case. If I was a patient intending to kill someone else and I contemplated seeking professional help to prevent me from doing so, I might be reluctant to do so if I knew that the professional was duty bound to share my dark secret immediately with law enforcement and even the target of my morbid plans.

6.42   Doctors might also be required by law to pass on confidential test results to public health authorities. In Canada, for instance, the results of a patient's tests for sexually transmitted illnesses will routinely be shared with the country's public health authorities. The reasons for this are – surprisingly, given the deontological nature of the profession's public promises on this issue – again of a consequentialist nature. The ethical justification lies in the need to protect the wider public's health interests. This is very much in line with the rationale developed by the California Supreme Court in the Tarasoff case. However, public health experts have warned that if doctors were duty-bound to disclose HIV test results to sexual partners of infected people, people at risk of HIV infection would have a serious disincentive to get tested, thereby undermining prevention efforts.

There are other instances where prima facie confidential information is 6.43 shared. In many countries private insurance companies will routinely access or receive private health information pertaining to their insured clients from these patients' doctors. However, typically this only occurs after patients have granted their doctors the right to share relevant information. It is questionable how voluntary such consent truly is. After all, what choice do they have if the condition of enrolment in a health insurance scheme is that the insurance companies have access to such information?

Mark Siegler suggested in a widely read article that the traditional con- 6.44 cept of confidentiality in medicine is a decrepit concept (Siegler 1982). He describes in a telling example how problematic the idea of confidentiality in modern medicine really is. One of his patients, admitted to his hospital for an elective **cholecystectomy**[16], threatened to leave the hospital unless he was guaranteed the confidentiality of his patient records. Siegler then tried to enumerate the number of professionals within the hospital that would have had routine access to his patient's records. He came up with a figure anywhere between a minimum of 25 and a maximum of 100. Unsurprisingly the patient did not find it reassuring that all these people needed to know his private health information, even though they were 'working for him', as Siegler puts it (Siegler 1982, 1519). His article is basically a plea for a more realistic approach to confidentiality, including clear information for patients with regard to who will have access to their records.

6.6 Conscience Matters

Many of us will have come across newspaper articles discussing legal cases 6.45 pertaining to conscientious objectors in the **military**[17], **medical profession**[18], and even the **civil service**[19]. They typically refuse to provide services that they are expected to deliver, on grounds of *conscience*, and that their patients or clients are entitled to receive. But what exactly is that, the conscience? Most of us who are not **sociopaths**[20] have a conscience. It typically expresses itself by triggering feelings of guilt when we do things our conscience tells us we should not be doing, like gratuitous lying, for instance. The medical ethicist Daniel Sulmasy describes conscience as something that seems to operate both retrospectively as well as prospectively; according to him it impacts on past actions and it impacts on how we evaluate normatively possible future actions. To his mind when we talk about conscience we are talking about both our conviction that we should act in accordance with our individual understanding of what morality demands of us, and of deliberately and voluntarily acting in accordance with what we consider to be morally good and right (Sulmasy 2008).

6.46   Most jurisdictions protect citizens' right to freedom of religion. How does this affect the relationship between health care professionals and patients though? It is a fairly straightforward matter when it comes to patients' religious convictions and the impact of those convictions on their health care. Decisionally competent **Jehova's Witnesses**'[21] refusals to accept blood transfusions, even if that means that they will foreseeably lose their lives, are typically respected. The ethical rationale underpinning this respect is, unsurprisingly, the right of adults with legal capacity to make binding decisions with regard to what does or does not happen to and with their bodies, as long as they understand the consequences of their actions, and as long as there is no coercion in play. In other words, it is respect for autonomous choices made by such adults and expressed in their refusal to provide informed consent to blood transfusions. In legal terms, the refusal by a health care professional to respect such a choice – and go ahead with a blood transfusion anyway – would amount to assault or battery (Petrini 2014). The obvious exceptions are legal minors, because they are considered incapable of making autonomous, respect commanding choices until they have reached the age of maturity or until they are considered mature minors, that is minors who show the capacity to make informed, considered choices with regard to matters of life and death.

6.47   Typically in medical ethics when there is talk about conscience, however, it is not about patient conscience, but about doctors refusing to provide particular medical services that are within their scope of professional practice and that are both perfectly legal and that eligible patients have a right to receive. Often, but not exclusively so, this affects patients seeking reproductive health services such as an abortion or sterilization, or end-of-life medical services such as aid in dying.

6.48   Asking someone to violate their conscience-based convictions in matters that are of great importance to them is to ask such people to accept a potentially fairly high psychological cost to themselves. Mark Wicclair has suggested that the unfettered refusal to accommodate conscientious objectors would constitute a significant threat to some of the affected doctors' moral integrity (Wicclair 2000). Christopher Cowley thinks that the threat to these professionals' integrity could be so severe that they might drop out of the medical profession altogether, or otherwise qualified people might choose not to become medical professionals because of it (Cowley 2016). Peter West-Oram and Alena Buyx offer other possible justifications for the accommodation of conscientious objectors. They write:

> The right to exempt oneself from the fulfilment of a generally held duty is typically justified on the grounds that such a right is vital for the preservation of freedom of conscience. The latter is itself argued to be a core value of pluralist, liberal-democratic states, and 'a moral right'. Further, the rights to freedom of conscience and conscientious objection are argued to be constitutive of liberty and autonomy, and to be necessary for the preservation of individual moral integrity. In promoting these goods, the rights are argued to be vital for the adequate toleration of different moral and philosophical perspectives in a pluralistic society.
>
> (West-Oram and Buyx 2016)

Opponents of the view that conscientious objectors in the medical pro-   6.49
fession have a moral claim to be accommodated raise a number of possible objections to arguments such as those described by West-Oram and Buyx, or those developed by Wicclair and Cowley. Their case is based on the following types of considerations: Doctors are *professionals*, patients visit them in that capacity, and not as individuals with their own idiosyncratic views of the universe. Professionalism entails the profession's **right to self-regulate**[22], but it also comes with clear societal expectations with regard to the delivery of professional services. Societies typically endow professionals with a monopoly on the provision of particular specialized services. The denial by individual doctors to provide the range of services that they voluntarily contracted to provide could well lead to a situation where patients are unable to access services that they are entitled to receive (Charo 2005). This concern is not of a purely theoretical nature. Francesca Minerva reports that about 70 percent of Italian gynecologists conscientiously object to performing abortions, which is arguably one of the reasons for high backstreet abortion rates in that country (Minerva 2015). Conscientious objection accommodation thus undermines one of the very reasons for why health care professions are established in the first place, namely to provide reliable, high-quality specialist services to eligible patients. Savulescu does not think much of Cowley's concern that otherwise qualified people might not join the medical profession. He points out that it is not clear that the medical profession and society at large would not be better off if conscientious objectors decided not to join a profession offering the range of services of which they object to. Their integrity would then not be challenged, and

patients would not be inconvenienced by conscientious objectors. He points out, there is no evidence that the convictions the objectors hold dear to their heart actually make them better doctors (Savulescu and Schüklenk 2017). Schüklenk, another opponent of conscientious objection accommodation, notes that court decisions across many jurisdictions have concluded that it would be inappropriate in secular societies to evaluate the plausibility of the normative convictions held by conscientious objectors. Given that it is also impossible to determine reliably whether a conscientious objector holds the convictions they claim to hold, the accommodation of essentially untestable conscientious objection claims seems bad policy to him, given their impact on the provision of patient care (Schüklenk and Smalling 2017).

6.50   Today in many jurisdictions a compromise position on this controversial issue has been reached. Health care professionals are often not obliged to provide the service they conscientiously object to, but they are obliged to transfer the patient on to a colleague who they know will provide it, and who is in reasonable proximity so that the patient is able to receive the service they have a moral and legal claim to. The obvious problem with this compromise solution is that it is not quite a compromise from the perspective of the conscientious objector. Say, if you believe that abortion is akin to murder, it is unlikely to be a satisfactory compromise that you do not have to commit the murder yourself but that you must transfer the assistance-seeking woman on to a health care professional who you know will commit the act you object to.

6.7 Duty to Treat

6.51 Doctors and other health care professionals might consider refusing to provide the care they are trained to provide for reasons unrelated to conscience. Life-threatening infectious diseases have led to renewed discussions about the risks to self that society can reasonably expect of their health care professionals. Sierra Leonians saw **about 10 percent**[23] of their – already scarce – doctors die as a result of exposure during the Ebola virus outbreak in 2014/15. Some of these doctors, of course, contracted the deadly virus socially, like their fellow country-men and -women, however, many died while providing professional care to those infected with the virus. During the SARS outbreak in Canada, **two nurses died**[24] as a result of occupational exposure to the virus, in Ontario, while caring for infected patients (Reid 2005). Notably, doctors and nurses who refused to attend

SARS patients in Canada faced no disciplinary sanctions (Ries 2004). It is uncontroversial that health care professionals have beneficence duties toward patients, the question is how far reaching those duties are. The ethical challenge is to determine where to draw a defensible line with regard to risks that society can expect health care professionals to accept on the job. It should not come as a terrible surprise that there is no professional or regulatory consensus on this difficult subject matter. Good arguments exist on both sides of the divide.

Some argue that the health care professions have a long history of heroic conduct in the face of catastrophic infectious diseases and that that should establish how health care professionals ought to conduct themselves today. There are two problems with this: firstly, tradition describes what has usually been done, but it tells us nothing about what ought to be done. A normative conclusion cannot be derived from describing how things always were. Secondly, that unqualified claim seems to overstate the matter somewhat. For instance, during the Roman plague many doctors barricaded themselves in their homes to protect themselves and their families. While it is true that the ideal of the physician as hero has been a frequent theme in world literature, such as for instance in Albert Camus' *The Plague,* it has never been the case that health care professionals accepted unlimited job risks for themselves. Compare that to **firefighters**[25] though, for instance those deployed during the attacks on the World Trade Center in New York City. They did not have the luxury to decide whether they would respond to that emergency or give it a pass. However, since the advent of antibiotics and powerful antivirals, as well as the existence of efficacious vaccines (for Hepatitis B, for instance), people joining the health care professions typically do not assume that heroic self-less risk-taking is what would be expected of them during their careers. 6.52

How then should we go about addressing this ethical question? Contractualists like Norman Daniels argue that a moral obligation to, for example, treat HIV-infected patients (prior to the advent of life-preserving drugs) could be attributed to doctors only if it can be established that they voluntarily agreed or consented to do so as part of their decision and commitment to pursue a career in medicine (Daniels 1991). The question of whether doctors would have an obligation to treat patients in an epidemic seems to be a function then of the codes of conduct that were in existence when particular doctors joined the profession. By this logic different doctors might have different sets of obligations depending on when they entered the medical profession. This view, if implemented, would entail 6.53

significant practical challenges for any health care system's management. However, there is nothing in Daniels' account that would prevent a profession from advising professionals joining it that its codes of conduct are subject to change and that the decision to remain in the profession implies acceptance of its up-to-date rules and regulations.

6.54   It is worth noting that the World Medical Association's version of the Hippcoratic Oath, namely its **Declaration of Geneva**[26], offers these promises, 'I SOLEMNLY PLEDGE to consecrate my life to the service of humanity' and 'THE HEALTH AND WELL-BEING OF MY PATIENT will be my first consideration' (WMA 2017). If that deontological document was taken to form the basis of the doctor-patient relationship, patient and societal expectations on doctors' risk-taking would justifiably be very high.

6.55   Consequentialists focus their concern on the outcomes of various possible policies. Comparing the consequences of a volunteerist policy versus a mandatory treatment-of-patients policy, and adopting similar empirical assumptions about risks as Daniels, Smolkin argues that the implementation of a policy of volunteerism would bring about a number of harms and injustices, namely: (1) the infection risk for the doctors who do volunteer would be greater than if treatments were evenly dispersed; (2) the unavoidable public knowledge of the policy would give HIV-infected patients incentives to conceal their HIV status, undermining the trust that the doctor-patient relationship is based on; and (3) that same incentive might impede the effective treatment of HIV, which requires prompt and full disclosure of relevant information and timely and reliable access to health-care services. This, along with broader social ill-effects of discrimination against people with HIV by the medical profession, could cause significant physical and psychological harm (Smolkin 1997). We will have more to say on this topic in the last chapter where we take another look at this question in the context of professional care obligations during the 2020 SARS-CoV-2 pandemic. (Schüklenk 2020)

6.56   None of these approaches provide clear, uncontroversial guidance on this difficult subject matter. It will ultimately be the responsibility of statutory, regulatory bodies and governments to decide what duties health care professionals have in case of public health emergencies.

Questions

Do you think doctors have a moral right to deceive patients if they believe that is in their patients' best clinical interest? Do doctors have a moral obligation to breach the confidentiality of patient information if other people who are not their patients are at risk? Do you think doctors have a professional obligation to act professionally when they are 'on the job', so to speak, or do doctors have a moral claim to refuse the provision of professional services when they have moral qualms about particular professional services? What are your reasons for your answers?

Website Links

1   https://asbh.org/
2   https://www.cmpa-acpm.ca/serve/docs/ela/goodpracticesguide/pages/communication/Informed_Consent/why_and_when_do_we_need_consent-e.html#lc1/
3   https://www.cmpa-acpm.ca/en/advice-publications/handbooks/consent-a-guide-for-canadian-physicians
4   https://www.cmpa-acpm.ca/en/home
5   https://www.who.int/mediacentre/news/releases/2012/dementia_20120411/en/
6   http://www.cdc.gov/ncbddd/birthdefects/anencephaly.html/
7   http://www.latimes.com/local/la-me-0104-banks-jahi-mcmath-20140104-column.html#axzz2pSYRfoPz/
8   https://www.cbc.ca/news/canada/toronto/hassan-rasouli-case-top-court-upholds-life-support-right-1.2125140
9   http://journalofethics.ama-assn.org/2007/05/cprl1-0705.html/
10 https://medlineplus.gov/ency/patientinstructions/000536.htm
11 http://www.ccboard.on.ca/
12 https://www.wma.net/policies-post/wma-declaration-of-geneva/
13 http://www.catholiceducation.org/en/religion-and-philosophy/catholic-faith/the-seal-of-the-confessional.html/
14 https://www.courtlistener.com/opinion/1175611/tarasoff-v-regents-of-university-of-california/
15 https://www.courtlistener.com/opinion/1175611/tarasoff-v-regents-of-university-of-california/
16 https://www.mayoclinic.org/tests-procedures/cholecystectomy/about/pac-20384818/
17 http://www.jpost.com/Israel-News/IDF-denies-Kaminer-conscientious-objector-status-460131/
18 http://www.newstatesman.com/politics/feminism/2016/07/how-conscience-objection-doctors-being-used-threaten-safe-access-abortion/
19 https://papers.ssrn.com/sol3/papers.cfm?abstract_id=2631570
20 https://www.healthline.com/health/mental-health/sociopath
21 https://en.wikipedia.org/wiki/Supreme_Court_cases_involving_Jehovah%27s_Witnesses_by_country

22   https://journalofethics.ama-assn.org/article/professional-self-regulation-medicine/2014-04
23   https://www.pbs.org/wgbh/nova/article/ebola-doctors/
24   https://www.ona.org/news-posts/day-of-mourning/
25   https://www.telegraph.co.uk/news/worldnews/northamerica/usa/10994227/911-death-toll-rises-as-cancer-cases-soar-among-emergency-workers.html
26   https://www.wma.net/policies-post/wma-declaration-of-geneva/

7

RESEARCH ETHICS

In this chapter we will be looking at some of the historical events that led to 7.1
the rise of research ethics primarily in terms of policies and regulations but
also as a research focus of bioethicists. We will proceed from there to a sum-
mary of the main methodological elements of clinical trials. This will permit us to look at a wide range of ethical issues, some of which we will discuss
in some depth in this chapter. We will start off with a quick review of ethical
issues in animal experiments involving sentient non-human animals. From
then onward we will focus on research involving human participants. Why
does informed consent play a critical role in research involving competent
trial participants? What does or doesn't count justifiably as a trial-related
injury that ought to be subject of compensation, even if informed consent
to risk was given? Is it ethically defensible to use placebo controls in trials
involving catastrophically ill patients? What are the ethical challenges in
research involving participants in trials undertaken in the global south?
What kind of benefits, if any, ought to accrue to them and their communities? Should the research undertaken there be designed to address local
health needs? Is it acceptable to benefit from the results of uncontroversially unethical research?

Researchers did – and occasionally do – gruesome things to research 7.2
participants. The Nazis, for instance, used prisoners in their concentration
camps for a whole range of vile experiments. The United States Holocaust
Memorial Museum notes that **these kinds of experiments fell broadly into
three categories**[1]. For instance, the Nazi scientists left prisoners **immersed
in icy water**[2] in order to test means to ensure that their pilots, shot down

This Is Bioethics: An Introduction, First Edition. Ruth F. Chadwick and Udo Schüklenk.
© 2021 John Wiley & Sons, Inc. Published 2021 by John Wiley & Sons, Inc.

over the English channel, could survive longer. Another category of investigation inflicted wounds on these concentration camp prisoners that mirrored wounds German soldiers would incur during battle or occupation. Other research falling into this category included infecting prisoners with infectious diseases such as **tuberculosis**[3] and testing various experimental agents on them with a view to fighting the infection. Last but not least, given the Nazi ideology's views on race and racial purity, twins among the prisoners were subjected to a wide range of cruel experiments. **Josef Mengele**[4] was a German doctor whose name is most closely identified with these sorts of experiments. Given that the Nazis believed that gay men were a threat to the Third Reich, homosexual men were interned in concentration camps. Many of them were subjected to medical experiments as a result of the Nazis' interest in finding a **cure for homosexuality**[5]. As the Holocaust Memorial Museum **points out**[6], 'these experiments caused illness, mutilation, and even death, and yielded no scientific knowledge.'

7.3   Whether or not the prisoners ultimately survived these experiments was of little concern to the researchers, given that they were meant to be murdered eventually.

7.4   Research ethics came into its own as an ongoing academic and regulatory concern in the aftermath of the **Nuremberg Trials**[7]. Knowledge of the Nazi experiments led to the first international guidelines stipulating basic ethics standards for research involving human participants (Trials of War Criminals before the Nuremberg Military Tribunals under Control Council Law, 1994 [1949]). For instance, the lack of first person voluntary informed consent in the concentration camp experiments led to a provision in the Nuremberg Code that stipulated that for medical experiments to be ethical it is a necessary – but not sufficient – condition that trial participants are volunteers, that they are properly informed and that their consent or refusal to participate is the result of their autonomous choice and must be respected. The ethical justification for this provision is based on the view that prospective trial participants have the inalienable right to make up their own mind about whether or not they would like to support a particular experiment as a participant.

7.5   Subsequent scandals – including but not limited to the **Tuskegee syphilis study**[8] – led to further, and improved ethics guidelines such as the World Medical Association's **Declaration of Helsinki**[9] (World Medical Association, 1964–2013) as well as such national regulatory documents such as the landmark **Belmont Report**[10] in the USA (National Commission for the Protection of Human Subjects of Biomedical and Behavioral Research,

1979). It is noteworthy that the Declaration did away with the Nuremberg Code's first person voluntary informed consent requirement, at least with regard to some participants. Apparently it had not occurred to the drafters of the Nuremberg Code that there are certain categories of prospective trial participants who are incapable of giving informed consent – or refusal, as the case might be – and whose trial participation could be very important. For instance, research on particular incapacitating mental illnesses that render those afflicted by them incompetent could not be undertaken with such patients, if the Nuremberg Code was taken as the final word on the matter of informed consent. Similar problems would arise in research involving very young children or elderly patients suffering from dementia or Alzheimer's disease.

What conditions must be met then for clinical research to be ethical? 7.6 Given what happened during the Nazi experiments and other during other unethical research in human history, it seems that we need to consider both what kind of research should and should not be undertaken, as well as the question of how is this research going to be conducted.

7.1 Elements of Ethical Research

Ezekiel Emanuel and colleagues published an influential article in the 7.7 *Journal of the American Medical Association* where they propose the following criteria that they argue are both necessary and sufficient conditions that clinical research must meet in order to be ethical (Emanuel et al. 2000):

1. value-enhancements of health or knowledge must be derived from the research;
2. scientific validity – the research must be methodologically rigorous;
3. fair subject selection – scientific objectives, not vulnerability or privilege, and the potential for and distribution of risks and benefits, should determine communities selected as study sites and the inclusion criteria for individual subjects;
4. favorable risk-benefit ratio – within the context of standard clinical practice and the research protocol, risks must be minimized, potential benefits enhanced, and the potential benefits to individuals and knowledge gained for society must outweigh the risks;
5. independent review – unaffiliated individuals must review the research and approve, amend, or terminate it;

6. informed consent – individuals should be informed about the research and provide their voluntary consent; and

7. respect for enrolled subjects – subjects should have their privacy protected, the opportunity to withdraw, and their well-being monitored.

7.8   We will look in the remainder of this chapter at some of these conditions, as well as a number of other important issues. Academic and policy analyses in research ethics are marked by reasonably clear dividing lines between clinical and non-clinical investigations, as well as between research conducted in developed countries and research in developing countries. A few issues cut across these dividing lines, such as concerns about academic misconduct like the falsification of data, arguments about legitimate claims to authorship of a scientific publication, and plagiarism (ICMJE, 2010). Most of the latter concerns have been successfully addressed in international guidance **documents**[11].

7.2 Clinical Research: The Basics

7.9 In order to understand better some of the ethical controversies surrounding clinical trials it is important to know **broadly the mechanics of clinical research**[12].

7.10   Simply put, there is one phase involving non-human animals, and three to four trial phases involving humans. Initially researchers try to establish animal models for particular human diseases with a view to replicating what is happening in our bodies in animals. Once they have succeeded on that frontier and the experimental agent works in animals, first trials in humans begin. Initially, in phase 1 trials, they involve a fairly small number of people testing voluntarily the toxicity of the experimental drug when it is given to humans. Often the volunteers undertaking the toxicity testing are not sick at all, because the concern is not whether the drug works but what its negative effects are on our health, if any. These volunteers are well informed about the nature of the trial that they are participating in, and frequently they are paid volunteers. Once it is established that the experimental drug is safe or reasonably safe to take, a larger number of people, over a longer period of time, takes the experimental agent in order to determine whether it works as a preventative or therapeutic drug. If no gold standard of care exists the drug is typically compared against a placebo control, i.e. a dud pill. The ethical justification for the placebo control is that in the absence of a successful drug we need to know whether the experimental agent is doing better or worse than what is at that time our standard of care. Where we have a successful standard treatment the aim is to improve on what that standard treatment has to offer to patients, either in terms of therapeutic benefits or in terms of the reduction of side-effects. Depending on the success or failure of this investigation the drug trial ends there or is extended to a much larger group of people in phase three clinical trials. Phase 3 clinical trials are long-term clinical trials involving large numbers of people.

The idea of clinical equipoise between different trial arms as an ethical pre-condition of a clinical trials was proposed by a Canadian bioethicist, Benjamin Freedman. There is some plausibility to this idea. If we have no good scientific reason to prefer one trial arm over another, it is not unfair to randomize trial participants into either of the trial arms (Freedman 1987). However, once we have clear evidence that the agent in one of the trial arms is superior over the agents in the other arms, we would knowingly enroll patients into trial arms featuring inferior treatment regimes leading to inferior outcomes, possibly irreversibly so. That might be difficult to justify in most circumstances. We will return to this issue in our discussion of the ethics of landmark HIV clinical trials. 7.11

We should mention the rise of what is called personalized medicine, that is the attempt to use modern genetics techniques to design medicines for a particular individual. Quite obviously this moves away from the premises underlying much of the clinical research enterprise as we have described it earlier. They were premised on the view that what we need to research are averages across large numbers of patients, hoping that what is true for them would also be true for future patients that are roughly like them. In reality drugs developed using this method fail a fair number of patients, because too often patients are not roughly alike. So, with new technologies involving **genomics**[13], **proteomics**[14] and **metabolomics**[15] efforts are undertaken to design drugs for particular patients. 7.12

You might want to read **an article**[16] about 71-year-old Queenslander Chris Payze, the patient-participant in a clinical trial where n = 1, namely Chris Payze. It also provides a good overview over the differences between randomized controlled trials and n = 1 trials (Orford 2019). 7.13

Let us briefly reflect on the use of non-human sentient animals for research purposes, before we proceed to having a closer look at ethical issues involving human research participants. 7.14

7.3 Animal Experiments

7.15 Attitudes toward the use of non-human animals in clinical research tends to be strong on both sides of the divide. Feelings often run high. As we have seen in Chapter 4, much of this has to do with the moral standing that we ascribe to non-human animals. In case you agree with either **Tom Regan's case for animal rights**[17], or Peter Singer's sentience-based utilitarian approach, one thing is certain, you would be almost implacably opposed to animal experimentation involving animals that could reasonably be described as being a subject-of-a-life or that are capable of experiencing pain and suffering. Many animals used in experiments are comparable to us in important respects, otherwise they would probably be unable to function as animal models of our human ailments. Regan's and Singer's respective rationales behind their approaches differ. Tom Regan would be opposed to using subjects-of-a-life as mere means to achieve ends that are not their ends and that they have not volunteered to support (Regan 1988). The Kantian approach, sans rationality as the threshold determining moral standing, to ethics comes through here quite clearly.

7.16   The utilitarian Peter Singer, on the other hand, focuses on animals' capacity to suffer (Singer 2011). Recall from Chapter 2 the utilitarian focus on minimizing suffering and maximizing well-being in the world. These dispositional capacities, as opposed to species membership, are what matters to utilitarians. A mammal then, belonging to a species other than our own, but capable of experiencing pain and suffering, in ways comparable to our own, should be ascribed an interest in avoiding such experiential states just as we would try to avoid or end them. Utilitarians have proposed that we ought to cease most, if not all, animal experiments and even that we ought to become vegetarians (Singer 2011, chap. 5). This would reduce the suffering inflicted on sentient nonhuman animals and so would contribute to the overall reduction of pain and suffering.

7.17   Some have argued that the lower developmental states of non-human higher mammals would justify using them both in animal experiments as well as for the purposes of food production. Such views are often based on the premise that sentient non-human animals are not persons, and that persons are the only entities with an uncontroversial right to life. Utilitarians counter this typically by pointing out that the argument is not about giving, say, great apes the right to vote but to give equal weight to their interest in not being hurt that we grant fellow humans with similar dispositional capacities for pain and suffering. If we do this, it would follow that most (if not all) experiments involving sentient non-human animals would be unethical. It is worth noting that similarly radical conclusions were reached by influential mainstream non-consequentialist ethicists and political philosophers, too (Regan 1988; Donaldson and Kymlicka 2011).

In many jurisdictions a pragmatic response to concerns about the moral   7.18 standing of non-human animals and controversy about the ethics of their use in experiments has been the introduction of the **three R's**[18]: Replacement by alternatives, reduction in number of animals used, refinement with a view to minimizing discomfort and pain.

As explained earlier, we will focus primarily on human bioethics in this   7.19 book, so let us move on to other important debates in research ethics.

7.4 Informed Consent

As we have already seen in Chapter 6, informed consent is a foundational   7.20 concept in health care ethics. The same holds true for research ethics, certainly since the Nuremberg Code. Let us briefly consider why it is so important in clinical or other research involving human participants. For clinical as well as non-clinical research it is widely accepted that it would be usually unethical to undertake either without voluntary informed consent by a competent prospective research participant.

How can this be ethically justified? Kant-inspired medical doctors such   7.21 as Samuel Hellman think that the use of competent people without their express voluntary consent violates the Categorical Imperative's dictum that we must never use persons as mere means to achieve other ends. Hellman argues that 'individual patients should not be used as a means to achieve even a societally desired end, if in doing so the individual right to medical care is compromised' (Hellman and Hellman 1991). Informed consent in the context of the participation of decisionally competent people in clinical trials is an attempt at addressing the ethical requirements of Kant's Categorical Imperative. How does that argument work? After all, on the face of it, don't we use trial participants as mere means to generate knowledge benefitting – hopefully – future generations of patients? The actual participants' well-being is not what primarily motivates clinical research. Surely that should make clinical research involving human participants morally suspect? Not quite. It is here where the moral significance of voluntary first-person informed consent to trial participation becomes apparent. Once well-informed and truly volunteering, trial participants are no longer mere means to achieve particular research ends. They become active participants in a research project, they make the goals of the project their own. It is for this reason that some writers in bioethics have proposed to replace the still often used 'research subject' with 'research participant', lamenting that the former renders mistakenly the research trial participant a passive means to achieve another objective while the latter indicates that the participant plays in active role in the research endeavor.

7.22   There are also consequentialist attempts at justifying informed consent, but they are inevitably more conditional than Hellman's argument. Consequentialists could argue that informed consent is a good means to foster trust in the researcher-participant relationship. Trial participants will be more likely to abide by the rules governing their conduct in the research project if they have made a voluntary, considered choice to do so. As a result of that the efficiency of medical research is increased.

7.23   Informed consent also has a legal function. It authorizes someone (the researcher) to use the trial participant's body within the parameters agreed on by both parties during the informed consent process. In the absence of that agreement using someone would in most jurisdictions be considered assault, if not worse.

7.24   Given that this authorization must be both voluntary as well as informed, there has been extensive debate about the question of what exactly constitutes voluntariness as well as about the question of what constitutes adequate information. The Nuremberg Code, for instance, required that there be no **'force, fraud, deceit, duress, overreaching, or other ulterior forms of constraint or coercion.'**[19] It also held that the prospective research participant should have 'sufficient comprehension' to make an informed decision.

7.25   Let us now turn to injuries that trial participants may acquire during the trial. One of the ethical principles guiding this kind of research is that the researchers have an obligation to minimize the worsening of a trial participant's baseline, that is the state they were in when they joined the trial.

7.5 Trial-Related Injuries

7.26   With that in mind, it is easy to see why prevention trials then pose their own set of ethical challenges. Let us have a closer look at HIV vaccine trials as an example. Central is the question of whether people who become infected during HIV prevention trials have good reason to claim that their infection is a trial-related injury that should be subject to some kind of compensation, or whether an infection they acquired during a vaccine trial is a clear case of harm to self. At the outset of HIV prevention trials – as in other prevention trials – the trial participants are not infected. That then is their baseline: They are HIV negative. The objective of these trials is to ascertain whether a vaccine candidate is better than doing nothing. You will recall that such a trial design is ethically justifiable if no gold standard of prevention (i.e. a working vaccine) exists. At the time of writing no preventative HIV vaccine exists, hence, in the absence of a gold standard vaccine, these trials are justifiably placebo controlled. For trial participants to acquire HIV they need to engage in unsafe sex, share unsafe injecting equipment or engage in other risky activities. It is their own conduct that results in the acquisition of the infection.

In developed countries participants in such prevention trials, should they   7.27
acquire HIV, would receive access to life-preserving medicines, quite unlike their counterparts in many countries of the developing world. Analyses of the ethical implications of this inequitable situation have focused on the question of whether such infections should be considered trial-related injuries requiring compensation in form of access to life-preserving antiretroviral medicines (Schüklenk and Ashcroft 2000). Diverging opinions variously insisted that the voluntary risk-taking of trial participants means that no ethical obligation to provide post-trial care to them exists, at least none that is based on the trial-related injury rationale. Rather this understanding of the situation sees this as a typical case of *volenti non fit injuria*.[20] The common law doctrine *volenti non fit injuria*,[21] loosely translated, maintains that no injustice is done to someone who agrees to a particular course of action that is arguably harming the person, as long as that is what that person wants, and as long as that person is competent and volunteering.

The opposing point of view pointed to a variety of the 'therapeutic mis-   7.28
conception', an empirical phenomenon affecting a significant percentage of trial participants in any given trial. People laboring under a therapeutic misconception are trial participants who, despite having been properly informed, believe that they are given a drug that will work against their ailment. The equivalent to the therapeutic misconception, in the case of prevention trials, is more of a preventive misconception, involving trial participants who mistakenly think they are (more) protected as a result of their trial participation than they would be if they did not participate in the trial (Simon et al. 2007). According to this argument, if trial sponsors and investigators knowingly keep a significant number of trial participants in

the trial that have mistaken beliefs about the efficacy of the trial medication and indeed the trial design, an ethical duty on the part of researchers and trial sponsors to care for infected participants exists. Indeed, most researchers, ethicists, activists, and policymakers now hold the view that ensuring access to HIV treatment and care should be offered to study participants who become infected during the course of the trial (e.g. Macklin 2006; Weijer et al. 2006; Lo et al. 2007). Ethical review committees evaluating applications for HIV prevention trials anywhere in the world today require that infected trial participants be given access to life-preserving anti-retroviral medicines while they can derive a clinical benefit from doing so.

7.6 Benefits

7.29 Drugs developed as a result of trials undertaken in developed countries will eventually be made available to patients in those countries. The same does often not hold true for trial participants in developing countries. There is a risk that trial participants in developing countries might not reasonably enjoy their fair share of the benefits that should accrue from their risk-taking, at least not in a way that is comparable to what their developed world counterparts would receive. Patients in developed countries might therefore become free-riders on developing world trial participants' risk-taking. Ensuring post-trial access to drugs developed during clinical research is today required by most international research ethics guidelines.

7.30   The following questions have been the source of much debate: How should we determine what levels and what kinds of benefits should reasonably be provided? What procedure should be followed with a view to determining reasonable benefits? Is it the responsibility of clinical researchers to find the resources to guarantee those benefits? Is it the responsibility of trial sponsors to provide such benefits? Should benefits be provided at the individual level or the community level? Should we draw a distinction between for-profit research and non-profit investigations?

7.31   An influential procedural approach to benefit-sharing argues that though there may be an international consensus that requires that impoverished trial participants in the developing world derive some benefit from their risk-taking, it is much less clear that the benefits should be in the form of medicines. Giving full effect to the concept of fair collaboration, local communities and international trial sponsors should negotiate what are considered fair benefits by the participating communities (Participants 2004). One of the practical challenges here is that often such communities are of an informal nature, so it is difficult to determine who could negotiate and speak on behalf of the people that make up a particular community (Schüklenk and Kleinsmidt 2006). Attaining ethically defensible community consent to a particular negotiated benefit then could turn out to be difficult if not impossible. Recent large scale research initiatives such as that undertaken by the Human Hereditary and Health in Africa research consortium **H3Africa**[22] have put significant energy and resource into community consultations on this particular issue and **produced substantive policies**[23] for its researchers on the issue of informed consent. Interestingly, assuming the challenges surrounding informed consent can be met, it is worth noting that these benefits need not be medical benefits and may include a school, health center or water well. Most of the ethical criticism of this approach has centered on its potential to precipitate a proverbial 'race to the bottom'. In our current globalized research context, where free market forces may be at work, well-resourced pharmaceutical company trial sponsors could potentially search the globe for the best possible deal, and in the negotiating process required by this procedural approach, treat desperate impoverished communities unfairly by playing them off against each other in protracted benefits negotiations (London et al. 2010). Although what constitutes 'exploitation' in an international research context is hotly debated, such a 'race to the bottom' would likely be considered exploitative regardless of whether one uses a traditional Kantian conception or one of the more modern conceptions of exploitation, such as that proposed by Alan Wertheimer (Wertheimer 2008). The originator of this procedural approach eventually declared that it 'suffers from a fatal flaw.' (Lie 2010) Given this acknowledged failure of the predominant procedural approach, what remains unresolved and subject to ongoing intense ethical debate is whether it is possible to arrive at a defensible substantive consensus on what levels, and what types, of benefits are owed to trial participants in the developing world (Ballantyne 2010).

A completely different issue, that has also to do with benefits, but with a   7.32
different kind of benefits, needs to be raised, namely the question of whether it is ethically acceptable for us to benefit from uncontroversially unethical research.

7.7 Benefiting from Evil

A good example of this is the earlier mentioned gruesome medical research   7.33
that Nazi scientists carried out on inmates in German concentration camps. Usually these experiments resulted in mutilation, disability and death.

Some have argued that Nazi research was scientifically unsound, but it is doubtful that this holds true for all of this research. As Proctor points out, 'Nazi inspired research was often idiotic, but not always' (Proctor 1999, 275). The ethical issues as they pertain to the use of research results garnered in this manner are to some extent straightforward. The research was evidently unethical, because the concentration camp prisoners were not volunteers, they did not give informed consent, and the risk-benefit ratio was unacceptable. More often than not those who survived the torturous experiments were murdered after the conclusion of the investigation. The verdict 'unethical!' is undoubtedly correct even though ethical review committees did not exist at that point in time.

7.34   Controversial is whether we should be permitted to benefit from the suffering of these victims of the Nazi scientists' cruelties. Various authors have struggled with the issue of whether it is ethically defensible to use data from the Nazi hypothermia experiments to develop new rewarming techniques for victims of hypothermia or to design new survival suits to protect shipwrecked sailors. Different ethical views as to whether researchers should be permitted to use these data have been expressed and defended (e.g. Moe 1984). It has been argued, for example, that utilizing such research results would encourage copycat criminals keen to be famous or notorious at all cost, and that this would be a sufficient reason to discard such research results. Others have argued that using such data would make researchers complicit in these atrocities. Some Jewish scholars and even some survivors of such experiments take a different stance on this. They argue that discarding valuable information gathered under these criminal circumstances does injustice to the victims of such crimes, because their suffering then would have been completely in vain (e.g. Cohen 1990).

7.35   Today, the consensus reached in guidance documents published by medical associations, and major medical journals, is that such research results should be utilized like any other information capable of improving the human condition, but also that academic papers about the research in question should either omit the name of the unethical researchers to reduce the risk of copycats, or that these academic papers should be accompanied by an editorial decrying the means by which these results were achieved. **Some editors of leading biomedical journals declared**[24] that they would cease to publish the results of unethical research, others publish unethical research while denouncing the method deployed by the researchers (Angelski et al. 2011). In practice biomedical journals tend to continue publishing the results of unethical research.

What do you think, how should academic journals, dedicated to publish-   7.36
ing the best research, respond to submissions of articles describing research
that is unethical? Let us turn now to another difficult issue, the participation of patients in trials who happen to suffer from catastrophic illnesses.

7.8 Ethical Issues Affecting Clinical Research Involving the Catastrophically Ill

Ever since the advent of the HIV/AIDS pandemic, research ethicists as well   7.37
as policy makers have been concerned with the question of whether or not
we ought to give catastrophically ill patients access to experimental agents
as a possible last-chance treatment (Schüklenk and Smalling 2017).
Surprisingly the **same question continued, decades later, to exercise
lawmakers in the USA**[25] as well as policy makers at the World Health
Organization with regard to the 2014 Ebola outbreak in West Africa
(Ademabowo et al. 2014).

In the **late 1970s**[26] a previously unknown virus that would eventually be   7.38
called human immunodeficiency virus, or HIV, began spreading rapidly
predominantly among gay men and IV drugs users in Western countries.
Fairly young, oftentimes well-educated people developed an immune deficiency as a result of the HIV infection that rendered their immune system
unable to respond efficiently to any number of otherwise harmless infections. The nature of this – at the time – lethal infection was that no gold
standard of clinical care existed that could have preserved the lives of those
infected. Doctors treated the patients' individual infections, but eventually
they would lose that fight. The clinical trials system that existed at the time
created a whole set of ethical issues that became public knowledge because
those dying AIDS patients did not consider the standard rules of the clinical research enterprise ethical or acceptable, and they were quite vocal
about that.

AIDS activists acknowledged at the time that no gold standard of care   7.39
existed, but many rejected outright the placebo proposition. They understood its methodological rationale, but they did not consider it ethical to
compel dying patients into participation in placebo-controlled randomized
trials. The HIV infected activists refused to participate in placebo-controlled trials because they did not believe that true equipoise existed
between the placebo and the active agent arm. This evidently matters a
great deal when the illness in question is life-threatening. They also had

other ethical concerns. Many insisted that they should be able to access experimental agents as a kind of last-chance treatment. They fully understood that the odds that the experimental agent would work were fairly small, but they thought that that still constituted better odds than the placebo control. These patient-activists knew that non-treatment meant death for those infected.

7.40   Some bioethicists argued that trial participants behaved unethically when they began to cheat to access experimental agents, for instance by investigating the content of the pills they were given to determine who received an active agent and who received the placebo, and by sharing the active agents and by discarding the placebo pills. To their mind HIV-infected trial participants who gave first person voluntary consent to participation in a randomized placebo-controlled trials had no right to subvert the trial design for their own purposes. John Arras wrote:

> No one is obligated to make promises, but once made they must be kept. Likewise, no one has a duty to become a research subject in the first place, but by entering a protocol, subjects enter into a moral relationship with researchers by promising (…) to abide by certain restrictions in return for the benefit of participation. Dropping out of an ethically designed study merely because one has to be randomized to placebo, pooling drugs, or taking unapproved remedies all amount to a violation of this promise.
>
> (Arras 1990)

7.41   Trial participants had a different take on that very same issue. They rejected Arras' argument that their participation was truly voluntary. They pointed out that they had no reasonable alternatives, given that at the time legal access to experimental drugs was limited to participants in clinical trials. Arras retorts, 'the question is not whether potential research subjects have "no choice," but rather whether AIDS researchers or "society" have an independent obligation to provide HIV-infected persons with better alternatives than in current protocols' (Arras 1990). Macklin and Friedland also suggested that 'those who agree to a placebo group do so, presumably without coercion and after being fully informed' (Macklin and Friedland 1986). **The courts in the United States**[27] decided eventually that dying patients have no legal right to access experimental drugs.

7.42   Activists argued at the time that one way to ensure that participants in these vital trials were true volunteers would be to offer experimental agents to anyone unwilling to participate in a placebo randomization. George Annas rejected this proposition. He wrote (Annas 1990):

Making unproven drugs available is poor policy, if unproven remedies are easily available, it will be impossible to do scientifically valid trials of new drugs. Those suffering from AIDS will be unwilling to participate in randomized clinical trials, and those who are randomized to an arm of the study they do not like will take drugs they 'believe in' on the sly, making any valid finding from the study impossible.

Compare this take on reality with that described by HIV-infected indi- 7.43 viduals at the time. Martin Delaney wrote (Delaney 1989):

> It is as if I am in a disabled airplane, speeding downward out of control. I see a parachute hanging on the cabin wall, one small moment of hope. I try to strap it on, when a government employee reaches out and tears it off my back, admonishing, 'You cannot use that! It does not have a Federal Aviation Administration sticker on it! We do not know whether it will work.'

Likewise trial participants fighting for their survival were anything but 7.44 trusting of principal investigators or trial designs. One of them wrote (Schüklenk 1990, 104):

> I hesitate taking them because I do not know if they do me any good, and I wonder if they may hurt me. ... I go for a while and take my medicine and then go for a while and not take it. ... I do not participate in drug research that involves a placebo because I want to know what I am taking.
>
> I hate to say it but K ... we are no more than lab rats to these people. ... As time passed by [in the study this patient participated in] my (antibody) counts eventually dropped to almost their original level and I gracefully bowed out of the study ... thank you Mr Lab Rat.

One of the consequences of many catastrophically ill patients' distrust of 7.45 HIV/AIDS clinical trial designs was that in large numbers they would drop out of trials once they discovered that they were randomized into placebo arms, they faked entry data to get into particular promising trials (aided often by their primary care providers) and they would resort to other means that compromised the integrity and eventually the predictive value of ongoing clinical research (Novick 1993; Dixon 1991). It turns out that these trial participants had reason to be skeptical about the impact of placebo-controlled trial designs on their individual well-being. Anthony Fauci, who was then in charge of HIV/AIDS research at the United States National Institutes of Health, reportedly conceded that 'the randomized clinical trial routinely asks physicians to sacrifice the interests of their particular patients for the sake of the study' (Hellman and Hellman 1991). Partly for this reason it matters that the consent to trial enrolment is forthcoming from patients who are truly volunteering.

7.46   It is worth noting that none of the experimental agents HIV-infected people turned to at the time actually preserved their lives. Those drugs resulted from successfully conducted randomized placebo-controlled trials.

Question

What do you think, should catastrophically ill patients be able to access experimental agents outside the confines of controlled clinical trials? What are the ethical reasons underpinning your conclusion?

7.47   We will now turn our focus on a number of important problems that arise when research is undertaken by researchers hailing from the global north in the global south.

7.9 Developing World

7.9.1 Utility of Research Question

7.48 A different set of questions pertains to the ethical justifiability of research that is considered to be undesirable in a developing world context, such as research that is not directly responsive to local health concerns or needs (London 2008). The criterion of locally appropriate research serving local health needs is frequently mentioned in international research ethics guidance documents, such as for instance the **research ethics guidelines produced by the Council for International Organizations of Medical Sciences**[28], CIOMS (CIOMS 2016). It would require of ethical review committees to not only investigate questions such as the reasonableness of the risk-benefit ratio and whether the proposed informed consent process is sound, but also to take an ethical stance on the question of whether the research itself is desirable. The latter requirement is arguably a qualitatively different proposition altogether. Different positions have evolved on this question. Some scholars have expressed the view that whether or not a research proposal is ethical depends exclusively on matters such as the risk-benefit ratio, the voluntariness of the participants' informed consent, and other mostly process-related questions that are intrinsic to a given trial.

Whether a research project is of value to anyone other than those asking the question is considered uninteresting on this account.

The earlier mentioned view, on the other hand, maintains that determin- 7.49
ing whether or not a particular research project is ethical also requires review committees to take a stance on the research question itself. It is not just the procedures undertaken in the study, but also the goals of the trial itself that must be ethically justified. For example, it would not be ethical, according to this logic, to undertake a trial that satisfies all procedural conditions an ethical trial would have to meet but that aims to develop a procedure that would neither benefit the trial participants nor people belonging to the same social class or ethnicity or sex of the trial participants. Equally a trial the results of which might put specific individuals or sections of society at a disadvantage or in harm's way could be deemed unacceptable. The voluntariness of the trial participants in its own right would not make such a trial ethical. The difficulty with this view is that ethical review committees would be tasked with the much more difficult question of evaluating the value of a proposed research project as such. They might have to address questions such as whether or not it is ethical to undertake genetic research on sexual orientation in a world that is often hostile to gay people (Schüklenk et al. 1997), whether research into the biology of intelligence is ethically acceptable (Reiss 2000) in a world where ethnicity-specific answers might give rise to racist abuse of such investigations. Traditionally these types of ethical questions have been taken to be beyond the purview of ethics review.

7.9.2 Standards of Care

It is arguable that the background of many of the ethical debates pertaining 7.50
to research ethical issues in the developing world can be reduced to a single word: Poverty. If most people in underdeveloped parts of the world were able to afford access to existing medication that those of us who live in developed countries can take for granted, many of the discussions that exercise research ethicists would become superfluous. Standards of care in clinical trials, post-trial access to newly discovered drugs, access to life-preserving medicine for those who became infected while participating in HIV prevention trials, and any number of other issues would cease to be problems. Try to keep this perspective in mind while you read what follows below. The concern about background justice constitutes a significant insight. If ethical arguments put forward in the context of debates about global health ethics and corresponding obligations would be heeded and acted upon, arguably

the controversies discussed below would either not take place or be of low practical relevance (Lowry and Schüklenk 2009).

7.51   One significant ethical controversy with real-world consequences occurred around the question of whether it is ethical to provide patients in developing world-based clinical trials with lower levels of care than the levels of care that would be provided to trial participants in developed countries. A case in point: is it acceptable to knowingly use a placebo control or to provide a lower standard of care, when an effective treatment for a particular ailment exists elsewhere in the world (often called the gold standard of care). We mentioned already, when a gold standard of care exists, any clinical investigation offering a control arm not featuring the best current international standard of care does not begin with genuine clinical equipoise between the trial arms. Patients randomized into the control arm providing knowingly a substandard level of care than the gold standard of care would be predictably worse off, and so, arguably, be harmed. Clinical equipoise as such does not exclude the possibility of placebo controls, but placebo controls are ethically acceptable only under certain circumstances. For example, use of a placebo control might be acceptable if there is no established gold standard of care, or it could be acceptable if study participants who receive the placebo will not be subject to any additional risk of serious or irreversible harm if they do not receive the best proven intervention (e.g. World Medical Association 1964–2013, 33: Use of Placebo).

7.52   The question arose whether these rules, given that they govern research in the developed world, should reasonably be applied to developing countries. Several counter arguments have been offered to justify the use of placebo controls in poorer parts of the world, even when a gold standard of care has been established elsewhere. Some have argued, with justification, that in a society where the gold standard of care is unavailable to the overwhelming majority of patients, it may be reasonable to investigate alternative, more affordable, or easier to administer means of medical care in a trial that involves the use of placebo controls (Levine, 1998). After all, such research would meet a criterion mention earlier, it would be locally appropriate research addressing local health needs. This point of view also stresses that no trial participant would be any worse off because of their participation in the trial; these participants would not have been able to access the gold standard of care in any case, typically due to their inability to afford the medicine in question. According to this view, research aiming to address local health problems needs to compare new and potentially locally-affordable treatment regimes with whatever constitutes the local standard of care as opposed to some elusive international gold standard. The research should aim to establish whether or not a new treatment regime would leave local patients in a better situation than they would have been otherwise. It should not aim to establish that a new treatment regime is better than a locally unaffordable treatment regime that is the gold standard in wealthier parts of the world. The ethical rationale underlying this analysis is consequentialist in nature.

Critics of this analysis have argued that the reasons for impoverished   7.53
patients' lack of access to even essential, life-preserving medication has frequently to do with the drug prices of patented medicine. They question whether economic reasons as opposed to genuine scientific clinical rationales provide a good ethical justification for continuing drug trials in the developing world. After all, drug prices can and have been reduced, and patents can and have been set aside when human lives are at stake. These critics also stress an important implication of the economic justification for allowing placebo-controlled clinical trials: Pharmaceutical companies could price impoverished patients in developed countries with two-tiered health care systems out of affordable access to their patent protected drugs in order to be able to continue placebo controlled clinical trials there, too. Accepting the logic of local standards of care could so have wide-ranging implications for trial standards in many developed countries, too.

Other issues in research ethics have to do with embryo research for the   7.54
purpose of cloning research as well as other genetics research, the ethics of paying research participants, as well as the establishment and use of largescale databases of medical information for research purposes. Of concern has also been the question of whether biochemical warfare research, of either the aggressive or the defensive kinds, should be considered ethically justifiable (Miller 2008).

Questions

If HIV negative people participate in a trial designed to test the efficacy of a preventive HIV vaccine candidate, and some of those participants get infected during the trial, is the infection in your view a trial related injury that should be subject to compensation? Do you think it is ethically justifiable to use sentient non-human animals in clinical research that aims to improve human health? Imagine a researcher had kidnapped and killed a family during a gruesome experiment that led unexpectedly to a cure for cancer. Should we be permitted to use the results of that research to cure current and future cancer patients? Give ethical reasons for your respective answers.

Website Links

1   https://encyclopedia.ushmm.org/content/en/article/nazi-medical-experiments
2   https://encyclopedia.ushmm.org/content/en/article/nazi-medical-experiments
3   http://www.ushmm.org/wlc/en/media_ph.php?ModuleId=10005168& MediaId=1413/
4   http://www.ushmm.org/wlc/en/article.php?ModuleId=10007060/
5   https://encyclopedia.ushmm.org/content/en/article/persecution-of-homosexuals-in-the-third-reich
6   http://www.ushmm.org/wlc/en/article.php?ModuleId=10005261/
7   https://www.loc.gov/rr/frd/Military_Law/Nuremberg_trials.html
8   https://www.cdc.gov/tuskegee/timeline.htm/
9   https://www.wma.net/policies-post/wma-declaration-of-helsinki-ethical-principles-for-medical-research-involving-human-subjects/
10   https://www.hhs.gov/ohrp/regulations-and-policy/belmont-report/index. html/
11   https://publicationethics.org/
12   https://www.nccn.org/patients/resources/clinical_trials/phases.aspx
13   https://www.england.nhs.uk/genomics/
14   https://www.sciencedirect.com/topics/neuroscience/proteomics
15   https://www.scq.ubc.ca/a-brief-overview-of-metabolomics-what-it-means-how-it-is-measured-and-its-utilization/
16   https://www.the-scientist.com/features/n-of-1-trials-take-on-challenges-in-health-car-66071/
17   https://animalstudiesrepository.org/cgi/viewcontent.cgi?article=1003& context=acwp_awap/
18   https://3rs.ccac.ca/en/about/three-rs.html/
19   https://history.nih.gov/research/downloads/nuremberg.pdf/
20   http://www.duhaime.org/LegalDictionary/V/VolentiNonFitInjuria.aspx/
21   http://www.e-lawresources.co.uk/Volenti-non-fit-injuria.php/
22   http://h3africa.org/
23   https://h3africa.org/wp-content/uploads/2018/05/H3A%202017%20 Revised%20IC%20guideline%20for%20SC%2020_10_2017.pdf
24   http:/www.biomedcentral.com/1472-6939/13/4/
25   https://theconversation.com/should-dying-patients-have-the-right-to-access-experimental-treatments-33884
26   http://www.avert.org/history-aids-1986.htm/
27   https://scholar.google.ca/scholar_case?case=12964037297767722899&hl= en&as_sdt=6&as_vis=1&oi=scholarr&sa=X&ved= 0CBsQgAMoADAAahUKEwjb_86d5-zGAhWKSZIKHdriBDE/
28   http://www.cioms.ch/publications/layout_guide2002.pdf/

8

GENETICS

8.1 Genetics and Genomics

8.1.1 Introduction – Genetics, Genomics and Bioethics: Is Genetics Special?

Stories about issues in genetics, whether connected to purported new 8.1 medical breakthroughs or to editing the genome, continue to make news. Genetics has had a big impact not only on society but also on bioethics itself. Sometime called gen-ethics, bioethics in this area has become increasingly specialized. Towards the end of the twentieth century, rapid developments in genomics and the **Human Genome Project**[1], saw the allocation of a dedicated budget to address Ethical, Legal and Social Issues (ELSI) in the USA. This was followed by an ELSA program (ethical legal and social aspects) in Europe and **GE3LS**[2] in Canada. What have also been noticeable are the ways in which scientific developments have posed challenges for ways of thinking about bioethical issues such as informed consent, leading to a considerable amount of work on ethical frameworks (see, e.g. Knoppers and Chadwick 2005, 2015).

In this chapter we will start by looking at whether there is anything 8.2 special about genetics, and then proceed to examine issues of testing and screening in clinical genetics. (As we saw in Chapter 5, genetic testing can be used for selection purposes in the reproduction context.) We will then look at issues of therapy: gene therapy and gene editing. Following that we shall explore genomic research, including biobanks and the development of personalized medicine. We will include a discussion of reproductive

This Is Bioethics: An Introduction, First Edition. Ruth F. Chadwick and Udo Schüklenk.
© 2021 John Wiley & Sons, Inc. Published 2021 by John Wiley & Sons, Inc.

cloning and conclude by briefly mentioning the wider use of genetic information in areas such as ancestry tracing and sport. You will notice that some of the arguments discussed in this chapter are also relevant to enhancement, to be covered in Chapter 9.

8.3   The thesis of **genetic exceptionalism**[3] holds that there is something special or different about the ethical issues in genetics. The reasons typically advanced for this are that genetic information is predictive and independent of time. Hence there is an ethical issue about, for example, a test in childhood that has the potential to reveal an individual's risk status for diseases that will only manifest themselves later in life. This may cause anxiety on the one hand, but allow an individual to prepare, on the other. The anxiety may of course be misplaced. If you have a 50 percent risk of developing a disease, that is not a certainty in relation either to developing a disorder or to its severity if you do. Another feature of genetic information is that it is shared with blood relatives and this can give rise to issues about confidentiality and disclosure. If I am at risk, my brother may be too. The thesis has, however, been criticized on the grounds that other types of medical information may share these features in varying degrees (See, e.g. Green and Botkin 2003): although the ethical issues in genetics may be particularly complicated, they are not in a wholly different category from those relevant in other areas of medicine.

8.4   In addition to genetic exceptionalism, another thesis we need to deal with is that of **genetic determinism**[4], the thesis that a person's genes determine a person's characteristics and abilities. When the Human Genome Project (see below) was completed it revealed that there are far fewer genes in the human genome than had previously been thought – closer to 25,000 rather than 100,000. This suggested to some that genetic determinism was dead. If there are so few genes in the human genome, genes cannot possibly explain the huge variety and complexity that we see in human beings. Genetic *factors*, as opposed to whole genes, are clearly influential but so are many other factors, such as gene–environment interaction.

8.5   In the previous chapter, you will recall, we talked about the historical background of the Nazi period and its influence on the development of research ethics. Genetic science was also misused in the early twentieth century, and not only in Germany. In the USA, for example, in the case of **Buck v. Bell**[5] (US 1927) it was claimed that 'three generations of imbeciles are enough' and this was thought to justify sterilization of Carrie Buck. The eugenics movement was strong also in the UK and although eugenic ideas, which commonly rested on a poor understanding of science, should be clearly distinguished from the science of genetics itself, this period had a significant influence on how debates became framed in the second half of the twentieth century, in particular in relation to the emergence of the **non-directive ethos**[6] in genetic counseling. Reaction against forced sterilization of those deemed 'unfit', such as Buck, led not only to concerns about the improper interpretation of scientific information and abuse of genetic science, but also to an emphasis on free choice in the genetics clinic; and a preference for environmental explanations and interventions at a social level. In the second half of the twentieth century, however, genetic explanations and promises regained popularity along with advances in both the science and associated ethical debate.

8.1.2 Issues in Clinical Genetics: Genetic Testing and Counseling

Within the genetics clinic, in relation to diseases recognized as having an 8.6
identifiable genetic component – for example, **Huntington's disease**[7], the ethical issues turn largely on the autonomy and confidentiality of the client in relation to testing, whether diagnostic of a current condition or predictive of a late onset one. Testing may take place not only of adults but also of children and fetuses. In the clinical context a genetic *test* (as opposed to *screening*) is typically carried out where there is some reason to think there may be a problem. A good example is the situation where there is a strong family history of breast cancer. Celebrities such as **Angelina**[8] Jolie have done much to draw attention to the decisions that individuals may be faced with – in the case of breast cancer, possibly a preventive mastectomy. Because these situations may be very difficult and distressing, it has been argued by some that there is a right not to know (see below) the result of a predictive test which may reveal that the individual may be at risk (see Chadwick et al., 2014).

8.1.2.1 Non-Directiveness

As indicated above, the abuses of genetics in the early twentieth century 8.7
together with the rise in individualism in society and in bioethics, led to the prevailing ethos in genetic counseling being that of non-directiveness, facilitating rather than directing the decision of the client (see, e.g., Elwyn et al., 2000). Non-directiveness may of course be difficult to achieve, in situations where there is a power differential between counselor and client; and some clients may actually want and expect to be directed or at least advised, but for present purposes the main point is that the ethos reflects the primacy of autonomy.

8.8   In some situations, there is a clear tension between the interests of the client and those of third parties. Some of the most discussed questions in the early 1990s concerned possibilities of disclosure to family members of the results of genetic tests on their blood relatives, and the conflict between the interests of those family members and the confidentiality of the person tested – for example, is it right to disclose to a woman's partner a finding of non-paternity where a genetic test on the fetus reveals that he could not actually be the genetic father? The balance between competing interests here is normally struck by the position that individuals should be encouraged to share their information. While there may be some cases at the extreme, where disclosure is permissible, the health professional needs to consider the power dynamics within the couple. Might disclosure of the result put the woman in a situation of physical, economic or emotional risk, for example?

8.1.2.2 Children

8.9   The genetic testing and screening of children has long been acknowledged to be a special case (BSHG 2010). In relation to children, the issues of autonomy are more complicated. It might be the case that it is the parents' wish to have a child tested, because *they* want to know. The possibilities of stigmatization and self-fulfilling prophecy are real issues for a child who is symptom-free but identified as being at risk of a late onset disorder. Hence there are strong arguments for the view that children should not be tested for late onset disorders until they are capable of deciding for themselves whether or not to be tested. The situation is different where there are potentially life-threatening or life-limiting disorders which can be treated in childhood, where the expectation would be that parents should opt for treatment as they would with any other illness.

8.10   In the case of prenatal testing however, as we have seen in Chapter 5, there might be difficult questions concerning termination decisions, in cases where a fetus is found to be suffering from a genetic or chromosomal abnormality. Relevant factors also include the context of social support, or lack of it, for persons with disabilities, which might affect a pregnant woman's decision. Developments in reproductive technology have provided opportunities for preimplantation genetic diagnosis and embryo selection, and this avoids the issue of abortion but raises issues of the criteria for selection of embryos.

8.1.2.3 Genetic Screening

In contrast to genetic testing, where there are factors relating to an 8.11 individual which suggest that testing is indicated, a screening program is carried out on a population where there is no specific reason to think, for any given individual, that he or she is at higher risk. In the 1990s there was considerable discussion about the principles underlying the introduction of a genetic screening program – adapting the 1968 **Wilson and Jungner**[9] principles, for screening in general, to the particular context of genetic screening (see **Nuffield Council**[10] on Bioethics, 1993). The first criterion is that the condition screened for must be important, or serious; another is that there must be an acceptable treatment – which was changed in the genetic context to 'scope for action', as the intervention in question may be a termination or change of lifestyle. There has been considerable but to some extent inconclusive discussion about what constitutes a condition sufficiently 'serious' to warrant a screening program. A classic example is **phenylketonuria**[11], for which newborns are screened and which can be controlled by a diet low in phenylalanine.

There have been cases of interventions at the population level to counter- 8.12 act high incidence of genetic disease, for example, in the case of thalassemia in Cyprus. In 1980 premarital screening was made compulsory by law in a program aimed at preventing the birth of affected babies. This example makes clear that genetics retains its connection with reproduction deci- sions of those who may be themselves unaffected, but carriers, and is not only concerned with individuals who either have a condition or are diag- nosed as being at risk.

8.1.2.4 Direct-to-Consumer Testing

Following the Human Genome Project commercial companies such as 8.13 **23andMe**[12] emerged, offering testing direct to consumers, where the find- ings could include information about genetic ancestry, and health related information. As regards the latter they gave rise to many concerns about the bypassing of professional counselling and advice in the delivery of the information, as well as criticisms regarding the accuracy and usefulness of the information provided. (There are also worries about the fact that such companies, by offering a service of genetic testing, thereby have access to large numbers of samples which can form the basis of a research database to be used for other purposes.) Whereas some people regarded it as an aspect of the 'democratization' of science to facilitate this kind of accessing of their genomic information, there were worries about the possible adverse effects of individuals acting on misleading information about themselves and their families. In December 2013 in the USA, for example, the **Food and Drug Administration**[13] (FDA) ordered the company 23andMe to halt its disclosure of health-relevant results to new direct-to-consumer testing clients. Early in 2015, however, the FDA authorized marketing of a direct-to-consumer genetic carrier test for **Bloom syndrome**[14] and announced the exemption of carrier screening tests from premarket review.

8.14   Let's turn now to the issue of treatment.

8.2 Gene Therapy: Somatic and Germline

8.15   One of the reasons why issues in genetics have been so high profile lies in the nature of genetic disorders and the options for treatment. Genetic disorders cannot typically be cured in the way that infectious diseases can, for example, by prescribing drugs. The boundary between genetic and non-genetic disease is not, of course, clear-cut: both common and infectious diseases have a genetic component. People will differ in their susceptibility and response to any disease in accordance with their own genomic variation.

8.16   It is important to recognize that there has been considerable controversy about what counts as a disorder. This is a live issue even without the genetic element: mental disorders are a case in point and testing for predisposition to such disorders is particularly sensitive. In the genetics clinic the question of what counts as a disorder has been a particularly difficult issue because of the fact that termination was one potential outcome of prenatal genetic counseling.

8.17   Disability rights groups objected to the identity and worth of people being reduced to a disorder, questioning the very label of disorder, and have feared the return of a form of eugenics. Arguments on the other side have attempted to draw a distinction between the conditions and the people who experienced them: between discrimination against a disorder and discrimination against persons with disabilities, with varying degrees of success.

8.18   Gene therapy has had by no means a smooth path but there have been some notable successes. An article in *Nature* in December 2018 talked about how the largest organ in the body, the skin, is an excellent target for gene therapy. It concerned the son of Syrian refugees who had fled to Germany. Hassan was born with junctional epidermolysis bullosa (JEB) which causes large painful blisters on the skin and internal mucous membranes. By the time he was seven Hassan's skin was almost entirely destroyed. However, he was treated with a technique which involved taking a sample of unblistered skin from Hassan's groin, culturing the cells and modifying them using a viral vector to introduce and express the missing gene. It was then necessary to grow enough sheets to return to the boy's body. By 2017 Hassan's skin had been virtually replaced (Arney 2018).

We chose this example because it is clearly a heart-warming success 8.19 story, concerning an innovative treatment on an indisputably desperately ill child. Consideration of this suggests that genetic modification, in this case by gene therapy, can deliver significant goods in terms of health benefits. So, from what points of view could this technique be controversial?

There are of course potential safety concerns. The innovative treatment 8.20 with Hassan worked but the early hype surrounding the promise of gene therapy was followed by a number of disappointments and indeed scandals. A key case was that of **Jesse Gelsinger**[15] in 1999 (Stolberg 1999). Jesse had a genetic disorder called ornithine transcarbamylase (OTC) deficiency. This prevents the body from breaking down ammonia. He had managed the disorder quite well throughout his life by following a strict diet but in young adulthood volunteered for a gene therapy trial which was designed to help newborns with the condition from which he suffered. The idea was to introduce a normal OTC gene, using a vector called adenovirus, into his liver. Four days after the injection Jesse died.

In both the Hassan case and the Jesse case a vector was used to introduce 8.21 the genetically modifying material. Subsequent examination of the facts of this case suggested that Jesse had not been adequately informed of the risks of the use of this particular vector. There were also issues of conflict of interest raised in so far as the lead scientist had a financial interest in the development of the vector in question.

In relation to gene therapy the safety of the vector has always been one 8.22 issue – another is the question of hitting the right target in the body. In the case of Hassan, the skin was modified, grown and then applied to the body, but if genetically modified material is introduced into the body in other ways it may be difficult to ensure that it is taken up and used appropriately. However, if practical and safety issues can be satisfactorily addressed, and there is a sound informed consent procedure, we might tentatively conclude that in principle gene therapy can be used to good effect.

8.23   Both these cases, however, concern gene therapy techniques applied to the bodies of individuals, so-called 'somatic' interventions without affecting reproductive cells. The issues become more complicated when we turn to the modification of the germline and thus future generations. We will now look at why modification of the human germline is argued to be a matter of concern. Several arguments have been brought forward against germline modification, which apply both to germline gene therapy and to germline gene editing.

8.2.1 Is There a Need for Germline Gene Therapy?

8.24   What are the possible scenarios in which germline modification might be a serious option? There are some circumstances in which a couple cannot avoid having a child with a genetic disorder, for example, they both have two copies of the same mutation. If on the other hand they are heterozygous for the same mutation – that is, they each have one copy of the mutated gene – they have a 25 percent chance of having a child with that disorder. It is argued by some, however, that there is no need for germline genetic manipulation because it is in most cases at least possible to achieve the desired result by other means. For example, individuals and couples who are worried about having offspring with a genetic disorder may be able to use artificial reproductive techniques, including donated gametes where necessary, preimplantation diagnosis and embryo selection.

8.25   But is it enough to say this? The fact that there is already a method for achieving a desired result is not in itself an argument against trying a different one. The progress of medicine is precisely concerned with finding safer, more effective and preferably affordable treatments.

8.2.2 Risks and Irreversible Consequences

8.26   One traditional concern related to germline genetic manipulation has been that unintended and undesirable consequences may also be irreversible. This is the safety concern 'writ large' as compared with its application in the somatic gene therapy case. The basic thought is that some change might inadvertently be introduced which is irreversible in future generations, either through the introduction of something disadvantageous or the removal of something which is advantageous, such as a feature which has a protective function against a disease.

8.27   Sheila Jasanoff has made the point that concerns about safety and risk tend to be framed in terms of individual risk, whereas there are also discussions to be had about social risk (see Bergmann 2019). Part of this relates to issues of access and social justice, but there is more to it than that, in terms of reinforcing prevailing perceptions and expectations of medicine in general and of genomics in particular, and there are also worries about effects on attitudes towards disability.

8.2.3 Future Generations and Lack of Consent

Another important concern in relation to germline genetic manipulation is 8.28
that it by its very nature affects future generations, who will not have been able to consent to what amounts to a genetic experiment upon them. While this is true, it is surely the case (as has frequently been pointed out) that all sorts of decisions we take in any generation will have effects on as yet unborn people not only in the near but also in the far distant future. As regards the next generation, parents take decisions about medical interventions on their children, which may well be irreversible. For the medium to long term, climate change is a case in point. There are many issues about our use of resources on the planet which will inevitably affect people of the future, for good or ill. By our actions we also inescapably affect who those people will be: not only explicit population policies but also economic trajectories affect who has children and how many.

Some people object to germline manipulation *even if* safety concerns are 8.29
satisfactorily addressed and even if we can set aside the anxieties about non-consenting future people. It is important to deal with the potential objection that there is something undesirable about germline genetic modification *in itself*. This might be a religiously motivated argument or one concerned with the impropriety of deliberately modifying the basic structures of life.

8.2.4 The Iconic Significance of the Germline

In 1995 Dorothy Nelkin and Susan Lindee referred to the gene as a cultural 8.30
icon (Nelkin and Lindee 1995). The ways in which conceptions of the gene and of DNA have permeated western culture in particular are legion. The germline, however, arguably has a special place within the domain of genomics. The significance of the germ cells is that they form the link between generations and thus offer continuity between the present and the future. It has been not uncommon to allude to the genome as the common heritage of humanity (see e.g., UNESCO 1997) and thus anyone who is concerned for the future of the human species has reason to be concerned

about the germline as well as about the planetary and cosmic environment in which the human species exists.

8.31   Until relatively recently the accepted view was that there is a clear dividing line between somatic and germ cells, which served to increase the specialness of the germline. Somatic cells could not pass information to germ cells and thus to future people. Nevertheless, there were some concerns that gene therapy intended to be a limited somatic intervention could *inadvertently* affect the germline. However, the advent of stem cell technologies has led to the use of technology to generate germ cells from somatic cells. If in theory any cell can become a germ cell the somatic/germ line distinction seems to be challenged, to say the least.

8.32   However the germ cells are themselves generated, the question arises as to what the main area of ethical concern is. It might be claimed that editing the germline constitutes 'Playing God' as discussed in Chapter 3. There are also potential concerns about social justice and an argument that it is incompatible with the autonomy of a human being that decisions about its make-up should be taken by a third party: we will examine these in the next chapter on enhancement, because genetic modification is a possible mechanism for enhancement.

8.2.5 Gene Editing

8.33   Whereas gene therapy has suffered traditionally from worries about lack of precision, the new techniques of gene editing offer the exact opposite, as well as speed. The term 'gene editing' covers a group of technologies, allowing genetic material to be added, altered or cut at specific locations in the genome in a very precise way. The technology best known is called **CRISPR-CAS9**[16] (short for clustered regularly interspaced short palindromic repeats and CRISPR-associated protein 9). The system is adapted from a naturally occurring genome editing system in bacteria. When a bacterium encounters a new virus, it will use an enzyme to cut out a small segment of the attacker virus's DNA and store it, to facilitate fighting it next time.

8.34   The first reported use of CRISPR-Cas9 to repair the DNA of a nonviable embryo took place in 2015. The point about non-viability is important because to modify a viable embryo and transfer it to a uterus would cross the line between somatic and germline modification. In 2017 there was a report that the technique had been used to edit a gene in some early embryos carrying a mutation known to cause hypertropic cardiomyopathy (also without transfer to the uterus).

An **International Summit**[17] held in 2015 on gene editing issued a   8.35
statement saying that there should be a moratorium on germline gene
editing. However, the **National Academies of Sciences, Engineering and
Medicine**[18] in the USA in 2017 gave cautious support for rethinking this,
saying that clinical trials using heritable genome editing should be permitted only within a robust and effective regulatory framework and only for
serious conditions for which there are no reasonable alternatives.

In 2018 the announcement that an experiment on gene editing of   8.36
embryos in China had led to the birth of twins with the CCR5 gene disabled
(apparently only one copy disabled in the case of one of the twins), in an
attempt to make them immune to HIV, provoked a huge amount and range
of comment and controversy. The protein CCR5 is implicated in the way in
which HIV infects cells, and disabling it should, in theory, enable cells to
resist those strains of HIV which make use of it.

The scientist involved, **He Jiankui**,[19] put forward two lines of argument   8.37
to justify the use of the experimental procedure. First, the father of the
twins had HIV and wanted to ensure that his children would not suffer as
he had. Secondly, he argued that CCR5 is a well-studied mutation and that
there were good medical grounds for using CRISPR to cripple it in order to
prevent HIV/AIDS. Having broken domestic laws He Jiankui was sentenced
in December 2019 to three years in prison as well as a 430.000 $ fine. **The
Chinese court ruled**[20] that the scientist had acted 'in the pursuit of personal fame and gain', that he had 'disrupted medical order' and that he had
'crossed the bottom line of ethics in scientific research and medical ethics.'

The interesting thing to focus on here, however, is why the China experi-   8.38
ment was viewed with such dismay. The fact that this is a disease that is now
highly treatable is one of the arguments used to suggest that the intervention was wrong. Other concerns include questions over the adequacy of
informed consent of the parents and safety issues affecting the outcome for
the twins. Overwhelmingly, however, commentary has focused on the fact
that this case involved an editing that affected the germline, widely regarded
as highly premature.

Peter Singer and Julian Savulescu are among those who argue that what   8.39
was wrong with the Jiangkui case was not that it involved manipulation of
the germline, although they agree that it fell short of acceptable standards
in ethics. "He Jiankui's trial was unethical, not because it involved gene
editing, but because it failed to confirm to the basic values and principles
that govern all research involving human participants" (Savulescu and
Singer 2019). Germline gene editing is not regarded by them as unacceptable

in itself. On the contrary, Savulescu and Singer argue for a translational (or implementation) pathway towards gene editing in humans as follows:

- Catastrophic single gene disorders such as Tay-Sachs.
- Severe single gene disorders such as Huntington's.
- Reduction in the genetic contribution to common diseases (e.g. cardiovascular disease).
- Enhanced immunity.
- Delaying aging.

8.40   Further into the future they are willing to countenance the possibility of using editing techniques to enhance traits such as intelligence (see Chapter 9).

8.41   The Nuffield Council on Bioethics in its 2018 **report**[21] *Genome Editing and Human Reproduction,* has made a number of recommendations for the acceptable implementation of heritable genome editing, including suitable governance arrangements, public debate, and consideration of social as well as medical risks.

8.42   It might be argued that if we are to support a pathway to translation, more consideration should be given to editing of the epigenome as a step on the way. Epigenetics refers to factors 'over and above' the genome which affect the ways in which the genome is expressed (see Chadwick and O'Connor 2013). Interaction between our genomes and the environment leads to epigenetic marks being placed on the genome which can be transmitted across generations. Epigenome editing works on the same general principles as genome editing but puts in place or erases such an epigenetic mark (Elsner 2018). Epigenome editing leaves the underlying DNA unchanged and is thus arguably "a more subtle and potentially safer strategy" (Zezulin and Musunuru 2017, 10)

8.3 Genomic Research

8.3.1 The Human Genome Project

8.43   The aim of the Human Genome Project (HGP) was to produce a complete map and sequence of all the genes in the human genome: genomics marked a shift of attention from genes to genomes, where 'genome' denotes the full set of genetic material. Until quite recently most of the bioethical discussion related to genomics concerned the genome in the nucleus of the cell, the nuclear genome, which was what was referred to in the HGP. We also have DNA in our mitochondria, however, which exist in the cell outside the nucleus. The sequencing of the mitochondrial genome, completed in the 1980s, passed almost unattended by any ethical comment, presumably because of how the role of the mitochondrial genome, which exists within the cell outside of the nucleus, was perceived. The analogy of a battery has been used, suggesting that the role of mitochondria is just to provide energy to the cell, in contrast to the nuclear genome which, together with other factors, has been regarded as influencing the characteristics of the phenotype, i.e. the individual in their perceptible physical form.

It is nevertheless the case that a defect in the mitochondria, which are   8.44 inherited through the female line, can have a devastating effect on the phenotype. The battery analogy, however, has been influential in making the positive case for **mitochondrial replacement therapy**[22] which involves removing mitochondria from a woman's egg and replacing them with those from a donor. The egg can then be fertilized by the woman's husband or partner. This has been described in some sections of the press as producing **babies with three parents**[23], but the supporters of the technique argue that it prevents potentially very great suffering by the prevention of mitochondrial disease which cannot otherwise be cured. (For an overview of the ethical issues see Dimond 2015)

8.3.2 Biobanks

In addition to trying to make sense of the information provided by the   8.45 outcome of the Human Genome Project itself, attention turned in the last decade of the twentieth century to population wide genomic research (see Gottweis and Petersen 2008). Biobanks were established in several countries, such as Iceland and Estonia. The purpose of a biobank was to collect both genetic material - DNA samples - and phenotypic information (e.g. data about their lifestyle, body measurements and diet) from participants, in an effort to establish links between genetic factors and the development of disease, and not only diseases classifiable as 'genetic diseases'. For example, the **UK Biobank**[24] was established with the aim of clarifying the factors at work in the common diseases that typically manifest themselves in midlife, such as heart disease and the cancers.

The focus of attention now turned to the study of variation in the   8.46 genome – the ways in which individuals *differ* from each other at the genetic level, leading to effects which may be due to a single base pair in the genome.

There had been earlier interest in variation, in the **Human Genome Diversity project**[25] but that had attracted considerable amount of hostility among different ethnic groups who had concerns about the motivation behind the study of diversity.

8.47   Biobanks, particularly in **Iceland**[26], were also initially very controversial and gave rise once more to discussions about whether there is anything special about the ethical issues involved. One prominent example concerned informed consent. As discussed in Chapter 7, the doctrine of informed consent had become a cornerstone of biomedical research in the twentieth century, but the establishment of biobanks required fresh thinking about this.

8.48   Participants asked to donate DNA samples to biobanks were asked to give their informed consent. The problem that emerged was that it was not always clear what they were being asked to consent to. Biobank operators were proposing to collect and store their samples, but for what? It might not be clear even to the scientists and researchers what they might want to do with the samples a few years down the line. The new context gave rise to the bioethical debate about the difference between 'narrow' and **'broad' consent**[27]. A person who gives narrow informed consent agrees to specific, detailed research purposes, as in a drug trial, whereas broad consent involves agreement to research for purposes that may not be specified or specifiable in detail the time. UK Biobank adopted a form of broad consent, asking participants to consent to being in the Biobank – or not.

8.49   There are different arguments in favor of broad consent in the biobank genomics context. First, the purposes for which biobanks are established are clearly, to some extent, undermined if there are restrictions on the research that may be done on the samples. This is not just an argument about scientific freedom: it is argued that this kind of population research is essential for future population health, in addressing the incidence of the common diseases. Another argument is that the kind of harm which may befall contributors to a biobank is very different from that involved in conventional medical research such as a drug trial. The physical intervention involved is limited to the taking of a blood sample: the potential harm arises largely from the possible access to and misuse of a participant's information, especially if the samples are linked to personal and phenotypic information of various kinds.

8.50   Biobank research has given rise to a considerable amount of new debate about the handling of genomic information, both as regards storage and access. Storage issues include to what extent and in what ways samples are linked, or not, to phenotypic information, by techniques of coding and anonymization. If samples could not be linked at all, then the value of the research is decreased. On the other hand, the greater the possibilities of identifiability, the greater the risk to the privacy of the individual participant. Increasingly it was realized, in any case, that where DNA samples are collected and stored the possibility of maintaining complete privacy is undermined, and it was argued by some that the better course would be to acknowledge this fact. This led to a call for 'open consent' where participants would donate in the knowledge that there was no guarantee of privacy, in the interests of research (Lunshof et al. 2008).

8.3.3 Feedback of Findings

In the context of genomic research including in biobanks, there are issues   8.51
about whether, how and to what extent research findings should be fed back to participants. Opposing arguments have been advanced in relation to this. On the one hand it is argued that participants should not be given information other than the general results of the research. In many cases the raw data that emerges will not be meaningful to individuals in any case. On the other hand, it is argued that if information specific to an individual (sometimes called 'incidental' or 'secondary' findings) emerges which could be relevant to their health, even potentially life-preserving, then there is an obligation to tell them. While there is an emerging consensus that in some circumstances participants should be given feedback about findings, there are ongoing debates about exactly what information participants in biobanks and genomic research should have access to. (For an overview of the issues see Mackley and Capps 2017.)

As mentioned above, debates in the 1990s had already considered   8.52
whether there could be a right not to know genetic information (Chadwick et al. 2014). The historical predominance of autonomy, choice and informed consent in the second half of the twentieth century, however, produced a default position that individuals had a right to information: what had to be justified was withholding it. Using what he called a 'thick' interpretation of autonomy, however, Jørgen Husted suggested that some information can potentially undermine an individual's conception of themselves and their life plan, and hence autonomy can be compatible with choosing not to know (Husted, 2014).

For a given individual or community, the results of genomic research can   8.53
disturb long-held beliefs about their ancestry or relatedness, leading to

considerable distress and upset in some well publicized cases, such as that of research on the **Havasupai**[28] Indians, who gave consent to the use of their samples in research on diabetes, which was a serious problem in their community. However, they subsequently learned that their samples had been used to study other things, and that publications on the results contradicted their history as they saw it and a lawsuit led to the payment of significant compensation (Lunshof and Chadwick 2011).

8.4 Personalized Medicine

8.54   Interest in the variation between individuals, explored in population genomic research facilitated by biobanks, has driven the quest for a new form of individual-centered medicine, so called personalized medicine, whereby treatment could be prescribed in accordance with the genome of the patient.

8.55   The argument for personalized medicine has made much of the fact that traditional medical practice and drug prescribing had a considerable problem of disease caused by medical examination or treatment, or **iatrogenic disease**[29]. There is a large burden of not only illness but also mortality arising from the side effects of pharmaceutical products. While it has long been known that any given drug would not be appropriate for every individual, in the past for the most part the only way to find out would be for that individual to take the drug – a trial and error approach predominant in prescribing. The theory behind pharmacogenomics was that it should be possible through genomic research to discover the associations between genetic factors and drug response. Implementation in clinical practice would of course have to have access to genetic information about the individual patient, and this would then inform the choice of drug, or the appropriate dosage. The promise is safer and more effective medicine – and also a reduction in time wasted through trying drugs that did not work for a given patient (see Nuffield Council on Bioethics 2003).

8.56   The label 'personalized medicine' has not proved totally beneficial, because the term 'personalization' may be very misleading to patients. It can be confused with treating the patient *as a person*, for example. Initially personalized medicine might have meant assigning patients to groups of good or poor responders to a particular drug on the basis of a targeted test – a fairly limited sense of personalization, which might more appropriately be called patient stratification. The term is now being challenged by terms such as 'precision medicine', as in former US President Obama's

Precision Medicine Initiative[30] (NAS 2011; ESF 2012), succeeded by the **'All of Us' research program**[31].

Developments in science and technology, from genome wide association 8.57 studies to next generation sequencing, have given a new meaning to personalization, ultimately involving investigating the whole genome sequence of an individual. (Some approaches to personalized medicine also include wider ranges of non-genetic data; e.g. NAS 2011; ESF 2013.) The metaphor of 'tailoring' has been used to describe the fit between the individual's genome sequence and the prescription of medical and lifestyle advice. The cost for such sequencing has also fallen rapidly and continues to fall.

There are also new challenges, however. While on the one hand it fits 8.58 into an individualistic paradigm in society that employs the rhetoric of choice, this has also led to one of the main criticisms: that on a wide scale it is only feasible in wealthy societies (despite the falling costs). Indeed, it has been called 'boutique' medicine by Abdallah Daar and Peter A. Singer (Daar and Singer 2005). They claimed that the underlying research could be beneficial for other purposes – what has been described as 'drug resuscitation' of products taken off the market because of adverse events in the west, to help underserved populations in developing countries, where differences in genomic factors might avoid the adverse effects. This discussion is part of a much wider debate about the sharing of the benefits of genomic research. **Benefit sharing**[32], already introduced in the previous chapter, and to be understood in a wide sense beyond commercial benefit, has become a standard ethical dimension of proposals for genetic and genomic studies, one that points to the greater consideration of equity and justice (HUGO 2000).

We will now turn to the topics of stem cells and human cloning. 8.59

8.4.1 Human Cloning – Therapeutic Cloning

Today we typically distinguish between two types of human cloning, **thera-** 8.60 **peutic cloning**[33] and **reproductive cloning**[34]. Therapeutic cloning research essentially hopes to make use of embryonic stem cells' pluripotent potential. The aim is to manipulate them into growing into various types of bodily tissue, including possibly organs, at some point in the future. Medical doctor cum bioethicist Soren Holm explains the medical benefits we might be able to derive from such research (Holm 2002, 496–497):

> The most immediate therapeutic gains are likely to be in the area of cell therapy. Many diseases are caused by, or accompanied by, loss of specific cell types. The

lost cell types could be produced in the laboratory and later implanted to cure or alleviate disease. Further in the future it may become possible to grow whole organs from stem cells and use these for transplantation, removing the need for organ donation; and even further into the future we may be able to use stem cells for rejuvenating therapies leading to an increased lifespan.

8.61   Therapeutic cloning research is undertaken on both embryonic stem cells and adult stem cells. At the time of writing it is unclear whether adult stem cells will ever be able to take the place of embryonic stem cells for research purposes.

8.62   Given the potential of this research to lead to revolutionary breakthroughs it would need some pretty powerful reasons for any society to prohibit stem cell research. It turns out to be the case that there is such a reason, if you give weight to some of the reasons put forward by opponents of stem cell research. Ethically controversial is, of course, the question of whether it is acceptable to destroy embryos in the process of such research. This controversy mirrors to some extent the controversies surrounding destructive embryo research during the research that led to the development of IVF. If one holds the view that embryos must never be utilized to achieve some objective other than reproductive success, this kind of research would be considered unacceptable. It is this view that typically led to legislation designed to limit women's access to abortion. Equally, however, most jurisdictions concede that embryos do not have the same moral standing as newborns or adults, or else access to abortion would be much more severely restricted than it is. The developmental status of embryos is typically taken to be of great importance when regulations are drawn up. For the purpose of our discussion it matters then that the stem cells that are required for embryonic stem cell research are harvested during the first few days after conception. At that point in time no central nervous system exists, and no capacity to experience pain. Utilitarians would consider the destruction of these embryos for research – or any other – purposes as unproblematic, because they would not actually be hurt in the process. It turns out to be the case that the embryos that are usually used for this purpose are surplus embryos from IVF procedures. It is not unusual for them to have been donated by their progenitors for medical research. Even in the absence of stem cell research they would eventually have been discarded.

8.63   A good representative of those opposed to embryonic stem cell research is former United States President George W. Bush. **He explains**[35] why he is opposed to public funding for destructive embryo stem cell research. Bush outlines two questions he was asking himself while he was contemplating

his response[36] to this ethical challenge: 'First, are these frozen embryos human life, and therefore, something precious to be protected? And second, if they're going to be destroyed anyway, shouldn't they be used for a greater good, for research that has the potential to save and improve other lives?' (Bush 2001) He answered both questions in the affirmative. In President Bush's words, 'I also believe human life is a sacred gift from our Creator.' During his presidency he prohibited the use of public funds for embryonic stem cell research requiring new embryonic stem cells; however, research relying on already existing embryonic stem cell lines was permitted to go ahead, because the embryos that gave rise to them had been destroyed already. As former President Bush put it, 'I have concluded that we should allow federal funds to be used for research on these existing stem cell lines, where the life and death decision has already been made.' This probably constitutes, from his perspective, a case of 'make the most of a bad situation.' The harm, on this interpretation has been done already, accordingly nothing should stop us from using the cell lines from these embryos to further important health research objectives.

Proponents of embryonic stem cell research usually reject the view that 8.64 embryos have (significant) moral standing. President Bush, for instance, justified his views with reference to his religious beliefs in a Christian God. You don't need to subscribe to these religious beliefs, however, to sustain similar conclusions. You could, for instance hold the view that embryos are members of our species and for that reason entitled to special protections preventing their use for this kind of research.

8.4.2 Reproductive Cloning

Reproductive human cloning has been outlawed in most countries. Why 8.65 would anyone want to reproduce by means of reproductive cloning if it were possible? One reason has to do with the possibility of having a genetically linked child while avoiding the pitfall of passing on a genetic illness from one partner in a relationship. Then there might be infertile couples – including same-sex couples – who might wish to have a genetically linked child. There could be other reasons that some might find more objectionable. Say, a model might wish to clone a child in their likeness. Various concerns have been raised about the specter of human reproductive cloning. Medical ethicist Gregory E. Pence has produced a whole book countering these concerns (Pence 1998). We cannot discuss all of these arguments in great detail here. A short survey of the pros and cons of reproductive human cloning must suffice.

8.66   Some arguments against reproductive human cloning rely heavily on a rhetorical tool we have come across in Chapter 3. Slippery-slope arguments have been deployed quite generously in policy debates on reproductive human cloning. Among them is the following argument advanced by Leon R. Kass, the chairperson of former President George W. Bush's bioethics advisory council, in an article published in *The New Republic* magazine. He writes (Kass 1997, 25):

> Yet we are urged by proponents of cloning to forget about the science fiction scenarios of laboratory manufacture and multiple-copied clones, and to focus only on the homely cases of infertile couples exercising their reproductive rights. But why, if the single cases are so innocent, should multiplying their performance be so off-putting? ... When we follow the sound ethical principle of universalizing our choice – would it be right if everyone cloned a Wilt Chamberlain' (with his consent, of course)? 'Would it be right if everyone decided to practice asexual reproduction?' we discover what is wrong with these seemingly innocent cases. The so-called science fiction cases make vivid the meaning of what looks to us, mistakenly, to be benign.

8.67   Pence encourages students to find the maximal number of reasoning errors in this excerpt (Pence 1998, 144ff.) Perhaps you want to give it a shot yourself before you read on. Let us just stick to one slippery-slope argument here: the universalizability argument. It doesn't appear to make a lot of sense. Just because some people might avail themselves of reproductive human cloning if it were available, doesn't mean that a lot of people, let alone all people, would do so. Even if they were, it is unclear whether Kass' worries would turn out to be justified.

8.68   Kass also considers reproductive human cloning repulsive. He concedes that what we considered repulsive just a few decades ago might not be considered repulsive today, but he seems certain that that fate would not befall reproductive human cloning. Governments across the world appear to agree with Kass' take on the issue; they have outlawed reproductive human cloning. Still, a gut response to a new technology is not a sound substitute for an ethical analysis.

8.69   Various opponents of reproductive human cloning warned of dire, inevitable consequences if reproductive human cloning were to be permitted. Some suggested that genetic diversity among humans might suffer, but that also assumes that people across the globe would flock to an expensive technology in lieu of sexual reproduction. Not a terribly likely scenario, yet another rhetorical slippery slope argument. Others expressed anxiety about the possibility that reproductive human cloning could lead to armies of clones deployed at the push of a button by ruthless dictators. This slippery slope argument was never terribly plausible either. How many dictators could wait for their armies to be gestated for 9 months and then grow up, like other children? By the time their armies would have come about they would have died of old age or would have been deposed by the people or some other dictator. It has also been argued that some particularly fanatic parents might wish to see a copy of themselves reproduced and that this would violate these children's right to an open future (Pence 1998, 135f.) We do not know, of course, whether there would be such parents, or if there were, how many parents availing themselves of reproductive cloning would fall into that category. However, you might find it disconcerting that these children might not be seen as an end in themselves but as mere means to achieve some other objective. In this case the objective being to be a copy of one parent. Of course, if you were that child, would you prefer to be that child as opposed to not being at all? Nothing would eventually stop you from living your own life just as any other child that was brought up by overbearing parents hoping for a child just like them.

A more serious argument against reproductive cloning notes that before **Dolly the sheep**[37] became our first known successfully cloned mammal there were very **many deformed fetuses**[38]. Some opponents of reproductive human cloning have argued that would be too high a price for achieving reproductive human cloning success. It also turned out to be the case that eventually successfully cloned animals tended to **die prematurely**[39]. Utilitarians and other consequentialists could well argue that even a higher number of deformed embryos would be a comparably small price to pay in order to achieve the overall societal benefits an efficient reproductive human cloning procedure might offer. Kantians might be concerned about the motives of some prospective parents of human clones, namely those who primarily or exclusively see their cloned off-spring as a mere means to achieve one or another of their desired objectives.

8.70

8.5 Other Issues in Genetics and Genomics

In this chapter we have considered a number of issues including genetic testing and screening, therapy and gene editing, and human cloning. We will conclude by briefly mentioning some other issues, which we don't have

8.71

the space to cover in detail, but which you might wish to follow up. Ancestry tracing has already been mentioned. Behavioral and forensic genomics raise ethical issues about responsibility, freedom and punishment in the criminal context – could there be a legitimate defense in court relating to one's genetic predisposition, for example? (see **Levitt 2013**[40]). Also giving rise to concern are the promotion of tests related to character and natural talents of children, and to pick out budding sports stars so that they can be given appropriate training. In some cases this overlaps with medical matters, as in the case of a predisposition to **sudden cardiac death**[41] which is clearly important for someone considering a sporting career. The main issues here remain the quality of the scientific basis of the information on offer and the tension between the marketplace and the professions as the medium through which genetic information should be conveyed or bought and sold.

8.72   Another area to consider in the era of personalization is **nutrigenomics**[42]. At first sight it seems analogous to pharmacogenomics. Just as the latter facilitates personalized prescribing on the basis of genetic information, so the former, in principle, makes possible personalized dietary advice which can also be extremely important in the health care setting, especially in the light of the purported obesity epidemic. However, nutrigenomics is very different from pharmacogenomics in that foodstuffs with multiple ingredients are far more complex and work on more aspects of the body than do drugs, which are designed to act on specific targets and pathways in the body. Establishing the associations on the basis of which useful advice can be given is therefore more challenging.

8.73   In terms of international approaches to the issues in genomics, you might want to look at the **Universal Declaration on the Human Genome and Human Rights**[43] (UNESCO 1997). While this Declaration lays down universal principles, other international instruments incorporate rules. At the level of the European Union, for example, the **General Data Protection Regulation**[44], in force from 2018, lays down parameters for transfer of data, including genetic data, across the Union and beyond.

8.74   It is important to recognize that cultural differences in various parts of the world influence how genetic material is understood. Public engagement has become increasingly important, partly as a necessary condition of a process of benefit sharing. **The Human Heredity and Health in Africa initiative (H3Africa)**[45], for example, which includes a number of different genomics projects funded by the UK's **Wellcome Trust**[46] and the **National Institutes of Health**[47] in the US, is addressing issues of public engagement and informed consent in multiple populations in different social contexts, both rural and urban.

The rapid advances in technology and prospects for implementation 8.75 offer the promise of considerable development in the relationship between science and bioethical debate in the years to come. One of the arenas in which these issues are played out is that of enhancement, to which we now turn.

Questions

Are people right to be concerned about their genetic information? Is there something special about genetics?

Do you think there is a moral difference between somatic and germline gene therapy and/or editing?

Website Links

1   https://www.genome.gov/human-genome-project
2   https://www.genomecanada.ca/en/programs/genomics-society-ge3ls
3   https://www.alrc.gov.au/publication/essentially-yours-the-protection-of-human-genetic-information-in-australia-alrc-report-96/03-coming-to-terms-with-genetic-information/is-genetic-information-truly-exceptional/
4   https://link.springer.com/referenceworkentry/10.1007%2F978-3-319-16999-6_2162-2
5   https://www.law.cornell.edu/supremecourt/text/274/200
6   https://www.genome.gov/genetics-glossary/Non-Directiveness
7   https://www.nhs.uk/conditions/huntingtons-disease/
8   https://www.health.harvard.edu/blog/angelina-jolies-prophylactic-mastectomy-a-difficult-decision-201305156255"
9   https://apps.who.int/iris/bitstream/handle/10665/37650/WHO_PHP_34.pdf?sequence=17
10 https://www.nuffieldbioethics.org/publications/genetic-screening
11 https://www.nhs.uk/conditions/phenylketonuria/
12 https://www.23andme.com/en-gb/
13 https://www.fda.gov/home
14 https://ghr.nlm.nih.gov/condition/bloom-syndrome
15 https://www.sciencehistory.org/distillations/the-death-of-jesse-gelsinger-20-years-later
16 https://ghr.nlm.nih.gov/primer/genomicresearch/genomeediting
17 https://www.ncbi.nlm.nih.gov/books/NBK343651/

18   https://www.nap.edu/read/24623/chapter/1
19   https://www.nature.com/articles/d41586-018-07545-0
20   https://www.bbc.co.uk/news/world-asia-china-50944461
21   https://www.nuffieldbioethics.org/publications/genome-editing-and-human-reproduction
22   https://www.hfea.gov.uk/treatments/embryo-testing-and-treatments-for-disease/mitochondrial-donation-treatment/
23   https://www.newscientist.com/article/2107219-exclusive-worlds-first-baby-born-with-new-3-parent-technique/
24   https://www.ukbiobank.ac.uk/
25   https://www.sciencedirect.com/science/article/pii/B9780080970868820371
26   https://www.bbc.co.uk/news/magazine-27903831
27   https://www.ncbi.nlm.nih.gov/pmc/articles/PMC4791589/
28   https://blogs.plos.org/dnascience/2013/08/08/hela-the-havasupai-and-informed-consent/
29   http://medind.nic.in/maa/t05/i1/maat05i1p2.pdf
30   https://obamawhitehouse.archives.gov/precision-medicine
31   https://allofus.nih.gov
32   https://www.uclan.ac.uk/research/explore/projects/assets/cpe_genbenefit_frameworks.pdf
33   https://archive.bio.org/articles/value-therapeutic-cloning-patients
34   https://www.bioethics.ac.uk/topics/reproductive-cloning.php
35   ttp://georgewbush-whitehouse.archives.gov/news/releases/2001/08/20010809-2.html
36   https://embryo.asu.edu/pages/president-george-w-bushs-announcement-stem-cells-9-august-2001
37   https://dolly.roslin.ed.ac.uk/facts/the-life-of-dolly/index.html
38   https://www.nytimes.com/2001/03/25/world/researchers-find-big-risk-of-defect-in-cloning-animals.html
39   https://www.independent.co.uk/news/science/early-death-of-dolly-the-sheep-sparks-warning-on-cloning-119040.html
40   https://link.springer.com/article/10.1186/2195-7819-9-13
41   https://www.bhf.org.uk/informationsupport/conditions/sudden-arrhythmic-death-syndrome
42   https://www.nutritionsociety.org/blog/nutrigenomics-basics
43   https://en.unesco.org/themes/ethics-science-and-technology/human-genome-and-human-rights
44   https://gdpr-info.eu/
45   https://h3africa.org/
46   https://wellcome.ac.uk/
47   https://www.nih.gov/

9

ENHANCEMENT

9.1 Introduction

In this chapter we turn to human enhancement. First, we will examine what 9.1
it might mean to enhance humans, both at the level of the individual and
the species as a whole. A variety of techniques that might be employed for
this – from wearable or implanted technologies, through drugs, to genetic
modification, for example. Then, we will discuss the ethical arguments
applied to issues of enhancement. This will in part extend the discussion of
genetic modification in the previous chapter. As the debate about human
enhancement is becoming increasingly specialized, we will introduce the
issues related to moral and cognitive enhancement, although each of these
could take a chapter in themselves. While there are of course also issues
about physical enhancement, moral and cognitive enhancement raise
particularly interesting and at times perplexing issues.

9.2 Enhancement and Superhumans

In 2012, a biomedical research charity, the **Wellcome Trust**[1] in London 9.2
mounted an exhibition called 'Superhuman: exploring human enhancement from 600 BCE to 2050, and used two familiar examples:

> ...we are already living enhanced lives and have been for a long time. Some
> devices are so familiar that we barely think of them as enhancement at all,
> such as spectacles or hearing aids.
>
> (Wellcome Collection 2012, 8)

This Is Bioethics: An Introduction, First Edition. Ruth F. Chadwick and Udo Schüklenk.
© 2021 John Wiley & Sons, Inc. Published 2021 by John Wiley & Sons, Inc.

9.3   The exhibition included smartphones as a form of human enhancement noting that these devices have in effect become extensions to our anatomy (ibid. 8). What many people are interested in from an ethical point of view, however, is *bioenhancement* – not just adding an extension but enhancing humans 'from the inside', at the biological level. This might involve linking biological means with other mechanisms. For example, the UK Ministry of Defence suggested in 2010 that by 2040 the use of information and communications technologies (ICT) is likely to be so pervasive that people may be permanently connected - through the mechanisms of wearable and implantable ICT (Ministry of Defence 2010).

9.4   When we talk about enhancing human beings as such, rather than by adding extensions to individuals, matters become more complicated, as we debate the possibilities of creating posthumans. In some discussions the distinction between self/species enhancement is glossed over. Baylis and Robert, for example, in their discussion of the view that it is inevitable that humans will be enhanced - at times appear to be discussing enhancement of humans as such; while at others they speak of enhancement in relation to 'the self':

> …the resulting alterations may be conservative (i.e., used to normalize the self), liberal (i.e., used to liberate the self) or radical (used to fashion a self that effectively challenges others' conception of oneself).
>
> (Baylis and Robert 2004)

9.5   There are of course questions to consider about what *counts* as making a change (whether enhancing or not) at species level rather than at individual level. Let's consider the example of a tail for humans. Evolution has, as we know, produced humans without tails. However, Japanese scientists are producing **robotic**[2] tails to help unsteady elderly people keep their balance. Maybe eventually the tail could be introduced for all humans over a certain age. At what point would making this change count as an enhancement of the species (assuming it has not been done before)? If not, would a certain number or proportion need to be changed? Or is it the quality of change rather than the quantity of change that counts? While this is a difficult issue because of the contested boundaries of the concept of 'species', we think that (although it would not be appropriate to talk of all enhancement only in genetic terms), for an enhancement to count as an enhancement of the species it would have to be heritable, i.e., transmissible down the germ-line.

Otherwise the respect in which it makes sense to speak of enhancement of the species remains obscure.

Before proceeding any further, however, we need to address the question 9.6 of how to understand the concept of 'enhancement'.

9.3 The Meaning of Enhancement

What do you first think of when you hear the word 'enhancement'? Even in 9.7 the case of physical enhancement, the concept is extremely difficult to pin down. The London Olympics and **Paralympics**[3] in 2012 afforded considerable material for thinking about the concept of enhancement and its use. Both athletes with disabilities (whether using enhancement technologies or not), and those without disabilities, surpassed the abilities of most people by quite a long way; and indeed, the television trailers for the Paralympics introduced the competitors as 'superhumans'. This example makes clear some of the difficulties of terminology.

9.3.1 Enhancement and Improvement

At first it might appear obvious that enhancement means making 9.8 something better. If we have our eyesight or hearing enhanced, we might naturally understand that to mean being able to see or hear better than we did before – an improvement. But we need to be careful of making it true by definition that enhancement is a good thing, in the sense of being morally desirable. Speaking of a 'culture of enhancement', Marilyn Strathern suggested that: '[T]he very term enhancement implies we are bound to want it, and this is where things begin to get out of hand' (Strathern 1995).

This is important because for some, enhancement does imply 'improve- 9.9 ment', making something better, and thus something that there are good reasons to pursue. Some might draw the conclusion that there are moral reasons to pursue it from this alone. If enhancement is understood in such terms, how could one possibly object to it? If we are to make any progress with the ethics of enhancement however, we should not presuppose that to enhance is to improve. Whether any particular enhancement intervention is an improvement, especially from an ethical point of view, is an open question. From a linguistic point of view the concepts of 'enhancement' and 'improvement' are distinguishable. Important questions to ask include: for whom will it be an improvement and in what way? We have to have regard to the *respects in which* something is enhanced.

9.10   To enhance an x with respect to characteristic y is not necessarily to make x better overall. It is possible for breast enlargement (assuming this to be an enhancement of the breast) to distort the proportions of the body, for example. Is there a case, however, for saying that to enhance an x with respect to characteristic y should be understood as introducing an improvement to x *with respect to that characteristic?*

9.11   For an enhancement to count as a characteristic-specific improvement it is necessary to understand the background conditions obtaining, including the purposes or desires being served by the change introduced. So, in order to assess whether any breast surgery is an improvement or not we need to know for what purposes it was carried out, and if those purposes are achieved, then it counts as an improvement. If, for instance, the intervention is sought in order to make the person more attractive, however, it is arguable that the judgment of success, or not, has to have regard to broader considerations than simply the breast alone, such as the new proportions of the body, by whom it is found attractive and so on.

9.12   There may be circumstances, however, in which a characteristic-specific intervention can be introduced which meets a particular purpose without changing anything else. For example, suppose I need to increase my hearing range in order to do a particular job and this can be achieved by taking a pill that has no side effects. In that case this might appear to be an improvement and thus, on this definition, an enhancement with respect to the purpose – and moreover, as everything else remains the same, an improvement overall.

9.13   It is necessary, however, to be very precise about the respect in which an improvement is introduced. In the hearing example it is necessary to allow for the possibility that an improvement in the hearing *range* could be accompanied by a diminution of hearing *discrimination*. So, the relevant characteristic cannot be 'hearing' but must be 'hearing range'. To define enhancement in terms of improvement is, then, at least potentially misleading, in that it may direct attention away from the need to ask what purposes are being served and complicate the issue of assessment of the intervention from a moral point of view. This is not necessarily decisive against such a definition, however, provided that it is clear that to define enhancement as improvement does not preclude an adverse judgment on its desirability. Given this, the definition of enhancement as an improvement is quite uninformative, because it implies a provisional qualitative judgment which is open to revision, all things considered. At the species level, it is far from obvious how we can assess making changes to human beings as such, especially ones that are irreversible. Of course, it may be argued that we do this all the time anyway: this is how humans have evolved and developed culture. Now, however, we have at least the prospect of tools of deliberate design.

9.4 Alternatives to the 'Improvement' Account

9.4.1 Therapy–Enhancement Distinction

An explanation of enhancement has frequently been attempted in the bio- 9.14
medical context via a distinction between enhancement and *therapy*. This might seem to have some intuitive appeal, for example in relation to cosmetic surgery to repair burn damage as contrasted with interventions to make someone appear more beautiful. On closer inspection, however, this appears to be less helpful.

While it is likely that interventions deemed to count as enhancements 9.15
may be brought about by using techniques that originally have been developed for therapeutic ends, what counts as therapeutic is itself a subject of considerable controversy. In the early days of a medical innovation, for example, is it always clear whether trying it on a patient should count as therapeutic or experimental? It might be thought that intention is relevant to deciding this question, but it is not clear that therapeutic intention is a necessary condition of something counting as a therapeutic intervention. Experience with placebos shows the wide variety of types of intervention that can have therapeutic *effects*, even if not intended.

The Wellcome exhibition mentioned above did not represent an under- 9.16
standing of enhancement as going 'beyond therapy'. As the exhibition showed, some proposed modifications ('enhancements') to human anatomy were not successful and were rejected by their 'users' – notably prosthetic limbs for children born in the UK, as a result the thalidomide episode. These did not prove to be helpful to affected individuals, who preferred that society should accept them as they were, rather than offer uncomfortable means of adjustment, so presumably these interventions, whatever the intention, were neither therapeutic nor enhancing.

Another question concerns preventive interventions: can they be enhanc- 9.17
ing? An example might be a boost to the immune system to protect against infectious disease (Holm 1994). Is it possible, also, for a preventive intervention to be therapeutic? What might count as an example of such? Let us

consider, as a possible candidate, preventive mastectomy in the case of a woman with a strong family history of breast cancer (as in the case of **Angelina Jolie**[4] mentioned in Chapter 8) – what, if anything, makes this therapeutic? Since we can't be certain certain that a patient would have proceeded to develop breast cancer had she not had the preventive mastectomy, there are difficulties in saying that it is therapeutic in *that* sense although there might be therapeutic effects in terms of *reassurance*. (cf. Eisinger 2007). Arguably, however, the main aim is to reduce risk – so, in what sense is that different from the enhancing immune system change? And yet intuitively (and quite independently of any aesthetic considerations) it seems counterintuitive to speak of a mastectomy as an enhancement. It seems that in order to understand the answer to these queries, we need more substance to the concept of enhancement than simply the 'beyond therapy' criterion.

9.4.2 Species-Normal Functioning

9.18 **Norman Daniels (2000)**[5] introduces species-normal functioning as a way of distinguishing between therapy and enhancement, and this has the advantage that it can be used either in the individual or the species case. In the latter, if we have an account of species-typical normal functioning it is possible to assess individuals as to how far short they fall of that: we can have a measure, with regard to the species, of normal life expectancy, for example. In the individual case, if an intervention restores a person to species-typical normal functioning it falls within the 'therapy' category; otherwise it counts as an enhancement. In the preventive mastectomy case, the point would presumably be that the intervention restores the individual to the population level of risk (although that would not, of course, be zero risk).

9.4.2.1 Quantitative Account of Enhancement

9.19 An alternative way of understanding enhancement is quantitatively, as increasing or adding [to] a certain characteristic, possibly in intensity (e.g. in color) or degree, rather than in amount. This has been called the 'additionality view' (Chadwick 2008).

9.20   As noted in the **US President's Council Report**[6] (2003) *Beyond Therapy,* the Oxford English Dictionary definition gives a quantitative interpretation of enhancement – to enhance x is to add to, exaggerate, or increase x in some respect. On this criterion, to increase the range or degree of immune response would count as an enhancement. But how should a preventive mastectomy be assessed on such a view? Rather than an increase or an addition, it appears to be a (quantitative) *reduction* in at least two respects – both in the sense that a part of the body is removed, and in the sense that the risk of developing breast cancer is reduced. Any reduction in risk, however, is at the same time an *increase* in the probability of remaining free from disease.

What this example makes clear, again, is the importance of specificity as 9.21 to the *respect* in which x is enhanced. While it may make sense to speak of enhancing x with regard to characteristic y, it is not clear what might be meant by enhancing x *over all*. Indeed, to enhance x with respect to characteristic y may be at the expense of some other characteristic z. There are trade-offs to be had. So whether a characteristic specific enhancement is also an overall enhancement is a separate matter.

9.4.3 Enhancement: The Umbrella View

It might be argued that it is not possible to find a definition of 'enhancement' 9.22 that fits all cases that might attract the label 'enhancement'. The term is used to apply to a wide variety both of changes and techniques. Such interventions include lengthening the lifespan, making people taller, increasing cognitive powers or emotional sensibilities, and facilitating greater sporting prowess, among others. In addition, techniques of 'enhancement' could include cosmetic, genetic, pharmaceutical, and prosthetic. This way of looking at the issue allows for the fact that some 'enhancements' may also be therapeutic; that they need not add anything (they can involve reduction); they may not constitute an improvement. Specific interventions would have to be assessed on a case by case basis – rather than a judgment on the acceptability or desirability of human enhancement overall.

The advantages of this approach would be that it would then be possible 9.23 to avoid the difficult issues of disagreement when some individuals wish to make changes to themselves that they regard as enhancements, but which seem to observers to be damaging (e.g. elective amputation). Whether or not it was an 'enhancement' would not be the issue; the specifics of the case would have to be considered in making an assessment. The disadvantage, however, is that there are debates to be had about whether the pursuit of enhancement, *per se,* is part of human nature. It seems that what is needed is a sense of enhancement which enables us to discuss this issue, while at the same time there is some truth in the view that particular interventions should be assessed on a case by case basis. The latter requirement suggests a sense of enhancement is needed which does not prejudge the issue of acceptability and desirability. With this in mind the 'improvement' view is not helpful. The sense of enhancement to be preferred, we suggest, is the additionality view, where an enhancement is an addition or exaggeration of a characteristic which may or may not constitute an improvement.

9.24   The fact that it is necessary to be able to deal with the possible counter-example that some individuals regard the removal of a limb as an enhancement makes it even clearer that attention has to be given to the respect in which there is a claimed enhancement. If there is *no* respect in which something is added or exaggerated, then such an intervention would not count as an enhancement *on this definition*.

9.5 Ethical Issues

9.25 A major reason why there has been so much discussion about the distinction between therapy and enhancement has been for the purposes of drawing lines over what is acceptable and what is not. For consequentialists, of course, the distinction is irrelevant, because it is outcomes that are important, however the interventions are categorized. Daniels, however, has suggested that the distinction has served as a 'moral warning flag' (Daniels 2000). So, we have been warned that there are ethical issues to discuss, let's look at some of the arguments.

9.5.1 Is Enhancement Necessary?

9.26 Some might argue, in the light of climate change and other threats to the human condition, that it is necessary to consider making deliberate changes to humans in order to ensure that the species has a future, so necessary that it is a moral obligation. John Harris has suggested that the human species may not have much time to spare before planning its own biological future. He writes:

> The problem is that progress via Darwinian evolution is extremely slow, and the direction unpredictable; all we know is that it will facilitate gene survival. It is probable that, in the interests of human survival and certainly those of human welfare and well-being, we may simply not be able to wait. For example, we will need to accelerate the development of better resistance to bacteria, disease, viruses, or hostile environments or of the technologies that will be eventually necessary to find, and travel to, habitats alternative to the earth.
>
> (Harris 2016)

These ideas have a longer history than you might expect. The science fiction 9.27
writer Olaf Stapledon, in *Last and First Men* (1930), wrote in a very prescient
way about genetic engineering as a step to try to ensure the future of humans.
Such debates today also have to deal with predictions that robots will, in the
not too distant future, outperform humans to such an extent that humans will
become at best second-class beings if we sit back and let it happen. There are
also arguments to suggest that it is a matter of urgency to enhance humans
morally, which we will examine towards the end of the chapter.

9.5.2 Enhancement is Inevitable

Even if not necessary, enhancement might be inevitable. Francoise Baylis 9.28
and Jason Scott Robert (2004) have argued that it is, and that this sets limits
to the range of useful questions that can be asked. The inevitability thesis is
a frequent guest at the feast when new technological possibilities are on the
table. While it might appear that a simplistic technological imperative is
implausible, and uninteresting if it simply means that someone somewhere will try it sometime, there are important questions concerning
what is considered to be inevitable and why. Robert Sparrow, for example,
in relation to nanotechnology, identifies three different strands of thought
about inevitability, tracing inevitability to techno-optimism – development
is self-evidently good; to an empirical claim about the impossibility of
regulation; or to a resigned techno-pessimism based on contingent political
circumstances, whereby regulation would in principle be possible but in
fact is not. The first of these, Sparrow argues, may, in turn, depend on an
innate human drive (Sparrow 2007).

Baylis and Robert do in fact posit a 'biosocial drive to pursue perfection' 9.29
as an essential characteristic of humanness. They do not put the purported
inevitability down to a science-friendly social and political context, or to a
kind of empirical slippery slope. They further suggest that the inevitability
thesis is a key step in the ethical debate:

> We maintain that accepting the inevitability of genetic enhancement tech-
> nologies is an important and necessary step forward in the ethical debate
> about the development and use of such technologies
>
> (Baylis and Robert, 2004, 25).

Keep in mind the 'drive to perfection' argument as an important influence 9.30
on the debate, which pushes towards an understanding of enhancement in

terms of improvement. Indeed, this is the account supported by Baylis and Robert, who by genetic enhancement technology understand 'any technology that directly alters the expression of genes that are already present in humans, or that involves the addition of genes that have not previously appeared ...for the purpose of human physical, intellectual, psychological, or moral improvement' (ibid). Although the 'drive to perfection' argument plays a significant role in the debate, it is not supported by all pro-enhancers (see for example, Harris 2007).

9.31   In assessing the extent to which enhancement is morally acceptable and/ or desirable, it is important, as already indicated above, to distinguish different levels at which enhancement can take place. First, there is individual enhancement: individuals may seek out ways of enhancing particular characteristics, by any number of means – not only genetic but also dietary, surgical, through exercise or interventions emanating from new technologies. At the other end of the spectrum, as already discussed, there are issues about the enhancement of the human species – introducing into the species characteristics that have not hitherto been available to individual would-be self-enhancers. In between here are enhancement questions that are specific to particular areas of life or practices, such as sport. A cross-cutting theme running through all these is the issue of the extent to which it is appropriate to use medical resources for these purposes.

9.5.3 A Compromise Position?

9.32 Human enhancement, especially when it involves modification of the human germline, is a topic that gives rise to both strong support and strong opposition. In the context of gene editing, Maria Sulekova and Kevin Fitzgerald (2019) have argued for a new approach that takes us beyond the dichotomy between what they call enthusiasm-based (as in the case of Harris) and caution-based perspectives. Drawing on the work of Teilhard de Chardin, they suggest that a philosophy of moving towards complexity such as he argued for can appeal to both camps. On the one hand he allows for the ethical use of technology to advance humanity beyond the limitations of natural biology, but in a way that differs from the concerns of the transhumanists who seek the perfection of individual humans. The ethical use of technology requires responsibility and a concern for the common good, to enhance the unity of humankind, whilst at the same time respecting diversity. They sum up de Chardin's position in the following: 'Human beings should make every effort to create a higher form of life represented by a more unified humanity instead of just surviving' (Sulekova and Fitzgerald 2019). Evolution is no longer about where we have come from but where we are heading, but it is important to have a clear understanding of the processes of biological stability before proceeding with gene editing interventions. Interesting though this suggestion is, one possible problem with proposing an approach that may appeal to both camps is that both may also dislike it because it concedes too much to the other side. So, let's consider some more of the competing arguments that are advanced in the debate.

9.5.4 Autonomy

If individuals wish to avail themselves of enhancing interventions, then the 9.33
argument from autonomy suggests that, other things being equal, that is morally acceptable. More difficult issues arise where other things are *not* equal, either because their choice has adverse consequences for others, or in cases where individuals are choosing not for themselves but for others, e.g., children. There is also an argument that goes beyond the mere absence of consent, from Jurgen Habermas, to which we now turn.

9.5.5 The Habermasian Concern

Jurgen Habermas has argued that it is incompatible with the autonomy of a 9.34
human being that a decision about its make up should be taken by a third party (Habermas 2003). This makes the very nature of that human being something that is created by another. Genetic alteration (as well as genetic selection) implies a new form of control over humans which needs to be resisted. This is what he calls the argument against alien determination. Such arguments conclude that enhancement (including genetic modification of the germline in general) is morally wrong in itself. There is a line of thought that human dignity is undermined by being designed by another (see, for example, Fukuyama 2003). On the other hand, as we have seen in the argument about necessity above, there are arguments for a moral obligation to enhance. Be mindful also, in the context of dignity related arguments, of what was said about conceptual problems with 'human dignity' in Chapter 3.

It has frequently been argued throughout the history of debates about 9.35
genetic intervention that we seek to mold and change people by social influences such as education all the time, without regarding this as problematic, so why should changing them by genetics be problematic

(especially if this is to cure disease – changing other characteristics might raise other issues, to which we shall return later)? Habermas explicitly rejects this analogy between socialization and genetic modification, saying that adolescents, for example, can respond to and reject socialization, but not to genetic modification. The genetic modifier is a producer or a 'bricoleur'. However, there is a view that to object to changing people by biological interventions but not to doing it by social policy amounts to an unjustifiable 'biological exceptionalism' (Cohen in Sparrow and Cohen 2015).

9.36   According to Habermas the knowledge that we have been determined from the outside results in a change in the ethical self-understanding of the species. As Daniel Henrich has argued (2011), however, this claim is open to a weak or a strong interpretation. According to a weak interpretation, it will be a matter of empirical fact that some individuals will experience challenges to their notion of autonomy, but others may not. According to a strong interpretation human autonomy as a whole, and human morality, comes into question. In that case, however, in order for us to be swayed by the argument, we need to be given a good reason as to why this should matter.

9.6 Social Inequalities and Social Justice

9.37 It might be argued that enhancement could be a means of redress for certain existing social inequalities. Let us consider an example. If it is the case that taller people have certain social advantages, making people of below average height taller may help them to access social goods. In fact, earlier in this century there were reports of **leg lengthening surgery in China**[7], which later moved to ban it.

9.38   Against this, first, there is the obvious point that any apparent advantages may depend on the fact that not everyone can access them. Second, to go down this route may reinforce the social conditions that create certain inequalities in the first place. And third, depending on how enhancement interventions are distributed and accessed, social inequalities might be widened rather than narrowed, if, for example, those at the higher end of a given spectrum wish to increase the advantage they already have (not necessarily in the case of tallness of course). It will always be the case that some people will be better able to access technologies that will give their offspring an advantage in society over those who do not have access to such resources. Those technologies that will involve the use of artificial reproductive technologies combined with genetic modification are likely to be an expensive and scarce social resource, for which only some people will be able to pay privately. There is a risk of creating a society in the future in which people are divided into groups of those who have been enhanced and those who have not, facilitating new forms of discrimination (for a discussion of justice and discrimination see Chapter 12).

9.6.1 Consequences for the Future of Humans

Robert Sparrow has argued that the debate about the use of genome editing is 'nothing less than a debate about what it will mean to be human in the future' (Sparrow, in Sparrow and Cohen 2015). He has also written of the risk of obsolescence of certain enhancements as circumstances change. Speaking in particular of enhancement produced by genetic modification, he writes: 9.39

> If the genetic enhancements granted to children get better and better each year, then the enhancements granted to children born in any given year will rapidly go out of date. Sooner or later, every modified child will find themselves to be 'yesterday's child'.
>
> (Sparrow, 2015; see also Sparrow 2019).

This turns on its head the social justice argument about a possible future where the societies are divided into the enhanced and the unenhanced, where it is presumed the former will have an advantage. 9.40

John Harris (2012) draws a distinction between those human ills we have an obligation to do something about by enhancement, and those we have not. You might want to think of examples. Is there, for example, an obligation to make people more attractive if they wish it, in order to improve their quality of life? An argument that relies on relief of the harms of disease and death might appear to reduce enhancement in effect to therapeutic aims, which is an interesting reversal of the attempt to define enhancement by distinguishing it from therapy. 9.41

In trying to assess whether the consequences of an enhancement might be an improvement overall for the human condition, how are we to assess that? How is it possible to set criteria for what enhancements will count as an improvement or not without any agreement as to ends or purposes? One option is to leave it to individual choice, but given the issues about inequalities and access, apart from any other considerations, it seems that more is needed to guide decision-making. Nicholas Agar has written extensively on 9.42

the issue of human enhancement and has argued that it is important to take the *degree* of enhancement into account in considering its acceptability (see e.g., Agar 2010, 2013). He has argued for moderate rather than what he calls radical enhancement. Radical enhancement involves changing humans in ways that greatly exceed what is currently possible for them. You might want to think about whether and in what ways the degree of change makes a difference to Sparrow's concern about obsolescence. You may recall, also, the 'pathways to translation' of Singer and Savulescu discussed in the previous chapter as an example of a gradualist approach to introducing editing the germline. In thinking about the deliberate planning of human modification it may be instructive also to compare debates about gene editing in animal species, where gene editing could help, for example, small-holder farmers in Africa by editing animals to be resistant to heat. Some have expressed the view that this should not be an excuse for keeping animals in over-crowded conditions and have stated a **preference for traditional breeding**[8] practices over the use of an invasive technology. The general point here is, should less invasive approaches be the method of first choice?

9.43   A contemporary example of change in human abilities and experience is communication, as social media change the ways in which we communicate both in interpersonal relationships and in the political and commercial arenas. Kevin Warwick has argued that normal human communication abilities are 'so poor as to be embarrassing, particularly in terms of speed, power and precision' (Warwick 2010), and has advocated an implant enabling direct communication between nervous systems. But what happens if people want to be disconnected? The long-term effects on relationships between individuals are impossible to predict, but it is certainly far from obvious that immediacy of communication is a benefit in general, rather than in specific circumstances.

9.44   The issues may become clearer by looking at another area of life – for example, the context of sport, which is one of the contexts in which much has been written about enhancement. **Aristotle**[9], of course, in his *Nicomachean Ethics*[10], pointed out that the diet that is appropriate for an athlete is different from what would be suitable for other people:

> If ten pounds are too much for a particular person to eat and two too little, it does not follow that the trainer will order six pounds, for this is perhaps too much for the person who is to take it, or too little – too little for Milo, too much for the beginner in athletic exercises. The same is true of running and wrestling
>
> (Aristotle 1908, 1106a17).

The relevant *ends* in question are different. There is an issue not only 9.45 about the ends of the individual but also about the point of sport in general (which affects, for example, the issues about the use of performance-enhancing drugs). For the individual there might be different purposes involved in maximizing performance – winning is an obvious possibility (which might be a means to other ends such as earning more money), but there are also others, such as pushing oneself to one's limits. When we talk about sport in general, however, there are further questions to answer. *Is* the point of sport primarily competition and winning? What about other elements, such as providing an opportunity for exercise of certain virtues (which will be different according to whether or not team-playing is involved); physical exercise; development of human potential; entertainment and so on (see Miah 2004). The point is that whether or not enhancement will count as an improvement is, first, relevant to the context of sport, and second, to the purposes for which sport is engaged in, both on an individual and a species-level. We might not agree on the good that is internal to the practice of sport, but at least it seems possible to understand the kinds of considerations that are involved in different models of sport.

When discussion turns to improving humans overall, however, it is a 9.46 much more difficult issue, because it is not clear where to begin in looking for relevant purposes. An attempt to appeal to a concept of human nature can also lead in different directions. From a conservative point of view, trying to enhance human beings as such might be regarded as an unacceptable tampering with human nature and inconsistent with human dignity, as opposed to a liberal view supportive of the freedom to enhance.

We will now turn to discussing moral and cognitive enhancement.   9.47

9.7 Moral Enhancement

Why should we think there is a need or obligation to enhance human beings 9.48 *morally*? Well, it is established practice to try to educate children morally, to enable them to participate fully in society. This involves bringing them to understand the difference between right and wrong and to appreciate the feelings of other people and take them into account.

What is understood by moral enhancement, however, goes beyond moral 9.49 education and could involve intervening at the biological level to bring about an enhancement. But what exactly is it envisaged would be enhanced? This raises questions about the very nature of morality itself. From one point of view it might seem that the target would be their sensibilities – for example, an increase in their ability to feel empathy. From another point of view, what is important is not the degree of empathy that is important but their ability to reason about right and wrong and what to do. This distinction mirrors the long-standing debate in ethics about whether reason or feelings should dominate in ethics. As you might recall from our discussion in Chapter 1, the question 'Why should I be moral?' has long been debated in philosophy. Why should I care about the interests of other people unless it is in my own interests, in which case I am arguably not doing it for moral reasons? David **Hume**[11] said that "reason is, and ought to be, the slave of the passions", so it looks as if unless I want to, there is no reason to be moral. Have a look at what Hume said in Section IX, Part II of his ***Enquiry Concerning the Principles of Morals***[12] (1912 reprint of 1777 edition). When we turn to **Kant**[13], reason, which enables an autonomous being to appreciate the moral law, is paramount. For him two things gave rise to awe: the starry heavens above and the moral law within. So, these two traditions in moral theory give rise to very different understandings of what we might need to enhance, for moral enhancement purposes.

9.50   Another possibility that might be canvassed is enhancing strength of will. Although weakness of will constituted a puzzle for **Plato**[14] among others, we are all aware of situations in which we know what we ought to do but do not do it. If we were able to find a control mechanism for strength of will perhaps that is what should be aimed at in moral enhancement? On the other hand, it might be helpful also for those hesitating about doing something likely to cause great harm.

9.51   Let us put this issue aside for a moment and ask why it is argued that it should be considered important to undertake moral enhancement. It has been argued that it is important because in today's world there are unprecedented opportunities for doing not only immense harm but 'ultimate harm' (Persson and Savulescu 2008). Technologies exist that could wipe the human species off the planet.

9.52   There are, however, several practical problems as well as principled objections to the idea of moral enhancement as a response to this situation. First, it only takes one person to press a nuclear button. How could we be sure we had enough coverage to bring about the required change? (see Harris 2012).

9.53   Second, there is a difference between making the average person have a greater moral sensibility and dealing with those who are 'amoral'. The phenomenon of the psychopath, the characteristic of whom is to be lacking empathy while having full intellectual comprehension of the wrongness of their actions, offers a problem. A considerable amount of research has been done into psychopaths and exactly what is the cause of their condition. If we were able to identify a switch in the brain, that could be flipped, would that not be a good thing? An immediate problem that arises is that a psychopath would be unlikely to consent to such an intervention. Psychopaths are typically not unhappy to be the way they are. It would seem strange, on the face of it, to go against established principles of informed consent in order to bring about moral enhancement. And who is to be the arbiter in this? Governments hardly have a monopoly on knowing what is morally acceptable and desirable.

This also raises the question of the *means* of moral bioenhancement in this area. Possibilities might include drugs or brain surgery, or the use of gene editing techniques for moral enhancement. Suppose there was a variant that is shown to correlate with moral sensibility and that this could be routinely inserted into embryos to produce moral people. Would that be a good idea? There is again the obvious practical problem that in the interim period not everyone would be so treated. 9.54

Arguably the only acceptable intervention that would involve universal application would be to put a morally enhancing drug in the drinking water, analogous to using fluoride in the drinking water to prevent tooth decay. Could there be a case for this if it was included in a political manifesto which received the assent of the electorate? 9.55

With any form of enhancement it is necessary to think about the potential downsides and side effects. **Michael Innes'**[15] novel *Operation Pax* (1951) portrays an attempt to make the population more peace loving, but has the undesired consequence that people lose their 'get up and go'. Analogously, it has been argued that people with some degree of psychopathic tendencies may be very successful in certain careers and thus maybe needed in society. It might be counterproductive to eliminate all psychopathic tendencies. 9.56

Another problem is, if we tried to increase empathy, how would we know how much is enough? There is research to show that an excess of empathy can be damaging, leading to burnout, for example, in the caring professions, where a certain emotional distance may be required as a coping mechanism (see Young, 2016). 9.57

Trying to change morality through reasoning power might be even more complicated. Psychopaths may be highly intelligent people who can reason very well. As Aristotle pointed out in the *Nicomachean Ethics*, cleverness can be combined with evil ends; what is needed is practical wisdom, which 9.58

involves thinking and feeling in the right way about the right object. It is difficult, to say the least, to see how this could be brought about by moral bioenhancement.

9.59   But suppose it were possible to intervene in a person's reasoning powers so that they think in a way that is regarded as more 'moral'. An obvious problem that then arises is that of free will. If we cannot avoid coming to certain conclusions because of the ways in which we are manipulated then is this any better than the kind of brainwashing that is objected to when it is used to train terrorists? Of course, there are problems with the very possibility of free will in any case, but if we are manipulated to think in a certain way, it certainly looks as if we would be less able to act freely than if we were not. Against this, it might be argued, what is the difference between moral education, which is widely accepted and practiced, and brainwashing? Where is the line drawn?

9.60   We may conclude that there are problems with the idea of moral enhancement, first because the people who need it most would be unlikely to consent to it. Some have considered the possibility of incentive-based schemes (Rakić 2014; Carter 2015), but the more intractable problem is disagreement about the nature of what it means to be moral.

9.8 Cognitive Enhancement

9.61   When we turn to cognitive enhancement, we have already seen that under some interpretations, moral enhancement might also require cognitive enhancement, where moral enhancement is deemed to involve rational thought. However, it should not be forgotten that cognitive enhancement might also be thought to require moral enhancement (see Persson and Savulescu 2008).

9.62   Beyond that, it might be argued that cognitive reasoning powers are what make us distinctively human, and that it is beneficial to people to have greater cognitive powers – they are likely to have more successful and lucrative careers, although possibly not quite so lucrative as top sportspeople or certain artists working in the entertainment industry. It is also good for society in general that there are people around with high cognitive powers to invent new technologies and so on. Techniques of cognitive enhancement discussed in the literature include cognitive enhancing drugs, brain implants and gene editing. Some of these are already in use. Others may be employed at a future date.

But we are going too fast. What exactly are we assuming could or would 9.63
be enhanced? **IQ**[16] has long been a favorite with eugenicists and could be a
contender for the proposed target of enhancement, and yet this is arguably
one of the most controversial and difficult indicators to make the object of
social policy. There is interest in enhancing abilities to focus and concen-
trate, particularly for those involved in academic work. There is some evidence to support the view that interventions are available that could enable
people to have greater powers of memory (Hamzelou 2017), and this may
be helpful to those suffering from Alzheimer's in particular, but is this true
in life generally? Selective memory may be an evolutionarily advantageous
way of protecting ourselves.

Having regard to the ethical considerations listed earlier in the chapter, it 9.64
might be argued that if individuals wish to enhance their cognitive powers, e.g.
by taking cognitive enhancing drugs, then they should be free to do so, other
things being equal. More problematic are proposals for intervening at population level. Bearing in mind the distinction between enhancement and improvement made earlier in this chapter, would it be an improvement if it were
possible, in principle, to enhance the level of IQ in a population, for example
by increasing the proportion of highly gifted individuals? Jenny Krutzinna has
argued that it is essential to consider empirical evidence: in this case we need
to have regard to the experience of highly gifted children who already exist
(Krutzinna 2016). Do they have better lives than those less gifted? There is
evidence to suggest that they may suffer above average degrees of loneliness
and unhappiness, even bullying. There are issues about whether it would be
right to use technology to enhance the already gifted to super intelligent levels
or whether to focus attention only on those who are held to be below average.
This directs our attention, again, to effects on social inequalities.

There is a long tradition that the point of morality is to respond to certain 9.65
features of the human condition: limitations in resources, limitations in
knowledge, limitations in sympathies and limitations in wisdom (Warnock
1971). Addressing the first of these is subject to external conditions, but the
associated problems can be ameliorated by the application of principles of
fair resource allocation. Other moral principles help us to overcome limitations in sympathies, by drawing our attention to the nature, needs and
interests of other human beings. Limitations in sympathies, knowledge
and wisdom, however, are internal to humans – so might not human
enhancement be a good thing?

This chapter has discussed arguments for the view that attention has 9.66
to be paid to the specific interventions and purposes at issue rather than

making it true by definition that an enhancement is a good. In assessing these from a moral point of view ethical considerations include the freedom of individuals to choose enhancing interventions when no harm is done to others. Interventions at population level, however, are more complicated. Even in a social context that purports to support the importance of individual choice it will be important to assess the ways in which choice will in fact be affected by an enhancement. The communication example above suggests that it may in fact be restrictive of the choice *not* to be permanently connected. The issue has to be considered both with regard to the choices of individuals directly enhanced, and the wider implications for individual and group choices. It is also necessary to consider the impact on social inequalities at the very least. Others would go further: on the one hand some seek to rule out deliberate human design as incompatible with their understanding of human dignity, and on the other some argue that it is part of human nature to seek to enhance ourselves and even a moral obligation in the light of the challenges we face as a species.

Questions

Do you think there are cogent arguments for enhancing the human species to help it to survive? If so, what are they?

Thinking of different types of enhancements, for example those which have been discussed in this chapter, are there any you would want to rule out? If so, why?

Website Links

1   https://wellcome.ac.uk/
2   https://www.reuters.com/article/us-japan-robotic-tail-idUSKCN1V411X/
3   https://www.paralympic.org/london-2012
4   https://www.medicinenet.com/angelina_jolie_mastectomy/views.htm
5   https://www.hsph.harvard.edu/norman-daniels/
6   https://biotech.law.lsu.edu/research/pbc/reports/beyondtherapy/fulldoc.html
7   https://www.theguardian.com/world/2003/dec/15/gender.uk/
8   https://www.bbc.co.uk/news/science-environment-47197896/
9   https://plato.stanford.edu/entries/aristotle/
10   http://classics.mit.edu/Aristotle/nicomachaen.1.i.html
11   https://plato.stanford.edu/entries/hume/

12   https://www.gutenberg.org/files/4320/4320-h/4320-h.htm#2H_PART92/
13   https://plato.stanford.edu/entries/kant/
14   https://plato.stanford.edu/entries/plato/
15   http://authorscalendar.info/minnes.htm
16   https://ghr.nlm.nih.gov/primer/traits/intelligence

10

MENTAL HEALTH

In this chapter we shall address the issues surrounding mental health: 10.1
first, the nature of mental illness and then the ethical issues surrounding
detention and treatment. Mental health as an issue is increasingly moving
center stage: you may be surprised by the statistics about the proportion of
adults on anti-depressant medication alone. If you watch Jack Nicholson in
the 1975 film *One Flew Over the Cuckoo's Nest*[1] it is not unreasonable to
feel alarmed about treatment of mental health conditions, with its depiction
of the treatments being used as mechanisms of control. Much has changed,
however, in mental health. Developments in medications and talking
therapies, together with a move to decrease the use of detention in mental
hospitals, have led to considerable advances. There remain ethical issues,
however, concerning the differences in treatment of physical illness and
mental disorders. First it may be helpful to look at the context of the
discussion. Mental health is one of the most challenging areas in health care
and one which has had something of a Cinderella status. Although mental
health issues are very prevalent, the status and funding accorded to mental
health care has historically not matched that given to physical illness. And
yet data from the **World Health Organization**[2] identify neuropsychiatric
disorders as the third leading cause of **disability-adjusted life years**[3]
(WHO 2014).

People with severe mental health issues also have higher rates of physical 10.2
illness (De Hert et al. 2011). In the United Kingdom members of the royal
family have done much to draw attention to this subject, including talking
about their own difficulties with mental health issues.

10.3   The principles most commonly appealed to in discussions of the ethics of mental health include autonomy and best interests. Justice is also important in so far as there are issues about persons with mental disorders being treated differently (and worse) than persons suffering from physical illness. Feminist bioethics has something to say about the ways in which mental health diagnoses have been used, historically, to control women's behavior.

10.4   When we give consideration to ethical approaches other than the principle based ones, Jennifer Radden and John Sadler have argued that virtue ethics may be particularly appropriate in a mental health setting. They are not suggesting that this is an alternative to principles: indeed, they rightly claim that virtue approaches can be accommodated in principle based ones and with role morality. They argue that '...within a professional setting that involves role-specific duties, any trait that is conducive to the goal or good of that practice – here health and healing – *acquires the status* of a moral virtue' (their emphasis) (Radden and Sadler 2013, 66–67). In mental health care, they suggest, empathy and trust are particularly important, so cultivating trustworthiness and imagination is desirable. Radden and Sadler also emphasize Aristotle's virtue of *phronesis*, or practical wisdom, which they define as, 'the set of capabilities that allow us to deliberate about things with ends or goals in mind, and to discern and enact right action, thus acknowledging the complexities involved in practical realities' (Radden and Sadler 2013, 67). These complexities frequently require sound judgment about the best course of action, including determining the least restrictive option (see below).

10.5   In the case of mental health, moreover, the law has taken an increasingly active role, as issues concerning deprivation of liberty may be involved. It is not surprising that this has led to the prominence of a principle based rather than a virtue ethics approach, the latter being difficult to incorporate in legislation. One point about terminology before we proceed further: those in receipt of treatment or detained in a mental health facility will be described as 'service users' in this chapter.

10.1 Mental Illness

10.6 Let's start with trying to get a sense of what mental illness is. Debate about the meaning of mental illness has a long history. Some commentators, labeled the 'anti-psychiatry' movement, have argued that there is no such thing. **Thomas Szasz**[4] in his 1961 book *The Myth of Mental Illness* (although he did not himself adopt the term 'anti-psychiatry' to describe his views) argued that the concept of illness applies, strictly speaking, to abnormalities of the body. The brain, as an organ of the body, can of course be diseased, but to say the *mind* is diseased is true only in a metaphorical sense. We use the language of mental illness to talk about behavior of which we disapprove or which does not accord with societal expectations. Szasz also criticized some of the practices of psychiatry such as detention, as well as the concept of mental illness itself.

Psychiatric labels have been used at different historical periods to control 10.7
dissidents in certain countries. You might want to have a look at the online account of the political abuse of psychiatry by **Robert van Noren**[5], (2012) who describes how there was a certain logic in the idea that people must be mentally ill if they opposed the best political system available. **Andrei Snezhnevsky**[6] developed the concept of **'sluggish schizophrenia'**[7] to describe such cases.

The work of Szasz was important in drawing attention to the ways in 10.8
which psychiatric diagnosis can be and has been used as an instrument of control, as has the concept of 'normality' (Chadwick 2016). The **Diagnostic and Statistical Manual**[8] (DSM) published by the **American Psychiatric Association**[9] (2013) has been very influential and it is often noted that homosexuality was classified in the DSM as a mental illness until the relatively recent past. It was only removed from the second edition of the DSM in 1973. Ronald Bayer describes how psychiatrists removed homosexuality as a mental illness from the DSM after bitter political battles with gay activists and after having to concede that homosexual people are no less well adapted and healthy than comparable heterosexual people (Bayer 1987). This came a good 100 years after a German psychiatrist, **Richard von Krafft-Ebing**[10] invented homosexuality as a mental illness, with the implicit objective to protect homosexual Germans from police prosecution at the time. His thinking, essentially, was that if German authorities accepted that homosexuality is a mental illness, a desirable consequence would surely be a more empathetic approach to homosexual people, less prosecution, and the like. It turns out that Krafft-Ebing only succeeded in pathologizing homosexuality and opening up to a century worth of often unethical research aimed at treating homosexual people so that they would become heterosexual. Some of that research involved hormonal treatment as well as varied attempts at brain surgery, leaving perfectly healthy homosexuals severely brain damaged for the remainder of their lives.

In the fifth edition – **DSM-5**[11], the so-called **'bereavement exclusion'**[12] 10.9
was removed from diagnoses of major depression, in response to the criticism that this would medicalize ordinary grief of those depressed following a bereavement (see Pies 2014). Although Szasz had a considerable

influence on the practice of psychiatry, several writers who might be described as 'pro-psychiatry' have tried to give accounts of mental illness which explain it as a real phenomenon which goes beyond problems of living. For example, drawing a distinction between illness and disease, explaining disease in terms of dysfunction, can apply in both mental and physical realms. Illness on the other hand referred to the person's experience of the disease. Chris Megone gave an account of illness as the 'incapacitating failure of bodily or mental capacities to fulfil their functions' (Megone 2000). Fulford, on the other hand, explained mental illness in terms of 'action failure' (Fulford 1987). The point is that all these accounts are trying to explain mental illness as something real, but not reducing it to a physical lesion (which could amount to agreeing with Szasz that for an illness to be a genuine illness it must have a physical cause, and then it becomes properly classified as a physical rather than mental illness).

10.10   The organization **Mind**[13] in the UK starts from trying to give an account of mental health: 'Good mental health means being generally able to think, feel and react in ways that you need and want to live your life. But if you go through a period of poor mental health you might find the ways you're frequently thinking, feeling or reacting become difficult, or even impossible, to cope with' (Mind 2017).

10.11   It might be argued that to try to portray mental illness as a myth risks leaving people in real distress and without help that they need. Szasz, however, did not deny that the phenomena of individuals with real problems needed addressing. The question is, how should these problems be classified? Although there may be few who would take a position as hard as Szasz on this question of classification, there remain disputes over particular conditions. Debate about specific disorders can be as contested as that over the concept of mental illness in general. There is some consensus over common problems such as depression and anxiety and less common ones such as schizophrenia and bipolar disorder, but there are disputes at the margins such as the classification of post-traumatic stress disorder (**PTSD**[14]). There are also issues about the borderline between treatable mental health conditions on the one hand and personality disorders, on the other.

10.2 Diagnosis

10.12   The issue of classification matters ethically because of the social and practical implications of a diagnosis for those diagnosed. In addition to the political abuse of psychiatry that has already been noted, there are ongoing issues about the stigma that can attach to mental illness, despite the facts that increasingly there are campaigns against this and that some extremely famous celebrities, artists and historically influential people have experienced it (for example, **Winston Churchill**[15] and **Samuel Johnson**[16] are both said to have suffered from depression). There are ongoing issues, however, concerning the ways in which some groups in society are more likely to be diagnosed as suffering from a mental disorder, possibly reflecting prevailing power differentials. Those in a position of relative power may have greater license to determine the standard of 'normality' so that behavior that is regarded as deviating from the normal in some way may be pathologized.

Women have historically been more likely than men to be diagnosed, 10.13 and questions can also be asked about the distribution of diagnosis according to class and ethnicity. Clearly in some cases there are good reasons why women are more likely to be diagnosed, such as **post-natal depression**[17] for example, but against this it might be argued, as it has been by feminist bioethicists, that the very condition of post-natal depression can result from social factors surrounding the process and expectations of childbirth and women's role. Similarly, historically diagnosis has been used as a means of control of women's sexual behavior.

The social disadvantage experienced by a given less powerful group in 10.14 society may itself be a factor contributing to illness; different groups may be more or less likely to seek medical help. Different causal factors may also be at work in specific contexts. The presence of facilities is another very significant factor influencing diagnosis. A service needs to exist in order to have patients, and where there is underfunding in a particular area, fewer patients are likely to be diagnosed and treated.

The **United Nations'** *Principles Regarding the Protection of Persons* 10.15 *with Mental Illness and the Improvement of Mental Health Care*[18] state that a 'determination of mental illness shall never be made on the basis of political, economic or social status, or membership of a cultural, racial or religious group, or for any other reason not directly related to mental health state.' The stigma that attaches to a diagnosis may arise from the fact that it is harder for someone who is not a service user to understand what it is like to suffer from a mental disorder, than it is to empathize with someone suffering from a physical disorder, at least in some cases. A phenomenon such as 'thought insertion', for example, where an individual experiences having the thoughts of someone else, is difficult to make sense of (cf. Chadwick 1994). As Kathleen Wilkes said, it is 'difficult if not impossible to see the world through the mind of the schizophrenic' (Wilkes 1988, p. 90), but 'the mentally ill ... are, since they belong to the same species, as like us [i.e. non-service users] as it is possible to be' (ibid., p. 98). In the case of depression, since we all experience some degree of feeling unhappy or depressed, it might be thought that it is easier to empathize, but for someone who has experienced only normal unhappiness it may be difficult to understand the kind of depression that leaves the sufferer unable to get out of bed, or depression that is 'treatment resistant'. Wilkes also suggested that we may be distinctive as a species in our capacity for mental illness, but there is evidence to suggest that other species – **horses**[19] for example – suffer from depression.

10.3 Autonomy and Capacity

10.16   When we turn to ethical issues of treatment, there is an immediate concern relating to the difference between physical and mental ill health. Whereas in the case of physical illness, in relation to adults at least, there is a starting assumption that individuals are free to exercise their autonomous choice to accept or refuse treatment, in the case of a user of mental health services the extent to which they have the capacity to make such an autonomous choice may be precisely what is in question. In some legal systems, at least, the law allows treatment to be given to an adult without consent if the adult lacks capacity to give that consent.

10.17   Two important points need to be noted from the start. The first is that the test of capacity is a legal test in various jurisdictions and medical practice must follow this legal test. Nevertheless, there are a number of philosophical and ethical principles which inform the legal test in question. The second point is that a determination of capacity is not a once and for all test, and not one with 'global' application: it relates to the ability to make a particular decision at a particular time. The capacity of an individual with a condition such as dementia, for example, is likely to fluctuate. Individuals should therefore be supported in making and communicating decisions, as far as possible. The fact that someone's decision appears *unwise* or *irrational* to onlookers is not sufficient to prove lack of capacity: individuals have the right to make bad decisions and we all do from time to time, especially when in situations of great distress or extreme tiredness, jet-lagged and so on.

10.18   We start, then, from the presumption that an adult is capable of making a decision about their interests unless proved otherwise. This is in accordance with the principle of autonomy. The lack of this capacity, prompting the diagnosis of a mental disorder, is the starting point for considering interventions of different kinds, treatment and detention. It is of course the case that mental health service users with capacity may consent to treatment, and this situation is not generally thought to give rise to challenging ethical issues. Difficulties arise when the service user refuses treatment. The 'threat' of legal powers being invoked must not be used to coerce consent (Mind 2017), but nevertheless the power to treat without consent, where lack of capacity has been determined, is something that service users should be aware of.

Nick Eastman has argued, appealing to the principle of reciprocity, that 10.19 the purpose of law in this area should be to ensure that where liberties are taken away, something is given in return, and this should include adequate treatment: 'civil liberties may not be removed for the purposes of treatment if resources for that treatment are inadequate' (Eastman 1994). The UN Convention on the Rights of Persons with Disabilities (2006) offers a challenge in this area. In Article 12 it provides that 'States Parties shall recognize that persons with disabilities enjoy legal capacity on an equal basis with others in all aspects of life.' Matthé Scholten and Jakov Gather have argued that this could have adverse consequences if applied in the mental health area:

> Consider a person who suffers from a severe psychotic episode. In many such cases, there is little reason to think that unreservedly respecting the person's current treatment choices will protect or further her interest in either autonomy or well-being.
>
> (Scholten and Gather 2018)

Temporary lack of capacity to make a decision may arise from causes 10.20 other than mental disorder. Alec Buchanan considered the following counter-argument to making the removal of liberty depend on the presence of mental disorder: 'If someone is, for whatever reason, unable to choose, why should their access to medical services be dependent on something as difficult to define as mental disorder? There are … many non-psychiatric causes of an inability to make a proper choice' (Buchanan 2014). Buchanan rejects this as too wide. It is a safeguard on individual liberties that there is an 'uncontroversial' objective of restricting the use of mental health legislation 'to cases where the inability to choose stemmed from mental ill-health' (ibid.).

10.4 Least Restrictive Option

A determination of lack of capacity, opening up the space for an interven- 10.21 tion, does not mean that anything goes. There are principles that guide what is acceptable, and there are debates about particular types of intervention, such as electro-convulsive therapy (ECT). This form of treatment, which involves sending an electric current through the brain, is used mainly for severe cases of depression which are not responding to other forms of therapy. It has been very controversial because of the way in which it was administered in the past, without anesthetic, and because of side effects such as memory loss. Today it is used less frequently and in ways designed to be a less unpleasant experience. Neurosurgery is another intervention, performed very rarely, and is not to be equated with the technique of lobotomy used in the past.

10.22   In determining the best course of action/intervention one principle that reflects the importance of autonomy in this area is the principle of the least restrictive option, which originated in the United States. The United Nations Resolution of 1991 (UN 1991) says that '[E]very patient shall have the right to be treated in the least restrictive environment and with the least restrictive or intrusive treatment appropriate to the patient's health needs and the need to protect the physical safety of others.' It is to be noted, then, that 'least restrictive' applies both to the environment of care and to the choice of treatment.

10.23   What constitutes the least restrictive option in a given case, however, is far from obvious. Health care professionals and service users are likely to have different views on this issue, but health care professionals have to make a judgment. There are, however, some general considerations to take into account. Taking the least restrictive option does not equate to letting the individual do whatever they want: the Resolution quoted above mentions two other factors: the health needs of the service user and the protection of the safety of others. Arguably the most difficult judgment call here concerns the individual's health needs, which may involve balancing 'best interests' against minimizing restrictiveness.

10.5 Best Interests

10.24   The ethical principle of beneficence reflects the importance of acting in someone's best interests, and the best interests test is enshrined in law in some jurisdictions (e.g. in the UK) for those who are deemed to lack capacity in relevant respects. While in many cases acting in someone's best interests may coincide with adopting the least restrictive option, this is not always the case. Taking a decision in the best interests of another individual is always fraught with difficulty and uncertainty, as we know from John

Stuart Mill's reasoning about the harm principle. As Mill said, the chances are that we will intervene in the wrong way (Mill 1859). Even though Mill had in mind people who could choose for themselves, the same caveats apply whenever we are in the position of choosing for someone else.

Within applicable legislation there is typically guidance available on the 10.25 sorts of factors that may be relevant to making a decision about what is in a person's best interests and which are not. Some of these are in accordance with ethical principles of avoiding discriminatory treatment on irrelevant grounds such age: it would be wrong to assume that something is best for a person just because they are of a certain age. In dealing with someone who is thought not to have the capacity for autonomous decision-making, it is important to have regard to what, if anything, is known about their past preferences, both from any records they might have made of their wishes, and the views of relatives and close associates, if any. It is also relevant to consider the likelihood of the individual regaining the capacity for autonomous decision-making at some future date.

10.6 Treatment and Detention

As noted at the beginning of this chapter, mental health has been a particu- 10.26 larly difficult area because of the use of controversial treatments and the possibility of non-voluntary detention of service users: psychiatry's use of detention formed part of Szasz's critique.

10.6.1 Detention for the Good of the Service User

In the case of mentally disordered people, those who have sympathy with 10.27 the anti-psychiatry movement may suspect that service users may be detained, not in their own interests at all, but for the convenience of society. But let us put that on one side and assume that those with the power to detain are acting in what they genuinely believe to be in the best interests of the service user. The kinds of considerations thought relevant to such a judgment include the provision of what is thought to be necessary treatment and/or the prevention of self-harm.

Let us take self-harm first, of which the most extreme example is suicide. 10.28 Should efforts be made to prevent people from taking their own lives? We do not, as Richard Lindley points out, think it right compulsorily to detain, 'in their own interests', people who smoke (Lindley 1978, p. 31), even if we think that choice poses a significant risk of shortening their lives. In a society which respects choice, based on the principle of respect for autonomous self-regarding choices, if people want to take risks with their health, then we should not force them not to. It is however becoming increasingly common that public health measures are put in place which are designed to 'nudge' people into taking particular choices regarding their lifestyle (Thaler and Sustein 2008). Reducing the available areas and thus opportunities, to smoke, constitute examples of this. Nevertheless, it is arguable that even though it may be, in one clear and specific sense, against people's interests to smoke, in another, wider, sense, it is in their own interests to be in charge of their own lives, as long as they are not doing it in an environment where harming others (e.g. by passive smoking) is an issue. So why might being suicidal provide support for a decision to detain? There is an obvious point that any one choice to have a cigarette has only a small probability of being the 'tipping point' that will lead to an early death, whereas any given suicide attempt has a much higher probability of resulting in death.

10.29   An argument for the value of prevention is that it allows for the possibility of a change of mind if and when the disorder is alleviated and thus of the future exercise of autonomous choices, whereas death is the end of autonomy as of everything else. So, there is, in fact, an autonomy-based argument that while it might be paternalistic, interference can be justified, at least in some cases, for the sake of future autonomy. Robert Young introduced an important ethical distinction here, when he suggested that it is possible to justify the overriding of occurrent autonomy for the sake of protecting dispositional, long-term autonomy (Young 1986). In other words, our valuing personal autonomy justifies the overriding of certain autonomous choices. There is a problem, however, about how far it is acceptable to take interference. Constant surveillance of a suicidal patient may be counterproductive, and as was pointed out above, issues of perception are important with regard to degrees of restrictiveness.

10.30   For Kant, the suicidal person's thinking exemplifies a contradiction in the will. The self-love which wishes to avoid unhappiness will itself be destroyed by the suicidal act. It is hard to agree with Kant here, however. It is not difficult to think of cases where, to a rational person, death might seem the most preferable of the available alternatives, for example, if you are facing capture by hostile forces known to practice brutal torture. Furthermore, people not regarded as suffering from mental disorder are free to commit suicide if they wish. (Assisted suicide is of course another matter.) Although by 2014 almost 1 million people committed suicide every year

(WHO 2014), being suicidal is not itself regarded as a mental disorder, but may be a symptom of a disorder. Aleman and Denys point out that up to 90 percent of suicides are by people with a diagnosable disorder, but argue that it should be itself defined as a distinct disorder and that governments should invest as much in prevention of deaths by suicide as in deaths due to road accidents (Aleman and Denys 2014, 421–422). This suggestion is problematic, however, as it brings many more people (the other 10%) into the category of persons diagnosed as suffering from a disorder. In those cases of suicide where the wish to end one's life seems perfectly rational it is difficult to understand that this would be a good outcome.

10.31 Not all cases of self-harm are suicide-related. The incidence of other types of self-harming such as self-cutting, are increasing, particularly among young people. Steve Edwards and Jeanette Hewitt have outlined three different strategies for dealing with self-harm: prevention, failing to prevent, and supervised self-harm (Edwards and Hewitt 2011). They argued against the prevention strategy for a number of reasons. One of them, from a consequentialist point of view, includes the negative consequences of an over-reliance on observation. Close observation can erode the trust crucial to the professional–patient relationship and potentially increase a patient's anxiety. Although it might seem to go against a natural response to try to prevent someone from doing physical injury to themselves, self-infliction of physical pain is a coping mechanism against psychological distress and to try to prevent it may have detrimental effects on a patient's mental health. On the other hand, simply standing by and leaving the individual to get on with it is not a good strategy either. This may have brutalizing effects on the professionals, and in fact leave the patient feeling unsupported, worthless and abandoned. As stated above, adopting the least restrictive option does not mean leaving the service user to do whatever they feel like. They therefore suggest that there are grounds for supervised self-harm, while at the same time implementing strategies to try to reduce self-harming behavior. This strategy appears to offer a compromise between the least restrictive option and promoting the service user's best interests.

10.6.2 Detention for the Protection of Others

10.32 The second part of the justification for detention concerns the protection of persons other than the service user. Those mentally disordered people who are detained on the grounds that they are dangerous to others fall into two categories: those who have already offended in some way, and those who are thought likely to offend. We do not normally think it justifiable in contemporary society to detain individuals simply on the basis that they *may* harm others. Under the criminal law, persons are innocent until proven guilty. Many of us live in societies in which liberty is greatly prized, and in which the wrongful deprivation of that good is seen as a great wrong.

10.33   In such a context, strong arguments are required for treating people with mental disorders differently. However, things are gradually changing, even outside the mental health context. Alongside scientific developments in areas such as neuroscience and genomics, with prospects of greater predictive possibilities, there is a view that it is indeed justifiable to 'pre-punish' persons, of whom it is believed that they will carry out a criminal act. This idea has been depicted in Stephen Spielberg's film *Minority Report*[20], based on a story by Philip K. **Dick**[21] and starring **Tom Cruise**[22]. It depicts the consequences of a department of 'pre-crime' where murders can be predicted and the potential perpetrators tracked down. This idea is also the subject of considerable philosophical and ethical debate.

10.34   Let us assume for present purposes that punishing people who actually have committed a crime, by detaining them, is morally acceptable. In a classic article, Christopher New has argued that it is morally acceptable to punish people not only after but also before they have committed a crime, provided we know or believe beyond a reasonable doubt that they will commit a crime. This is the 'temporal neutrality thesis' (New 1992). Given the current state of scientific development, however, in most if not all circumstances we lack sufficient evidence to be certain that a given individual will commit a crime, and in the mental health context, as we have seen, a diagnosis of mental illness may be far from certain. It could be argued, however, that even in the case of punishment with respect to past actions, certainty is not required. The standard of proof of 'beyond reasonable doubt' is deemed sufficient, so why should that not be sufficient with regard to pre-punishment and detention in mental health cases? Saul Smilansky has argued against New that such a view fails to respect persons as moral agents, because it is open to an agent to make a different choice, however much we think we can predict what they will do (Smilansky 2007). It is of course true that preventive detention is used by some regimes around the world, and that in some cases individuals are punished for planning crimes which are not actually carried out. The latter can be explained not as pre-punishment, however, but as punishment for planning as a crime in itself.

10.35   If pre-punishment of pre-crime is problematic, the question remains concerning what grounds, if any, can be used to support a moral distinction between preventive detention of persons diagnosed with a mental disorder, and those not so diagnosed. There are, of course, some cases where persons suffering from communicable diseases are detained in quarantine. Quarantine, in so far as it entails restriction of liberty, also requires ethical justification. If those quarantined have a disease that poses a severe risk, if there are no other protection measures available, and if they are properly informed and well-treated, however, it can be argued that it is justified as protecting the greater good.

Analogous reasoning can be applied in the case of mental disorders. The judgment that a person poses a threat to others needs to be supplemented by the judgment that the person is actually suffering from a mental disorder in order to justify detention. It is the diagnosis here which makes the difference from the pre-punishment case, and makes it more like the quarantine case. It is arguably also in the service user's own interests to be prevented from causing harm to others.   10.36

In considering protection of third parties from those deemed to present a danger, it is worth reminding ourselves of the discussion of confidentiality in the Tarasoff case in Chapter 6. There are circumstances where the mental health professional has to consider the duty to protect the public as well as the duty of confidentiality to a client.   10.37

It is at least partly due to the anti-psychiatry movement that mental health care has moved as far as it has from its coercive past. Although disagreements remain about the classification of mental disorders and while a diagnosis of mental disorder along with a determination of lack of capacity can have consequences for an individual's liberty, the realms of physical illness and mental illness have moved closer together in the principles that govern them and continue to do so. Although liberty may be removed, the least restrictive option should be chosen. And as we have seen, the possibility that individuals who pose a risk to others may be pre- punished without having a diagnosed mental disorder and lack of capacity is not completely off the table.   10.38

Questions

To what extent do you think mental health issues and mental health service users can justifiably be treated differently from people with physical health problems?

In the light of the issues discussed in this chapter, what do you think are the challenges of applying the principle of autonomy in this area?

Website Links

1 https://www.imdb.com/title/tt0073486/
2 http://www.who.int/en/
3 http://www.who.int/healthinfo/global_burden_disease/metrics_daly/en/
4 https://www.psychotherapy.net/interview/thomas-szasz/
5 https://www.in-formality.com/wiki/index.php?title=Psikhushka_(FSU)
6 https://www.nytimes.com/1983/01/30/magazine/the-world-of-soviet-psychiatry.html
7 https://psychology.wikia.org/wiki/Sluggishly_progressing_schizophrenia
8 https://www.psychiatry.org/psychiatrists/practice/dsm/history-of-the-dsm/
9 https://www.psychiatry.org/
10 https://www.britannica.com/biography/Richard-Freiherr-von-Krafft-Ebing
11 https://www.psychiatry.org/psychiatrists/practice/dsm/
12 https://www.ncbi.nlm.nih.gov/pmc/articles/PMC4204469/
13 http://www.mind.org.uk/
14 https://www.mind.org.uk/information-support/types-of-mental-health-problems/post-traumatic-stress-disorder-ptsd/#.Wj_h_bYlddg/
15 https://theconversation.com/winston-churchill-and-his-black-dog-of-greatness-36570/
16 https://www.britannica.com/biography/Samuel-Johnson
17 https://www.nhs.uk/conditions/post-natal-depression/
18 https://www.who.int/mental_health/policy/en/UN_Resolution_on_protection_of_persons_with_mental_illness.pdf
19 https://lockergnome.com/2012/09/13/depression-symptoms-similar-in-horses-and-humans/
20 https://www.rogerebert.com/reviews/minority-report-2002/
21 https://www.britannica.com/biography/Philip-K-Dick
22 http://www.tomcruise.com/

11

END OF LIFE

In this chapter we will have a closer look at the ethical case for and against 11.1 the decriminalization of assisted dying. This will give us also an opportunity to revisit some of the kinds of problematic arguments that we discussed in Chapter 3, including examples of various types of slippery-slope arguments, as well as a different kind of argument, one best described as an argument from tradition or from authority.

11.1 Do You Want to Live Forever?

Dying is something that most of us would avoid if we could. Typically two 11.2 reasons are given for this: On the one hand it is the uncertainty that some people experience with regard to the question of whether or not there is an after-life that is causing distress, on the other hand a significant personal challenge in this context, is the quality – or lack thereof – of our dying itself that worries many of us. While little can be done to resolve the former question, there is strong empirical evidence to suggest that the latter concerns are justified. The *Economist* magazine's *Intelligence Unit* has **compiled a report**[1] into the quality of death and dying in a number of countries (EIU 2015). It does not make for comfortable reading even if you live in a country belonging to the comparably better-resourced global north. A crucial problem, but by no means the only one, is the sketchy availability of high-quality palliative care. What is palliative care? There is plenty of confusion surrounding the concept of palliative care. Many believe, mistakenly, that it

This Is Bioethics: An Introduction, First Edition. Ruth F. Chadwick and Udo Schüklenk.
© 2021 John Wiley & Sons, Inc. Published 2021 by John Wiley & Sons, Inc.

is linked necessarily to end-of-life care. Palliative care is not necessarily end-of-life care, and it does not constitute a form of assisted dying. Here is how the WHO defines palliative care (**WHO n.d.**[2]):

> Palliative care is an approach that improves the quality of life of patients and their families facing the problem associated with life-threatening illness, through the prevention and relief of suffering by means of early identification and impeccable assessment and treatment of pain and other problems, physical, psychosocial and spiritual.

11.3   Palliative care began as a deliberate clinical effort aimed at controlling pain in late-stage cancer. This has changed. Today palliative care is required in circumstances involving chronic diseases such as dementia, kidney disease, as well as heart and lung disease. Even in Canada, a country that ranks in the top 10 in terms of the quality of death and dying, palliative care is often unavailable to patients who could benefit from it. Particularly badly fare, reportedly, pediatric patients. A recent study notes, 'only 5 percent and 12 percent of the children who might benefit from the services of a paediatric palliative care program actually received these services' (Schüklenk et al. 2011, 17).

11.4   Let us get a handle on some further salient facts about the changing demographics of our death and dying. The population on our planet is aging pretty rapidly. For the first time in human history we have more people above the age of 65 than under the age of 5. We are living ever-longer lives requiring ever more expensive medical care toward the end of our lives. The vast majority of us, after the age of 65, experience chronic disease conditions requiring cost-intensive medical attention. Reflect on the following facts from a Canadian report. The picture painted there is not dissimilar to that faced by most advanced nations (Schüklenk et al. 2011, 11).

11.5   The pressure on the health care system stems from the substantial increase in health care needs and expenditures once individuals reach age 65. Seniors (people aged 65 and older) represent 12.7 percent of the population and account for roughly 30% ($36.3 billion) of the total economic health care burden. This population has the highest hospital care expenditures at $10.2 billion. Seniors account for 22.8% ($2.7 billion) of physician care expenditures, 20.2 percent ($2.5 billion) of drug expenditures, and 33 percent ($11.0 billion) of mortality costs.

11.6   Greater reporting of long-term disability costs and the greater number of elderly people with chronic conditions account for the large difference between long-term and short-term disability costs. Leading factors responsible for long-term disability are musculoskeletal conditions, followed by cardiovascular conditions, nervous system conditions, and injuries. Seniors alone account for over 33 percent of the long-term disability for cardiovascular diseases. With respect to prescription drug expenditures, seniors account for 54.3 percent ($963 million) of expenditures for cardiovascular diseases, followed by endocrine and related diseases (34.8%), musculoskeletal diseases (25.8%), digestive diseases (25.4%), respiratory diseases (15.4%), and mental disorders (13.4%). Seniors account for almost 50 percent ($413 million) of Canadian prescription drug expenditures for hypertension and arthritis ($129million), and for nearly 66 percent for ischemic heart disease ($331 million).

We will be looking at some of the resource allocation justice problems   11.7
this stark picture creates in the next two Chapters (12 and 13). Given the expense and limited resources available, might the elderly actually have a moral obligation to call it a day as it were. Perhaps we might not want to go as far as the makers of the movie **Soylent Green**[3] proposed – there, in a futuristic world bereft of natural resources, the solution to the food crisis was that people would be killed toward the end of their natural lives and their bodies recycled into a food product, **Soylent Green**[4]. However, as we have just seen, just as in the fictional world of this movie, our world also suffers from a reality where resources, including health care resources, are finite. The question arises whether access to resource intensive end-of-life care should be limited for those of us who had a fair innings, especially if there are others who otherwise would be left without the necessary health care resources to achieve a fair innings.

This is an argument put forward by John Harris. He writes: 11.8

> Anyone who does not reach 70 suffers, on this view, the injustice of being cut off in their prime. They have missed out on a reasonable share of life: they have been short-changed. Those, however, who do make 70 suffer no such injustice, they have not lost out but rather must consider any additional years a sort of bonus beyond that which could reasonably be hoped for. The fair innings argument requires that everyone be given an equal chance to have a fair innings, to reach the appropriate threshold but, having reached it, they have received their entitlement.
>
> (Harris 1970)

Harris concedes that there will be many people who have had a fair   11.9
innings who will have the same desire to continue living a good life than others who are younger. To this he replies:

Each person's desire to stay alive should be regarded as of the same importance and as deserving the same respect as that of anyone else, irrespective of
the quality of their life or its expected duration. This would hold good in all
cases in which we have to choose between lives, except one. And that is where
one individual has had a fair innings and the other not. In this case, although
there is nothing to choose between the two candidates from the points of
view of their respective will to live and both would suffer the injustice of having their life cut short when it might continue, only one would suffer the
further injustice of being deprived of a fair innings - a benefit the other has
received ... The fair innings argument points to the fact that the injustice
done to someone who has not had a fair innings when they lose out to someone who has is significantly greater than in the reverse circumstances.

(Harris 1970)

11.10   John Hardwig reached a similar conclusion to Harris, but his reasons are
quite different (Hardwig 2000, 119–200). He caused quite a bit of a stir
when he argued in a 1997 article in the *Hastings Center Report* that he, and
by extension, other elderly people like him, could well have a moral obligation to die, even in the absence of terminal illness and impending death.
Here is his reasoning[5]: Hardwig suggests that our continuing existence
could become so burdensome on our loved ones as to result in a moral
obligation on us to die. He does think that elderly people are entitled to
certain sacrifices of their family members in terms of care provided to
them, but there are limits as to what can justifiably be expected. To him it is
clear that there can be a point where our demands on others would be so
significant as to become unreasonable. When that point is reached we
might have to recognize that it is on us to end our lives in order to avoid
selfish demands on our loved ones.

11.11   What possible ethical counter arguments could one deploy to fend of
such a conclusion? A preference utilitarian might say that losing one's life
could be such a significant sacrifice as to outweigh the burdens typically
placed on others by us during our last life years. Of course, as so often with
consequentialist arguments, much would depend here on determining
what kinds of burdens are experienced, and by whom, before we would be
able to assess this claim. Hardwig insists that there can be circumstances
where what would be a huge sacrifice by ourselves would be outweighed by
a more significant sacrifice our loved one's would have to make if we insisted
on continuing living while requiring sacrifices from them to enable us
to do so. He uses the following case to support this point:

An 87-year old woman was dying of congestive heart-failure. [...S]he had less-than a 50 percent chance to live for another six months. She was lucid, assertive and terrified of death. She very much wanted to live and kept opting for rehospitalization and the most aggressive life-prolonging treatment possible. That treatment successfully prolonged her life (though with increasing debility) for nearly two years. Her 55-year-old daughter was her only remaining family, her caregiver, and the main source of her financial support. The daughter duly cared for her mother. But before her mother died, her illness had cost the daughter all of her savings, her home, her job and her career. This is by no means an uncommon sort of case. Thousands of similar cases occur each year. Now, ask yourself which is the greater burden:

a. To lose a 50 percent chance of six more months of life at age 87?
b. To lose all your savings, your home, and your career at age 55?

Hardwig's provocative view does look a lot less counter-intuitive now, doesn't it? One question that arises here, and that Hardwig does not address himself to, is whether a good society would force individuals to accept such sacrifices to themselves instead of providing support services that would permit the 87-year-old patient to continue living while her 55 year old daughter would equally be able to continue her life without the sacrifices mentioned in his scenario. However, when you consider the data provided earlier, and you keep in mind that for the next few decades the situation will get worse, before it gets better in terms of the imbalance of elderly versus younger people, it might be impossible even for wealthier societies to provide the kinds of services required for the very many patients that might be in need of them. 11.12

Ezekiel J. Emanuel, a medical doctor cum bioethicist in the United States, agrees also with Harris and Hardwig's conclusions, but he provides us with a third kind of rationale. Harris was focused on intergenerational resource allocation justice. Hardwig was specifically concerned about being an undue burden on family members. Emanuel, in an article published in the magazine *The Atlantic*[6], tells his readers that he does not wish to live beyond the age of 75. His reasons are entirely based on evidence on the quality of life he would likely be able to experience after that age has been reached. To his mind the quality of life that most people experience at that stage of their lives does not make it worthwhile undertaking all the necessary health care efforts to sustain their existence for a few more years, when death is inevitable no matter our medical 11.13

interventions. He quotes a researcher at the University of Southern California, Eileen Crimmins, who found that while we are successful in increasing people's lifespans, it is not an increase in life years with a good quality of life. Rather, what we are getting, Crimmins writes, is an 'increase in the life expectancy with disease and a decrease in the years without disease. The same is true for functioning loss, an increase in expected years unable to function' (Emanuel 2014).

11.14   Here is what this means practically for Emanuel personally. He thinks societal policy ought to look very similar:

> At 75 and beyond, I will need a good reason to even visit the doctor and take any medical test or treatment, no matter how routine and painless. And that good reason is not 'It will prolong your life.' I will stop getting any regular preventive tests, screenings, or interventions. I will accept only palliative – not curative – treatments if I am suffering pain or other disability. This means colonoscopies and other cancer-screening tests are out – and before 75. If I were diagnosed with cancer now, at 57, I would probably be treated, unless the prognosis was very poor. But 65 will be my last colonoscopy. No screening for prostate cancer at any age. (When a urologist gave me a PSA test even after I said I wasn't interested and called me with the results, I hung up before he could tell me. He ordered the test for himself, I told him, not for me.) After 75, if I develop cancer, I will refuse treatment. Similarly, no cardiac stress test. No pacemaker and certainly no implantable defibrillator. No heart-valve replacement or bypass surgery. If I develop emphysema or some similar disease that involves frequent exacerbations that would, normally, land me in the hospital, I will accept treatment to ameliorate the discomfort caused by the feeling of suffocation, but will refuse to be hauled off.

11.15   Emanuel derives two policy prescriptions from this: One is that society should not measure the quality of their health care systems by simply looking at increases or decreases in average life expectancy. The other is that biomedical research should focus its attention on alleviating the quality-of-life impact of diseases of aging rather than focusing on prolonging our dying.

11.16   Let us leave the question of whether there is a duty to die behind us for the time being and move on to a question that has traditionally occupied most of the ethical controversies that arose at the ends of our lives. Many pro-choice activists phrase the question this way: Do we have a right to die? The answer to this question is not very controversial among most secular bioethicists. Of course, we have a right to end our lives when we see fit, as long as we are competent, and as long as our decision is informed and voluntary. The widely accepted reason for this is that in important ways we not only *are* our bodies but also that we *own* our bodies. This entitles us to treat ourselves as we see fit. In fact, the common law doctrine **volenti non fit injuria**[7] confirms this. It maintains that no injustice is done to someone who agrees to a particular course of action that could be seen as harming that person, as long as that is what that person wants, and as long as that person is decisionally competent and not coerced. However, at the same time, most of the monotheistic world religions have issued bans on suicide, which in turn could be seen as morally binding at least on their followers. Still, the reason why suicide is not criminalized in many, if not most, jurisdictions has to do exactly with the view expressed earlier: we own our bodies and we are entitled to live and die as we see fit – that is, as long we do no harm to other parties in the process.

Why then is there a long and ongoing ethical controversy about the *how* of our dying? This controversy has to do not so much with our general right to die, but with the question of *how* we bring our deaths about in particular. While suicide may not be a criminal offense in most countries, assisting someone else to kill themselves is usually considered a criminal offense, and so is the killing of someone else, even at their request. This is what we will be turning our attention to after we have undertaken a bit of necessary terminological ground-clearing work. **11.17**

11.2 Terminology

Here is a quick overview of relevant terminology that is frequently used in debates on the ethics and politics of assisted dying. We will be guided here by definitions used in a major report on end-of-life issues that an international expert panel produced for the Royal Society of Canada (Schüklenk 2011, 5–6). **11.18**

Advance directives are directions given by a competent individual concerning what and/or how and/or by whom decisions should be made in the event that, at some time in the future, the individual becomes incompetent to make healthcare decisions. An example is a woman who has signed a document that states that, should she fall into a persistent vegetative state, she does not wish to receive artificial hydration or nutrition. Or, as another example, a man who has signed a document that states that, when he is incompetent, he wishes his wife to make all healthcare decisions on his behalf. There are two kinds of advance directives: *instruction directives*, which establish what and/or how healthcare decisions are to be made; and *proxy directives*, which establish who is to make healthcare decisions.

Assisted suicide is the act of intentionally killing oneself with the assistance of another. An example is a woman with advanced amyotrophic lateral sclerosis (ALS, or motor neuron disease) who gets a prescription from her physician for barbiturates and uses the drugs to kill herself.

Competent means capable of understanding and appreciating the relevant information and the nature and consequences of the decision to be made. It is important to note that competence is decision-, time-, and place-specific and that individuals may be competent for one decision (such as what to eat and drink) and not another (such as whether to refuse surgery) and may be competent one day and not the next.

Voluntary euthanasia is an act undertaken by one person to kill another person whose life is no longer worth living to them in accordance with the wishes of that person. An example is a man bedridden with many of the consequences of a massive stroke whose physician, at his request, gives him a lethal injection of barbiturates and muscle relaxants.

Non-voluntary means without the knowledge of the wishes expressed by a competent person or through a valid advance directive.

Involuntary means against the wishes expressed by a competent person or through a valid advance directive.

11.19   Traditionally ethical arguments on end-of-life decision-making centered around the positive case in favor of decriminalizing assisted dying, as well as the question of whether or not rational agents could reasonably want their own death, whether they are entitled to make such choices, but also whether assisted dying is compatible with the role of health care professional. Since then other questions have emerged, including most prominently varieties of slippery-slope arguments. We have seen already in Chapter 3 why slippery-slope arguments are kinds of arguments we should be wary about when we come across them. In the case of assisted dying slippery-slope arguments typically aim to show that we cannot protect the most vulnerable against abuse once we start decriminalizing assisted dying. Let us have a look at these issues now.

11.3 Case for the Decriminalization of Assisted Dying

Unsurprisingly, the paradigmatic argument for the decriminalization of 11.20 assisted dying is essentially the pro-choice case. It maintains, very much in line with enlightenment values, that the autonomous individual – that includes every competent adult and possibly even some mature minors – is sovereign with regard to important self-regarding actions. If such a person, after being made aware of the relevant facts of their particular circumstances, reaches the conclusion that their life is not worth living any longer, as individuals and as a society we are not permitted to interfere with their self-regarding actions. It is true, of course, that nobody ending their life can truly claim that their actions are purely self-regarding. Just think of the family members that are left behind, or the hotel personnel finding you in the hotel where you might have chosen to end your life, and so on and so forth. One would have to balance the inconvenience, grief and possibly even distress that such an act arguably causes to such third parties against a person's interest in ceasing to exist. It seems implausible to many that throughout our lives we should be able to live our lives as we see fit, and that may well include activities such risking our lives while scuba-diving in shark-infested waters, climbing dangerous mountains, or engaging in dangerous sporting activities, but when it comes to determining how our lives should end, we are told that we must not make such decisions if they violate other people's views on how our lives ought to end. This is strange, because the liberal democratic ideal on which Western democracies are build takes it as a given that one of the fundamental roles of the State is to protect our ability to make and to execute self-regarding actions. Our right to determine our own life is at the core of what living in a liberal democracy is all about.

Independent of this autonomy-based take on end-of-life choices, it is 11.21 worth noting that other ethical considerations could well be deployed to defend such choices, if we were to assume that the autonomous individual has some explaining to do in the first place. Utilitarians and other consequentialists could note that most people would only make choices as drastic as seeking to end their lives if the quality of their life, and their future prospects, are so dire as to make their lives not worth living any longer *to them*. The utilitarian calculus might then well support the choices of people seeking to end their lives. Kantians are more conflicted about this, but at the end of the day, they are strongly concerned about persons being enabled to make their own choices with regard to how they wish to live (and end) their lives. After all, with Kant, the enlightenment's credo was to free the autonomous individual of their self-inflicted ignorance about the state of the world. It would arguably contradict such values if we then turned against the emancipated citizen who has made a decision as important as wanting to see their life terminated. There would not be much point to the enlightenment if we freed the historically other-directed individual and gave her the tools to transform herself into a truly self-ruling person, only to then ignore the decisions she makes on such a fundamental issue as the end of her life. You could also belabor Kant's Categorical Imperative. After all, we could easily want it to become a universal rule in society that every competent adult who considers her life not worth living any longer, and who is fully informed about her state of health and her future prospects, should have the right to end her life. Kant's philosophy was also fundamentally about respect for persons, and how could we reasonably respect persons if we ignored their most important of all choices, namely their life and death decisions.

11.22   The case in favor of self-determination is pretty straightforward in the context of liberal democracies. Of course, nothing is ever as clear-cut in ethics and politics as it looks like on a first glance. You will have noticed that we used the phrase 'autonomous individual' to describe the person we typically think has the right to self-determination. In legal terms that is relatively straightforward inasmuch as anyone of mature age who has not been legally declared incompetent is such an autonomous individual. That is true even for people who might be significantly distressed upon learning that they are suffering, for instance, from terminal cancer. In ethical terms it is less clear which kinds of actions should count as autonomous. A purely procedural account of autonomy would simply protect any self-regarding choices made by people considered legally competent. But perhaps we ought to aim for a higher standard, given what is at stake. Should we say that someone is autonomous if and only if they express logical and reason-based decisions? If we did this, depending on how strictly we define logic and reason, many religious people's choices might fall by the wayside because of their beliefs in an afterlife or the soul. So, perhaps such a restrictive account of autonomy is not what we should be aiming for. How about an account of autonomy where our course of action must reflect our longstanding considered views of the world and our longstanding core values. After all those long-held values could reasonably be held to be constitutive of our identity as persons. They are what makes us who we are. In other words, only choices that are demonstrably authentically our own would then matter. The problem with this account is that our decision-making in face of a terminal illness, or that in case of a chronic illness that severely reduces our quality of life, might not be in line with our long considered values. In fact the challenge posed to our values by such an event constitutes arguably a strategic inflection point of a kind. It could well lead to us making choices quite different to what our long-held values would have predicted we would do. A **strategic inflection point**[8] was described by Andy Grove, Intel's co-founder, as 'an event that changes the way we think and act.' It is pretty obvious that something as profound as death and dying will constitute for many of us just such a strategic inflection point impacting on our values and crucial life choices. Surely it would be difficult to accept paternalistic interventions under such circumstances, at least on the grounds that we changed our mind about what it is that actually matters to us in face of a life-threatening illness. The fact that we change our mind on important issues affecting our lives does not necessarily make our decisions any less autonomous.

Perhaps what we should reasonably aim for is a conception of autonomy 11.23 that is based on a legally competent person's voluntary informed consent or refusal. Which takes us to yet another conundrum. What level of information and comprehension should be required in order to accept that a decision made is truly an informed decision? Various disclosure standards have been proposed. It is worth considering each of them briefly in turn – you will already be familiar with some of them as we came across these standards in Chapters 6 and 7: A *reasonable-doctor standard* is a level of disclosure that provides patients with the kind of information that a reasonable doctor would appreciate and be able to comprehend. This standard would arguably provide patients with the best, as in most-in-depth, level of information of any of the models considered in today's debates. The drawback of this model is obviously that most of us who are not clinicians would not actually understand what is being communicated to us. Informed consent or refusal would be impossible on such a standard. Unsurprisingly, the next model is the *reasonable- patient standard*. Here the level of information disclosed provides the kind of information a reasonable (as in average) patient should be capable of comprehending. It would explain to the patient, in terms we can understand as non-specialists, what our prognosis is, what courses of action would be available to us, and what material risks attach to each possible course of action. This standard, in fact, is the most widely used today. An alternative to this is standard is the *individual-patient standard*. It was born out of a concern that the reasonable-patient standard takes insufficiently into account the wide range of different educational and cultural backgrounds of individual patients. It requires of doctors to provide individual patients with the kind of information necessary for patients to make their own choices. A practical problem with this approach is that doctors might not usually have the time to familiarize themselves in-depth with their patient's educational and cultural backgrounds to achieve what otherwise would surely be a desirable objective.

11.24   Let us return to the pro-choice argument again. Once we have determined that a patient is competent, that she has been properly informed, that she comprehends the information salient to her situation, and that she does not consider her life worth living when she takes into account her current quality of life, and what is known about the likely course of her disease progression, there is no good reason to interfere with her decision to see her life end once she has concluded that that is her wish.

11.25   Well, you might rightly say that this is all very well, but even *if* we were to grant the pro-choice argument, how does this translate into an obligation of society – or of an individual health care professional – to pro-actively assist such patients in achieving their objective, that is to end their lives? Different answers to this question have been offered. Some have argued that society and its health care professions have a moral obligation to assist citizens in ensuring that one of their last self-regarding choices in a life that was predicated on being self-determining, will be realized according to their wishes. It is the ultimate form of societal respect for its autonomous citizen's decisions at such a crucial juncture in their lives. Others have argued that society does not actually have such a responsibility. However, it must do nothing that would prevent its autonomous citizens and those volunteering to assist them, from acting on their self-regarding decisions. In other words, society should decriminalize assisted dying for decisionally competent citizens and those volunteering to provide assistance to them. Society would have an interest in ensuring that abuse of such a system is minimized. For that reason many jurisdictions have tasked health care professionals with the provision of life-ending health services. This seems prudent, because the health care professions are very tightly regulated. Keeping an assisted dying system within the health care profession confers additional patient protections against abuse.

11.26   The remainder of this chapter will focus on arguments usually brought forward against the decriminalization of assisted dying. Over the last few years the nature of these arguments has changed quite significantly. Traditionally these arguments were strongly motivated by religious concerns, comprising views such as that God has created us and it is not our decision to take our own lives. These arguments have mostly been replaced by various public-reason based rationales. It is these rationales that we will be focusing on now.

11.4 The Case Against the Decriminalization of Assisted Dying

Typically arguments against the decriminalization of assisted dying fall into two categories: either they suggest that there are strong in-principle reasons why patients asking for assistance in dying should not be obliged by health care professionals or other experts or they suggest that while there might be individual cases where we could consider supporting those requesting our help, a general policy permitting assisted dying would lead to seriously harmful consequences that would inevitably occur if we decriminalized. The latter kind of argument is a slippery-slope argument. You were briefly introduced to these kinds of arguments in Chapter 3. Please do familiarize or re-familiarize yourself with the content provided under the heading 3.10 Slippery Slope Arguments before you continue reading. 11.27

11.4.1 In-Principle Reasons Against Assistance in Dying

What kinds of in-principle reasons are often offered to deny moral claims for assistance in dying? A prominent argument can be traced back to Immanuel Kant's prohibition of suicide. He famously argued that we have an obligation to ourselves as rational beings not to commit suicide, because doing so would deny our rational nature. How should we understand this argument? Kant rightly noted that most of those committing *rational* suicide do not commit such an act because they truly want to cease existing, but rather because they want to escape overwhelming suffering. This desire, you might recall from our brief description of Kantian ethics in Chapter 2, eliminates our rationale as a rationale that carries ethical worth. Worse, by eliminating the person in the process of trying to avoid suffering, we act unethically, at least according to Kant. Kant denies here that suicide could be the expression of a rational and informed person's choice, rather he insists that such a choice is a choice driven primarily by inclination. The latter would make it not a moral choice rightly demanding our respect. 11.28

11.29 There is another aspect to Kant's argument. He also argued that someone who chooses to die in order to put an end to their suffering is treating themselves as a mere means to achieve another end, namely to eliminate their suffering. That, as you might recall, is an act prohibited by Kant's Categorical Imperative. Kant put it this way (Kant 1993, 36):

> If he destroys himself in order to escape from a difficult situation, then he is making use of his person merely as a means so as to maintain a tolerable condition until the end of his life. However, a human being is not a thing and hence is not something to be used merely as a means; one must in all one's actions always be regarded as an end in itself. Therefore, I cannot dispose of a human being in my own person by mutilating, damaging or killing him.

11.30 J. David Velleman, a current-day Kantian supports Kant's 1785 prohibition of suicide (and as a corollary of that view, assisted dying), when he writes (Velleman 1999, 624):

> The self-interested choice of suicide cannot be an exercise of rationality, because it entails treating oneself as an instrument of one's interests, which is incoherent. That's why this choice is not morally protected. One's value as a rational being cannot require that others defer to one's irrational disregard for that same value.

11.31 Not all Kantians agree with Kant's own take on this matter. Frances M. Kamm, for instance, thinks that patients' autonomous choices are choices that are protected. Kamm argues that it is true that for us to be persons entails a right to life, but equally a right to waive that right, which in turn 'releases others from a duty not to kill' (**Kamm 1997, 232**[9]).

11.4.2 Slippery-Slope Reasons Against Assistance in Dying

11.32 We have written a bit about the structural problems with slippery-slope type arguments in bioethics and biopolicy in Chapter 3, so there is some overlap with what follows. The next few paragraphs can probably be best understood as an application of the criticisms and concerns raised in Chapter 3 on the assistance-in-dying matter. Remember that we suggested that more often than not slippery-slope arguments in bioethics fail. Let us see how this unfolds in a real-world bioethics argument.

11.33 As mentioned in Chapter 3, different types of slippery-slope arguments exist. In assisted-dying debates we tend to see different varieties of these kinds of arguments, too. Do keep in mind that slippery-slope arguments can deny, but they do not have to deny, that there could be particular cases of assisted dying that are defensible. So you could come across an opponent of assisted dying who presents a slippery-slope argument against the decriminalization of assisted dying who could genuinely agree with you that in a particular case scenario you present assisted dying would be a great thing to have available. However, they would likely argue that as a society we would still be better off not to decriminalize assisted dying, because of a particular slippery-slope that we would inevitably and unintentionally slide down toward unjustifiable cases of assisted dying, if we decriminalized. Such a slippery-slope would lead to sufficiently significant harm as to provide us with good reasons not to decriminalize assisted dying in a given society even if that meant that some people who would definitely benefit from decriminalization would be worse off as a result of maintaining the status quo.

An influential kind of slippery-slope argument that you will encounter in 11.34 end-of-life discussions offers empirical claims about what would happen if decriminalization occurred. John A. Burgess cites a good example of such a slippery-slope argument. William Reichel and Arthur J. Dyck came up with it. They wrote:

> If euthanasia were legalized, might we not then regard certain individuals as unworthy of life? Such a concept laid the foundations of the euthanasia movement that began in Germany before the National Socialist movement and before Hitler's rise to power. ... To those who say, 'It cannot happen here', we reply: Imagine the easy marriage between respect for autonomy [...] and the need for greater cost containment – i.e. the patient's care is disproportionately expensive. What begins for the patient's own wishes, may later be endorsed for economic reasons.
>
> (As cited in Burgess 1993, 169)

You also frequently come across claims suggesting that 'vulnerable people' 11.35 would see their lives ended either against their explicit wishes or without even being asked. Fairly common is also the suggestion that cash-strapped governments might use the availability of assisted dying as a means to reduce investment in good-quality palliative care (Burgess 1993). The logic here is that governments would reduce palliative care resources, thereby triggering an increase in the number of requests for assisted dying. This, in turn, would lead to the intended reduction of health care expenditure. If you scan the literature carefully you will likely find other such claims. These are slippery-slope claims that even proponents of assisted dying would find difficult to counter if they were actually true. Much depends then on the question of whether these claims are supported by empirical evidence. If there was evidence that assisted dying truly led to the murder of vulnerable people or if there was evidence that it would make the availability of palliative care more difficult, surely proponents of assisted dying would have a case to answer for. This would be the case, even if it is true that simply maintaining the current status quo is also not cost-neutral either, given that it results in the unnecessary suffering of many people toward the ends of their biological lifespans.

11.36   John Burgess raises in an influential article on slippery-slope arguments another problem with these types of arguments. He writes:

> Unfortunately, purveyors of the Great Argument [slippery-slope arguments] rarely ever work it into a detailed slippery-slope argument. They rest content with the sketchiest of formulations, leaving the detailed work to their opponents: 'we have shown you (sketchily) that it might happen; now show us (in detail) that it couldn't.'
>
> (Burgess 1993, 169)

11.37   Let us have a closer look now at how slippery-slope arguments turn out in the rough and tumble of two published journal articles on assisted dying. We could have chosen any number of articles for this purpose, but as it happens, there exists an excellent exchange between the two sides that is worth having a closer look at. The authors are, respectively, Jose Pereira (2011), a palliative care professor at a Canadian hospital, and Jocelyn Downie (2012), a health law professor in Canada, and her Belgian colleagues. All contributors are respected academics in their respective universities. Pereira is a vocal opponent of assisted dying, Downie and colleagues are equally vocal proponents of the decriminalization of assisted dying. Their articles were published in a small Open Access publication called *Current Oncology*. We strongly encourage you to read the articles by **Pereira**[10] and **Downie**[11] and colleagues prior to continuing reading this chapter. Based on what you have learned about slippery-slope type arguments, try to identify slippery-slope type arguments in Pereira's article and decide whether you think Pereira's slippery-slope claim is sound, or unsound, and for what reason.

11.4.2.1 Pereira v. Downie

11.38 Pereira writes in his article, 'In 1998 in the Netherlands, 25 percent of patients requesting euthanasia received psychiatric consultation; in 2010 none did.' The slippery-slope claim here implies that once strict standards of psychiatric evaluation for patients requesting euthanasia are not maintained over time. As a result vulnerable psychiatric patients' lives are put at risk. However, as Downie and colleagues note in their response, Pereira actually uses a reference from 1994 as evidence for his assertion. Evidently, no researcher was able to know in 1994 what would or would not have happened on that count in the Netherlands between 1998 and 2010.

Pereira makes another claim of fact in his article. He writes, 'In Switzerland   11.39
in 2006, the university hospital in Geneva reduced its already limited palliative care staff (to 1.5 from 2 full-time physicians) after a hospital decision to allow assisted suicide; the community-based palliative care service was also closed.' He implies here a slippery-slope whereby the introduction of assisted dying resulted in reductions in patient access to palliative care. Downie and colleagues note in their response: 'The Chief of Palliative Medicine of the University Hospitals of Geneva has stated that "there was no direct or indirect relation between the palliative care staffing/provision of community-based palliative care services and the hospital taking a position (on the advice of its clinical ethics committee) on the provision of assisted suicide within the institutional walls." Furthermore, in the period referred to by Pereira, "the number of physicians full-time equivalents in palliative care increased from 3 to 3.5 and that number has subsequently increased to 7.5".'

Here is a final slippery-slope claim from Pereira's article. He writes: 11.40

> In 30 years, the Netherlands has moved from euthanasia of people who are terminally ill, to euthanasia of those who are chronically ill; from euthanasia for physical illness, to euthanasia for mental illness; from euthanasia for mental illness, to euthanasia for psychological distress or mental suffering – and now to euthanasia simply if a person is over the age of 70 and 'tired of living'.

This constitutes a standard slippery-slope argument. The argument   11.41
implies that once euthanasia is available in a jurisdiction, say for the terminally ill only, it will rapidly be made available for people who might just be chronically ill, or even for people who are 'tired of living.' Downie and colleagues investigated this claim, too. This is what they found:

> The Netherlands did not start with the limit of terminal illness, and it does not allow euthanasia where a person is simply over the age of 70 and 'tired of living'.

We can learn several things from the exchange between Pereira and   11.42
Downie. One important lesson is that we should be skeptical of claims of fact that are made even in the peer reviewed scientific literature. Make sure you satisfy yourself whether the evidence provided actually supports the claims

made. If a particular ethical analysis relies on the truth of empirical premises, it is important to ascertain whether these claims of fact are actually true. Another question to keep in mind when you think about these sorts of slippery-slope claims is to ask yourself whether they prove what they claim to prove, assuming the factual claims are correct. In each of the cases Pereira mentions, he has not actually demonstrated that what is of concern to him is caused by the decriminalization of assisted dying. Correlation does not equal causation. Last but not least you need to ask yourself whether what the slippery-slope claims to be true would be of concern to you. Consider Pereira's empirical claim about how the Netherlands allegedly increased the kinds of conditions under which people would be able to access assistance in dying. In addition to investigating whether these claims are true, you also need to ask yourself whether you would have ethical concerns if they were true. You might, for instance, think it is ethically defensible to provide assistance in dying to elderly people tired of living. If that is the case, Pereira's argument would not yield the kind of response from you that he was hoping for when he wrote down the argument that he presented.

11.43   A different type of slippery-slope argument is encapsulated in the suggestion that if we decriminalized assisted dying today, for decisionally competent people, soon we would see decisionally incapable people killed. Think of the elderly people with dementia who have not left behind valid advance directives, or severely disabled newborns, patients with significant irreversible brain damage, etc. This case is more complex to address. First, we must, of course, see again whether it is borne out by empirical evidence from jurisdictions that have decriminalized. That is, in the countries where assisted dying is available, has this slippery-slope occurred anywhere? Let us assume, for the sake of the argument, that there was a country that decriminalized assisted dying for competent people who request it voluntarily after they received the relevant information about their life's prospects. Let us assume furthermore that this country, years later, had decided, after an extensive public consultation, and after a parliamentary vote, that it would indeed permit the lives of, for instance, particular kinds of severely disabled newborns to be terminated as part of its assisted dying legislation. The policy has broad support among the voting public of that society. The rationale for extending the range of people able to access assisted dying had to do with these newborns' terrible quality of life and the fact that they would die within a short period of time after birth a pretty painful death.

11.44   If the experience with the availability of assisted dying in that society led to its citizens being comfortable with it, and its safeguards, a deliberate societal act of widening the criteria under which assisted dying is available does not constitute a slippery-slope. Here the ethical arguments for and against the proposed changes to existing policies were made, and heard. Then a political decision was made, presumably it was contested in the country's highest court, and it was eventually sustained. At issue here is that while it is true that a particular outcome predicted by those claiming a slippery-slope occurred, the policy leading to this outcome was changed quite deliberately. Such an event does not then constitute a slippery slope type situation.

The already mentioned **Royal Society of Canada**[12] panel comments on   11.45
this particular slippery-slope argument (Schüklenk et al. 2011, 48):

> The conceptual slippery-slope argument against assisted suicide and volun-
> tary euthanasia takes the ambiguity of the concept as the premise of an argu-
> ment that practicing assisted dying on incompetent people is unavoidable.
> The argument takes the form of what in philosophy is called a *sorites para-
> dox*: for every competent person, there will be one just slightly less compe-
> tent, where the difference between the two hardly seems significant enough
> to ground the claim that one is competent whereas the other is not. But then,
> there will be a person just slightly less competent than the second, and then
> another just slightly less competent than the third, and quickly, medically
> assisted dying is being practiced on patients of whom it would be very diffi-
> cult indeed to claim that they are competent. Frequently the specter of the
> Nazis' murder of intellectually disabled people is invoked in order to indicate
> where this slippery-slope would inexorably lead any society that decriminal-
> ized assisted dying in some form or shape.

What is important to recognize with regard to slippery slope claims is   11.46
that often they represent genuine anxieties about things that could go wrong if we were to introduce new policies or technologies. On occasion these claims point us to things that could actually go wrong if we are not careful. In a sense slippery-slope claims then could be important kinds of red flags that alert us to potential dangers certain envisaged policies could entail. It would then be up to society to ensure that those dangers are addressed by means of regulations, monitoring and transparent reporting.

11.5 Violation of Health Care Professional Values and Traditions

A different line of reasoning against health care professionals assisting peo-   11.47
ple in dying argues that participation in such kinds of activities violates the traditional professional standards health care professionals should abide by.

This argument, presented in different forms and shapes in public debates of the issue, usually is both correct and questionable at the same time. Here is why.

11.48   When you look at traditional guidance documents used by health care professionals, such as for instance the **Hippocratic Oath**[13], or the World Medical Association's stance on this matter, it is clear that the tradition is on the side of those opposed to physician-assisted dying. The Hippocratic Oath, for instance, stipulates in no uncertain terms, 'I will not give a lethal drug to anyone if I am asked, nor will I advise such a plan.' The reasons for this strict prohibition are not given in the Oath, but they likely can be derived from the Oath's foundational principle that doctors must not harm their patients. On closer reading it isn't clear whether the primary (historical) target of this prohibition really was euthanasia or whether the concern was about doctors who provide lethal drugs to others for assassination purposes. The historian Heinrich von Staden notes that 'the rich ancient lore about the poisoning of adversaries and rivals, the occasional use of poison as a means of suicide […] and the ancients' early awareness of the potentially harmful effects of certain natural substances used as simple drugs […] confirm that physicians knew only too well that part of their formidable pharmacological arsenal could be put to harmful and even fatal use' (von Staden 2009, 354). The **World Medical Association**[14] offers its own categorical statement, 'The WMA reiterates its strong commitment to the principles of medical ethics and that utmost respect has to be maintained for human life. Therefore, the WMA is firmly opposed to euthanasia and physician-assisted suicide.'

11.49   Of course, neither of these two examples gives us good reasons for why doctors should not participate in assisting patients in dying. They merely admonish them not to do so. This is not unusual for ethical guidance documents. More often than not such documents provide guidance but lack justification for the guidance provided. What should we make – more generally- of arguments from tradition then? Arguably we should not make much of them. It is true that arguments from tradition have been – and are being – used in political discourses to support particular sets of values. Just think of the Catholic traditionalism under the leadership of **Archbishop Lefebvre**[15]. Lefebvre proposed that religious services should return to the format of the **Tridentine Mass**[16], a format used by that church between 1570 and 1962. It included features such as the exclusive use of Latin language. Traditionalists also typically hold views about women's proper place in society that are incompatible with the values held today in modern secular multi-cultural societies.

We are mentioning this example not to suggest that reference to the traditions of medicine is necessarily incompatible with the majority values held in modern twenty-first century societies. However, the ethical desirability of these traditions is not self-evident. Accordingly, it is necessary for defenders of these traditions to go beyond merely noting that these are the traditions and that we ought to abide by them, because they happen to be the traditions of a particular profession. What needs to be demonstrated is that we have good ethical or prudential reasons to follow tradition-based guidance. After all, in human history there have been any number of traditions, including cannibalism, slavery and the refusal to permit women to vote or to stand for election in democratic elections, to name just a few. If the mention of tradition was sufficient to justify particular conduct, all of these traditions would then be defensible. The absence of a normative justification and mere reference to something that is, namely a tradition, runs the risk of committing a variety of the naturalistic fallacy that we have discussed in Chapter 3. Nature is replaced here by tradition, but the error is essentially the same. Someone derives mistakenly from a description of how things are a normative conclusion of how things ought to be.

11.50

Questions

Do you think that the decriminalization of assisted dying is ethically (in)defensible? What are your ethical reasons for your answer?

Website Links

1   https://eiuperspectives.economist.com/healthcare/2015-quality-death-index
2   http://www.who.int/cancer/palliative/definition/en/
3   http://www.imdb.com/title/tt0070723/synopsis/
4   https://www.youtube.com/watch?v=8Sp-VFBbjpE
5   http://web.utk.edu/~jhardwig/DutyDie.pdf
6   https://www.theatlantic.com/magazine/archive/2014/10/why-i-hope-to-die-at-75/379329/
7   http://www.e-lawresources.co.uk/Volenti-non-fit-injuria.php/
8   http://www.investopedia.com/terms/i/inflectionpoint.asp/
9   https://bostonreview.net/books-ideas/fm-kamm-right-choose-death

10   http://www.current-oncology.com/index.php/oncology/article/view/883/645/

11   http://www.current-oncology.com/index.php/oncology/article/view/1063/913/

12   http://onlinelibrary.wiley.com/doi/10.1111/bioe.2011.25.issue-s1/issuetoc/

13   https://www.nlm.nih.gov/hmd/greek/greek_oath.html

14   https://www.wma.net/policies-post/declaration-on-euthanasia-and-physician-assisted-suicide/

15   https://www.britannica.com/biography/Marcel-Francois-Lefebvre/

16   https://www.learnreligions.com/what-is-the-tridentine-mass-542958/

12

JUSTICE AND HEALTH CARE

12.1 Introduction

Throughout this book you will have come across references to justice, and 12.1
to issues of resource allocation in health care. Justice is a huge topic and
arises in many different areas of life, notably crime and punishment, but
also in the workplace. You might want to look at Michael Walzer's *Spheres
of Justice* (1983).

Most, if not all of us, will have experienced the burning sense of 12.2
injustice when we feel we have been treated unfairly: it is one of the most
basic of moral intuitions, but explaining the concept of justice is far from
straightforward. In this chapter we will confine ourselves to the issues of
justice that arise in relation to health and health care. In this context one
of the principal issues concerns allocation of health resources, but justice
in health care is not confined to this. We shall begin therefore by exploring
different types of justice such as justice in distribution, procedural justice
and justice in relation to discrimination. Justice is commonly said to be
connected with equality, so we will proceed to examine in what ways
justice and equality might be connected, before linking the discussion of
justice with ethical theories discussed elsewhere in this book. This will
include a discussion of the extent to which health, or health care, is a proper
subject matter of justice at all. We will conclude by briefly considering
some special cases.

This Is Bioethics: An Introduction, First Edition. Ruth F. Chadwick and Udo Schüklenk.
© 2021 John Wiley & Sons, Inc. Published 2021 by John Wiley & Sons, Inc.

12.2 Types of Justice

12.2.1 Justice and Discrimination

12.3   Issues of discrimination such as ableism, sexism and racism are among the most widely discussed, not only in ethics texts but also in society. Justice in relation to discrimination concerns the ways in which treating people differently on the basis of some characteristic can be justified, or not. The presumption is that individuals and groups should be treated in the same way unless there is a relevant difference justifying different treatment. As in other areas of social life, in health(care) there is potential for unjustified discrimination against particular patient groups, for example, on grounds such as age, disability, sex, sexual orientation, or ethnicity where those characteristics are irrelevant to the provision of the health care in question. This discrimination may be direct or indirect. For example, if research on a new drug is carried out only on a particular type of patient (e.g. men between the ages of 20 and 40), those who do not fit that profile will not stand to receive evidence-based medicine (EBM) as far as that drug is concerned. This may be of concern to feminist bioethicists in particular. Wendy Rogers, for example, has written about the ways in which EBM may not serve the interests of women (Rogers 2004a, 2004b). It may be argued, on the other hand, that they may have been excluded from trials for what are considered to be good scientific or medical reasons (e.g. concerns about pregnancy in women), so that there may be no intention to discriminate against a given group directly: it may be rather a case of indirect discrimination, where the result is discriminatory as a matter of fact. It is important to be clear about when a characteristic is relevant and when it is not. You will no doubt be able to think of examples where factors such as age, ethnicity and gender are relevant to health care, and examples where they are not.

12.4   A relatively recent addition to the list of groups in relation to which discrimination in health care is being discussed is that of transgender people. There are issues not only about the right to health care for those who reject binary classifications in relation to sex and gender difference, but also about the right to health care of a certain kind. There may be controversy, for example, over the types of therapies offered and the stage of life at which it is appropriate to offer gender reassignment.

12.2.2 Justice in Distribution

In health care the type of justice most commonly considered, as already 12.5
indicated, is distributive justice. This concerns how resources are distributed
between different individuals and groups, and becomes an issue when
resources are scarce. In health care it is only too obvious, from media and
political debate, as well as from experience, that they are *always* scarce. Think,
for example, of the waiting lists for transplant organs, or access to intensive
care beds during the recent coronavirus pandemic. Beyond this, it is an
ongoing cause for concern that life expectancy varies markedly between
different regions of a given country. Questions arise as to the part played by
different contributory factors including poverty, environment, and lifestyle
choices, as well as the availability and accessibility of health care. However
plentiful the latter resources, there will always be more that could, in principle
at least, be offered, and advances in medical research create new demands
and expectations, just as the appointment of a consultant in a new specialism
will create another waiting list. However, it is not always made clear in debates
on this topic that the issues of distribution apply not just to expensive medicines, but also to things which may be overlooked such as the *time budget* of
professionals such as nurses. Sometimes spending time with/listening to a
patient might be the intervention that makes the most difference.

Justice in distribution requires criteria for resource allocation, sometimes 12.6
called 'priority setting'. Distribution of resources, however, is an issue not
only within but also between countries. This can be seen starkly in the
situations where pandemics emerge, but even without these occurrences,
global inequalities make themselves felt in health and life expectancy differentials, as we will see in Chapter 13.

Justice in discrimination and justice in distribution are not unrelated. 12.7
Issues of discrimination arguably have effects at a deep level in terms of the
social and economic structures that enable inequalities to continue, and
which are prior to specific allocation decisions, whether at a macro or micro
level. Recall perhaps John Hardwig's arguments in Chapter 11. A societal
decision not to provide sufficient resources to care for the elderly suddenly
makes caring for elderly parents a problem for their children. Macro level
allocation is concerned with how much of the health care budget is allo-
cated to, for example, cancer as opposed to cardiovascular disease. Micro
level allocation is concerned with questions such as who gets a kidney when
one becomes available for transplant. There are also decisions to be made

about the proportion of GDP in a given country that is spent on health care as opposed to defense, prior to the macro level allocation mentioned. This last point makes it clear, again, that health care allocation decisions are intertwined with political commitments.

12.2.3 Procedural Justice

12.8   It is important in health care to consider also procedural justice. Just as in the legal system, every individual has the right to a fair trial – to be subject to the same legal process as anyone else – so in other areas of life people should be treated in the same way, and be 'processed' in the same way, subject to the same recognized procedures, which have been established for a reason, and this has applicability to the health care context also. This is likely to vary in different clinical contexts but there are procedures to be followed, such as keeping accurate records, which are very important to the provision of appropriate care. Procedural justice is arguably underrepresented in bioethical debates, but is relevant to debates about 'queue jumping' and triage situations, where decisions have to be made about who should be treated first, e.g. in emergency situations.

12.9   Procedure is also important in relation to how people can access their share of social resources, particularly if they are economically disadvantaged and have to claim benefits. Margalit has argued (Margalit 1996) that it is part of having a 'decent' society that such claimants should not have to go through procedures that are humiliating – something that may exacerbate existing disadvantage.

12.2.4 Justice and Exploitation

12.10   Another sense in which issues of justice arise in health care concerns exploitation of people who might be unusually vulnerable. While 'exploitation' has a neutral sense to mean the use of resources, in the context of justice exploitation is the action of benefiting unfairly from the work or resources of someone else, to their disadvantage. Using adults and children as slave labor is an extreme example of this. In the reproduction context exploitation has been a concern in the employment of surrogate mothers to carry fetuses. In health care however, issues of exploitation have been discussed largely in relation to research, for example abuse of certain populations by using them as scientific 'guinea pigs' or taking tissue samples. However, the context in which it is delivered is constantly changing. We live today in the era of 'big data' – health and other information is being constantly collected, for example from smart watches that we choose to wear, and placed into large data sets, to be used for different purposes and possibly for the financial benefit of people other than those from whom the data originate. This is arguably one of the big bioethical issues of our time.

Where use of personal information is concerned, the question arises as to whether or not it retains personal identifiers. If information does not retain personal identifiers, then the ethical issues are fewer, but at the same time the data are less useful – which is an ethical issue in itself. Where information *does* retain personal identifiers there are clearly issues about the extent to which it can justifiably be used, and by whom.   12.11

A key ethical issue in the current context is that large companies such as Facebook, Google and pharmaceutical companies derive financial benefit from the collection of large data sets while those individuals who have contributed their data, whether deliberately, knowingly or not, do not. In research the cases of **John Moore**[1] and **Henrietta Lacks**[2] have given rise to much discussion, but in both cases the issues turned upon the collection of bodily tissue leading to profitable research and development. Where data alone are concerned, the issues are different. Do most people even realize that when they employ a wearable technology to monitor their physical activity, their data are being collected and analyzed elsewhere? It is a matter of justice, then, when one party, which has power, obtains financial benefit from the contribution of another party, without power, especially when the latter party derives no financial benefit.   12.12

It might be argued that the exploitation in these situations is not quite as bad as it might seem. Individuals who do not read privacy policies of large organizations, it might be held, have only themselves to blame. While it may be true today, however, that in principle everyone has the opportunity to read privacy policies, in practice this is unlikely to be realistic. Too much information in literally small print arguably does not meet the requirements of good information practice. On the other hand, the benefits of participating in the practices, such as social media, which make possible the collection of information, are considerable and may be thought to outweigh the risks by users of the services.   12.13

So, we can see that questions of justice in health and health care arise in different ways and in different contexts. We will now look at what the concept of justice means and in what ways, if any, it is connected with equality.   12.14

12.3 The Concept of Justice and its Connection
With Equality

12.15 Although it is widely held that justice and equality are connected, justice has been described as an 'essentially contested concept' (Gallie 1955) because there are several different interpretations of justice, which are in constant and irresolvable conflict, and which will apply in different ways to the issues of distribution. These must now be considered.

12.3.1 Justice and Equality: Equal Treatment
and Equal Consideration

12.16 We have already seen in the section on discrimination above, that the starting point is a presumption of equality and if we want to depart from that, it has to be justified in some way. How the connection between justice and equality should be spelled out, however, is not clear. Amartya Sen has argued that there is in fact no logical connection between justice and equality (Sen 1996). Rather, he says that the requirement of equality 'derives largely from the political regularities that have emerged over time in the beliefs and convictions of people' (ibid., p. 308). This has led to a situation where every theory of justice that is given serious consideration does demand equality of some kind. The question for justice then becomes, as Sen notes – equality of what? Equal consideration? Equal treatment? Equal rights? Equality of opportunity?

12.17 Let's take equal treatment as an example. The presumption is that people should be treated equally, unless there is a difference between them that is relevant to the treatment in question and which justifies different treatment. For example, in distributing food, there is a relevant difference between a two-year old child and a grown man that justifies us in departing from the principle of equal shares. So not all inequalities are necessarily unjust: the issue is when inequality becomes *inequity*.

12.18 In fact, it might be argued that, if we interpret 'justice as equality' correctly, the above example does not represent a departure from the principle. In order to treat people equally, it does not necessarily mean that we should treat people in *exactly the same way*. Rather, we ought to give equal consideration to equal interests, or needs. In the food example, one person's needs are greater than the other's, but the needs of both are satisfied. So they have, in a sense, been treated equally in that their needs have been given equal consideration.

Problems arise when the needs of some people are given less weight than   12.19
others for reasons that are irrelevant. The point in question is how some
individuals may be treated worse than others, because of irrelevant factors,
whether or not this amounts to discrimination on the basis of a group characteristic, as discussed above. One may in some circumstances unjustifiably
be treated worse as an individual without that amounting to racism or sexism or any other -ism.

The example of food allocation above showed that treating people   12.20
exactly the same when there are relevant differences between them
would not give the right result and that what we should focus on is not
equal treatment but equal consideration. Different theories have different
answers as to how to do this. For the utilitarian 'each counts for one and no
one for more than one' – this is an interpretation of equality. Suffering is
bad whenever and wherever it occurs. We will see in Chapter 13 that this
view has far reaching implications for the issue of global health obligations.
For Kantian ethics, on the other hand, each individual person has an
inherent worth. In health care, however, as in the area of other public
services that are in short supply, it is not always possible to treat everyone
in the way that we might want. Even if it is bad for anyone to suffer, and
even if every individual has inherent worth, choices have to be made,
priorities have to be established if the resources are insufficient to meet
everyone's needs, and that is why we need principles of distributive justice
to explain when and how we can give people equal consideration but also
justifiably depart from equal treatment.

12.3.2 Justice, 'Deserving', and Personal Responsibility

A popular way of interpreting justice is in terms of what people 'deserve'.   12.21
Think, for example, of how strong this intuition can be in the criminal
justice context. This view is frequently aired in contemporary health care
debates: for example, in the view that liver transplants should not be
available to alcoholics, who may be perceived as responsible for their own
health problems. Justice, it might be said, is a matter of getting one's 'due'
where this is interpreted in terms of merit. This is what justifies a departure
from equal treatment, on this view. There are two senses in which it might
be argued that not all patients are equally deserving. First, some people's ill
health may be due to some feature of their lifestyle that could have been
avoided – smoking, overeating, drinking heavily or sexual promiscuity, for
example. We will have a closer look at this issue in Chapter 13. Do such

individuals deserve the same level of care as the fitness conscious person who 'out of the blue' is struck down by a tragic disease?

12.22   The flip side of the coin of the idea that individuals should be held responsible for their lives, including their health, is that it is in fact just to try to counteract the effects of bad luck in people's experience. It could be argued that we are not giving people equal consideration if this is not taken into account. Holding people responsible might be all very well in areas of life where individuals can be said to have control, but there are others where they do not. The view known as **luck egalitarianism**[3] takes this approach (Segall 2009).

12.23   The view that individuals should take more responsibility for their own health, however, has become increasingly influential in public policy in recent years, in part because of the perceived spiraling demand for health care resources. From smoking to obesity, from alcohol consumption to exercise, there is a constant outpouring of advice. Wearable technologies, allowing people to measure their heart rate and exercise, are increasingly widely used. But whatever we might think of the connection between justice, desert and responsibility, to operate a health service on the basis of such criteria would be impractical. If, for example, there is a statistically greater risk of serious injury for car drivers (who freely choose to take this risk) as compared with pedestrians, does it follow that pedestrians should take priority in health care? To implement such a policy would not be feasible. There is also a deeper objection to the desert argument. The desert model of justice rests on the assumption that, as autonomous persons, we are all responsible for the choices we make. But however much we might support autonomy as an ideal, it is essential to recognize that as a matter of fact, the social context in which people live often restricts the extent to which they can exercise their autonomy, or at least the extent to which they feel that they can. Feminist bioethicists, for example, will be concerned about the structural inequalities and constraints that affect the contexts in which people make decisions. You may recall this was alluded to in the discussion of reproductive choices in Chapter 5. It may be very difficult for individuals to exercise certain choices in particular situations. These may include factors as different as the availability of different and affordable foods, peer group pressure, as well as feelings of self-esteem which may be undermined by social inequalities. Economic difficulties, perhaps arising from unemployment, can all have a bearing on the exercise of autonomy.

12.24   The second way in which some people might be said to deserve less than others is where they may be thought to have already had more than, or enough of their fair share – you might recall the metaphor of the 'fair innings' that we discussed in Chapter 11, where Harris argued that younger people may deserve priority (see John Harris 1985). This sentiment might be bolstered by the thought that younger people have potentially more to contribute to society, or at least more time in which to do so. On the other hand, it may be argued that older people who have paid their taxes throughout their working lives 'deserve' to get some return on this. Thus we can see that there are different interpretations of 'desert' at stake.

12.3.3 Justice is Giving People What They Need

Another conception of justice in distribution suggests that resources should 12.25 be distributed according to need. Again, starting from a presumption of equality, people who have equal needs should be treated the same, but those whose need is greater should be given priority. You will find discussion in Chapter 13 about some difficulties in putting this into practice. There are strong supporters, however, of the view that need is specially pertinent as a criterion in health care. **Bernard Williams**[4] argued that as a matter of *logic* health care should be distributed on the basis of need (Williams 1973). There are goods logically internal to an area of practice and goods that are external. Ability to pay is an example of a criterion that is not logically connected with distribution of health care: it is not relevant to considerations of justice in distribution and is thus an 'external' good. It is not possible in this volume to take into account the detail of different ways in which health care delivery is managed in different countries, but we can note that, for example, the U.K. National Health Service has traditionally operated on the principle that care should be free at the point of delivery and distributed according to need, quite different from some systems elsewhere in the world.

We have briefly outlined different ways in which justice might be con- 12.26 nected with equality and in which it is claimed that departures from equality might be justified. We will now look more closely at justice in different ethical theories discussed in this book.

12.4 Theories of Justice

12.4.1 Utility and Well-Being

When we turn to a utility-based theory of justice, we are inevitably being 12.27 directed towards consideration of consequences and outcome. The question is, how is that outcome to be measured? The extent to which life can be extended is obviously an issue. But what about the quality of that life? Much effort has gone into trying to develop tools to measure outcome successfully. Utilitarianism as an ethical theory, as we have seen, includes both a concept of well-being and a principle of maximization: in other words, it is essential not only to know what outcome is being aimed at but also to produce as much of it as possible.

12.28   The most well-known concept of well-being that has been developed in the context of health care distribution is the QALY (**quality-adjusted life year**[5]), although there are variants of it such as the DALY (**disability-adjusted life year**[6]). The QALY was one of the earliest tools for evaluating interventions and it measures not only quantity of life achieved but also quality. This reflects the view that it is not only how long we can extend life for that is important.

12.29   The essence of a QALY is that it takes a whole year of life expectancy to be worth 1, but regards a year of unhealthy life expectancy as worth less than 1. Its precise value is lower, the worse the quality of life of the unhealthy person (this is the 'quality adjusted bit') If being dead is worth zero, it is, in principle, possible for a QALY to be negative., i.e., for the quality of someone's life to be judged worse than being dead (Williams 1995, 222).

12.30   The QALY's advantage, apart from providing a tool of measurement, is that it can offer a mechanism for making a decision: if intervention X will produce three QALYs, but intervention Y will produce 5, then intervention 5 is the right choice.

12.31   Decision-makers tasked with showing that a new development is cost-effective may find QALYs particularly useful, and they have in fact been used as the principal decision-making tool by the **National Institute for Health and Care Excellence**[7] in the UK (NICE). They may be of particular help in those situations where 'life' and 'quality' are both at stake, but where these two point in different directions, as may be the case in some cancer treatments. Treatment interventions may prolong life but have a negative impact on its quality for the patient.

12.32   The QALY has had many critics, however, who have pointed out its weaknesses. The main difficulty concerns how the QALY is measured: who decides what a certain state of health is worth? Perceptions of value have to feed into the establishment of QALYs and into rival tools such as the DALY. There are, however, several problems regarding the methodology for assessing the quality element. People who have a particular condition are likely to have a different view of it from those who have not experienced it. There is also a view that different types of features of quality are *incommensurable*, for example, physical as opposed to mental suffering (Evans 2013). If the information is based on the preferences of individual patients, furthermore, there are clearly difficulties in collecting health-related quality-of-life information from some groups of patients, such as children and persons suffering from mental disorder.

NICE in the UK based its QALY measurement on public preferences   12.33
across the population. Although in the UK NICE used cost-utility as a methodology, the unit of measurement being the QALY, with £20,000 per QALY being considered good value for money, until 2012, after that time there was a turn to cost- consequences and cost-benefit analysis, to take into account the wider picture in terms of effects of society and health, as well as those factors that are included in a QALY calculation (see the **briefing**[8] on the NICE website).

A second serious ethical objection to the use of QALYs relates to con-   12.34
cerns about equity. It might be assumed that an additional QALY has the same weight regardless of the other characteristics of the individuals in question. This is a reflection, in QALY terms, of the utilitarian principle that each counts for one and no one for more than one. A QALY counts the same no matter whose life it is. This, however, is not a position with which all members of the public are likely to agree (remember, for example, issues about 'desert' above) and it is significant that in developing other measurement tools, such as the DALY (disability-adjusted life-year) age based considerations have been included (Vergel and Schulpher 2008).

It might appear that applying QALYs to distribution issues is bound to   12.35
result in a preference for interventions benefitting young people, partly because more life years can in all likelihood be achieved, but also because of perceptions of quality of those years in later life as compared with youth and indeed midlife. You might recall what Ezekiel Emanuel had to say on this matter in Chapter 11. In addition, health care for the elderly is likely to be high in cost. Nevertheless, when cost per QALY is calculated some interventions benefitting older persons, such as hip replacements, may compare favorably with very expensive interventions on younger people.

It is important to note that age may be argued to be a relevant character-   12.36
istic not only in relation to treatment for people in the later stages of life: it has also been used, at different times and in varying ways, to put a ceiling on eligibility for reproductive technologies, for example, and to establish a threshold for the permissibility of gender reassignment.

There is an argument that ageism is different from other forms of   12.37
discrimination because every one of us, if fortunate enough to survive, will

become old, whereas it is not the case that, absent special circumstances, we will become a member of the opposite sex, or become a member of a different ethnic group. Of course, there are fuzzy boundaries in relation to these other isms – for example, in relation to genetic ancestry tracing there have been re-categorizations of people's line of descent in some cases. The main point however, as you will recall, is that treating someone differently on the basis of a characteristic that is irrelevant to the treatment in question is wrong. So the question then becomes, *is it* irrelevant to the treatment in question? Some may feel that if a person does not have long to live then that *is* relevant to the treatment in question, in a situation of scarce resources.

12.38   There are disagreements, however, about how we should take age into account. Should we be addressing the allocation issue across whole lifetimes, or taking an approach relevant to a specific slice of time? This might give us a different picture. Can you think of examples of how this might make a difference?

12.39   Another objection to the use of the QALY and other such decision tools arises from the view that such a procedure fails to give due weight to the individual. Each person has only one life which is of unique importance to them, and to use QALYs to take health care decisions involves, it is argued, weighing lives against each other. However, the fact of scarce resources suggests that weighing lives is unavoidable (Ventakapuram 2011, 185). It is true, however, that the use of the QALY is subject to the same objection frequently levelled at utilitarianism in general – namely that it is concerned with aggregation (in order to achieve its maximization aim) rather than with fairness in distribution. Decisions about people's treatment and lives become a numbers game.

12.4.2 *Respect for Persons: Rights to Health and Health Care*

12.40   A Kantian-inspired 'respect for persons' approach to justice in health care might take a number of forms: we have already noted the emphasis on the inherent worth of the individual. It might be argued, based on this line of thought, that there is a right to health or, at a minimum, to health care. What might this mean? What content could be given by to such a right? As indicated above, in the face of increasing pressure on health resources, it has been argued that individuals are expected to take more responsibility for their own health and this could in fact be understood as respecting the individual as a person who is accountable for their own choices. Especially in the light of the purported shift towards personalized medicine, however, there are questions about how far we should be expected to go in monitoring our vital signs, the number of steps we talk, our calorie intake, and so on.

To argue for a right to health is difficult: first, there are the ongoing dif- 12.41 ficulties of providing an acceptable definition of health to give content to such a right; and second, to say that there is a right to something implies that someone has a responsibility to provide it, and 'health' is not something that can be guaranteed. Health care, however, is a different matter. It at least appears to make sense to speak of a right to health care. But then there are difficult questions about how much health care – attempts to define a minimum acceptable level are not without controversy. Also, this might be interpreted in a context specific way, dependent upon available resources. This has the potential to reinforce existing geographical inequalities.

12.4.3 *John Rawls and Norman Daniels*

John Rawls' theory of justice, as you may recall from Chapter 2, depicts 12.42 rational agents coming together behind a 'veil of ignorance' to choose principles of justice for society, including the principles for distribution of 'primary goods'. He divided primary goods into 'natural goods' and 'social goods', the former being mental and bodily attributes; while the latter include income and wealth along with liberties and opportunities. He argues that rational contractors would choose two general principles: (1) Each person has an equal right to the most extensive liberties compatible with similar liberties for all (the principle of equal liberty; (2) Social and economic inequalities should be arranged so that they are both (a) to the greatest benefit of the least advantaged and (b) attached to offices and positions open to all under conditions of equality of opportunity. Rawls in *A Theory of Justice*, however, famously described health as a natural rather than a social good – and thus not an object for justice in distribution (Rawls 1971) – but the ways in which social factors can affect health is now widely recognized, so it is important to consider whether health is a matter for justice in distribution.

It is certainly true that we are all born with different genetic potential 12.43 (there may even be differences in the number of copies of a genetic factor between identical twins), and we know an increasingly large amount about the ways in which our genomes make us unique individuals. It is also true that for some genetic disorders there is no known cure. Although these differences in our make-up exist, however, that does not mean that we have to accept that nothing can be done to rectify the imbalances in the 'natural' order of things. Nor does it mean that issues of health justice do not arise. Much depends on how the concept of health is understood so we need to address this briefly.

12.44   Health defined as complete physical mental or spiritual well-being, as suggested in the constitution of the **World Health Organization**[9] is an ideal but in practice unattainable goal for society. Thus, it cannot be an end point for justice. If the circumstances of justice include limited resources, then to define as a goal something which would require unlimited resources is a non-starter. Something more modest is required, something which takes into account the relative nature of health and its context dependency. Once this is accepted, it becomes a suitable topic for justice.

12.45   If health is interpreted as the absence of disease, then it might appear that health cannot be provided for persons born with a genetic disorder. We know today that everyone has in their genome variations that are less than advantageous, and that whatever our 'natural' genetic endowment, we will all succumb to ill health, and death, at some point, discussions about life-extension enhancements notwithstanding. This model is flawed, however, in so far as it implies that health is a state of the individual, rather than a result of the relationship between the individual and the environment. And yet we know that our environment has a huge impact, most notably but not exclusively in relation to infectious diseases in different contexts, which any given individual may not have contracted had they remained in a different environment.

12.46   So, if health is interpreted in a different way, e.g. as adaptation to one's environment, including the social environment, then in principle, at least, adjustments can be made to the environment which make the individual count as someone who has a state of health. The developing science of epigenetics is also providing more information about how environments, including the environment of the womb, can impact upon the health of an individual and indeed upon their descendants. In turn these considerations allow for issues of justice to arise, as there may be social and political decisions, outside of the individual's control, that produce environments not conducive to health.

12.47   **Sridhar Ventakapuram**[10] has argued that there are four different categories of determinants of health, including biological, individual, social and environmental. Just as in disability studies it has been successfully argued that disability is at least in part a social construction, similar points can be made about the wider category of health. Environmental toxins such as **lead**[11] and **air pollution**[12], are all known to have a detrimental effect on health. You might want to look at the 2019 **report**[13] by the WHO on environmental health inequalities in Europe. More insidious threats are the social ones of stress, **poverty**[14] and so on. Power differentials and the vulnerability of certain groups play a very big part in issues of justice and discrimination – as feminist bioethicists have pointed out. We noted in the Chapter 10 the ways in which women historically were at times diagnosed with mental health disorders if they overstepped what were perceived as the appropriate boundaries.

Nevertheless there remain proponents of the view that it is health *care*, 12.48 rather than health *per se,* that can be the subject of justice, as of rights. Health care is more overtly something that can be and is distributed. Once we get into talking about health care the issues of distribution are easier to address, conceptually at least, if not practically.

Norman Daniels has developed a Rawlsian approach to justice which 12.49 adapts it to enable it to apply to health care (Daniels 2008). For Daniels what is important is the restoration of people to normal species functioning so that they have access to the 'normal opportunity range' in society. Daniels took one of Rawls's primary goods, fair equality of opportunity, and interpreted it as fair equality of opportunity to pursue a normal opportunity range of life plans for a society. Poor health can clearly have an adverse impact on ability to do this, so individuals should have access to health care. A just distribution will be judged by its impact on fair equality of opportunity. Although it might appear that it is unclear how this should be applied in making resource allocation decisions in health care, Daniels adjusted his theory to take social determinants of health into account and specified a list of six health needs (Daniels 2010). On Daniels' revision of Rawls, rational individuals behind the veil of ignorance would want to ensure that these were satisfied.

12.4.4 The Capabilities Approach

The capabilities *approach* is so-called because it is said not to be a complete 12.50 theory of justice. Its distinguishing characteristics are that it involves a focus on what people can be and do rather than what they have. Developed by Amartya Sen and Martha Nussbaum (Sen 1996; Nussbaum 2011), the capabilities approach in terms of health will aim to provide a space, metaphorically speaking, in which people can realize their capabilities. From this perspective it is not well-being that is important, or the distribution of any resource such as health care *per se,* but the recognition of what individuals require in order to flourish. Ventakapuram, building on the capabilities approach, has argued for a vision of health justice that focuses on a capability to be healthy (CH) (Ventakapuram 2011). The CH is described as a 'meta-capability' to enable individuals to achieve the capabilities that Nussbaum identifies as elements of a fully human life. The advantage of this approach, according to him, is that it takes into account multiple determinants of health and has wide-ranging implications in what is required in terms of a social response. Distributing health care is insufficient: 'providing or supporting threshold levels of CH entails social action through influencing the social bases of the causal components of each Capability' (ibid., p. 156). The social action required is likely to differ according to social context: 'when considering the spread of HIV/AIDS it becomes easy to see that in the absence of an HIV vaccine, avoiding infection requires having control over one's body and behavior over the entire life course. Prior to global experience with HIV/AIDS and the women's health movement, it was commonplace to think that healthcare is necessary and sufficient to address health concerns' (ibid., p. 157).

12.51   A challenge for the CH approach lies in the very fact that it is so potentially wide. Interpreting justice in health care as requiring social action in relation to the social determinants of health suggests obligations on an indefinite number of actors and institutions, not only health care institutions and health professionals.

12.5 Special Cases

12.52   There are issues about particular areas of health care and whether they give rise to special consideration as regards justice. One person's perception of need may be regarded as a luxury by others. Examples of this include cosmetic surgery, reproductive technologies, and tattoo removal. You will surely be able to think of other examples.

12.53   We have discussed the right to reproduce in Chapter 5. Even if it is accepted that there is a right to have a child, however, even within this category it may be argued that some *means* are more contentious than others. Significant variables include the extent of invasiveness, the probability of success, what alternatives are available, and the expense. Beyond this the 'yuk' factor also may play a part in the extent to which an intervention is regarded as something to which people ought to have access where public funding is involved.

12.5.1 Personalized Medicine and Justice

Personalized medicine may have consequences that are difficult to justify if   12.54
it is more or less only available in resource-rich environments, and so creates problems in terms of global justice. Its association with individualism is problematic for some, but as we have seen in Chapter 8, one important caveat is that personalized medicine may in fact be more about patient stratification rather than individualization, which potentially raises issues of justice of another kind.

The issue of neglected diseases is an important one worldwide. Traditionally   12.55
there has been little economic incentive for big pharmaceutical companies to develop treatments for diseases from which few people suffer, or diseases from which many people suffer who are unable to afford a potential future drug. Clearly in an era when pharmaceutical companies want to develop blockbusters, small, potentially impoverished disease communities are not an attractive target. In the era of personalized medicine, however, blockbusters have been said to be a thing of the past, and it has been envisaged that there may be special opportunities here for under-served populations in emerging economies.

The 'contest' about the meaning and application of justice in health and   12.56
health care goes on. Even if we take justice to have a close link with equality, Sen's question 'equality of what?' continues to have many competing answers. Social and political factors are at work in the move towards personalization and greater demands of personal responsibility, and have to be taken into account.

At the heart of the dispute about distributive justice there is a disagreement   12.57
about what is to be distributed. If the issue is the distribution of health care then there is a question about criteria for distributing that. If focusing on distributing health care is too narrow, however, in view of all the evidence about social determinants of health, nationally and globally, then the questions of justice become much wider. Added to that are all the issues about different kinds of discrimination at work in different societies, apart from the environmental factors that require social action. Underlying all these questions there remains an ongoing question on how we are to understand the concept of health itself.

Questions

Think about the ways in which justice has been connected with equality. Which, if any, seems most plausible to you, and why?

Is it possible, in your view, to find a way of justly allocating health resources?

Website Links

1   https://law.justia.com/cases/california/supreme-court/3d/51/120.html
2   https://www.hopkinsmedicine.org/henriettalacks/
3   https://plato.stanford.edu/entries/justice-bad-luck/
4   https://plato.stanford.edu/entries/williams-bernard/
5   https://yhec.co.uk/glossary/quality-adjusted-life-year-qaly/
6   https://www.who.int/healthinfo/global_burden_disease/metrics_daly/en/
7   https://www.nice.org.uk/
8   https://www.nice.org.uk/Media/Default/guidance/LGB10-Briefing-20150126.pdf
9   https://www.who.int/
10   https://www.kcl.ac.uk/people/sridhar-venkatapuram
11   https://www.who.int/ipcs/assessment/public_health/lead/en/
12   https://www.who.int/sustainable-development/cities/health-risks/air-pollution/en/
13   http://www.euro.who.int/en/publications/abstracts/environmental-health-inequalities-in-europe.-second-assessment-report-2019
14   https://www.health.org.uk/infographic/poverty-and-health/

13

POPULATION HEALTH

13.1 Global Health Issues

Population and global health ethics are concerned with population-level 13.1
and international health issues. Diseases do not cease to exist at our national
borders, infectious diseases, for instance, easily migrate across borders
while many non-communicable diseases also affect humanity globally.

We will start off this chapter by having a closer look at two different ethi- 13.2
cal questions: The first question is this: given global health needs, is anything owed, in terms of health aid, to those of us who live in dire poverty in
countries of the global south, and, if health aid is owed, who owes it. The
second question we will investigate is this: given that demands on global
health aid are likely to outstrip the amount of aid that is made available,
how should we best prioritize the allocation of health aid? Some of the
consideration you are now familiar with from Chapter 12 will help us in
addressing this question.

We will proceed from there to discussing the meanings of population 13.3
and public health. Having gained a better understanding of the concepts
that underlie the idea of public health, we will analyze in greater detail some
of the ethical challenges a communicable illness like HIV or SARS-CoV2
pose for us as individuals as well as for policy makers. Areas that we will
also take a closer look at include difficult questions surrounding the
ethics of compulsory vaccination, public health promotion campaigns, and
obesity prevention.

This Is Bioethics: An Introduction, First Edition. Ruth F. Chadwick and Udo Schüklenk.
© 2021 John Wiley & Sons, Inc. Published 2021 by John Wiley & Sons, Inc.

13.2 Health Aid Obligations

13.4 Globalization has succeeded in lifting millions of people in the global south out of dire poverty. The United Nations reports that one of its **Millennium Development Goals**[1], namely to cut the number of people who live in extreme poverty globally by half, **was reached around 2010**[2]. That translates into 1 billion people having left extreme poverty behind. The average global life expectancy has significantly increased during the last few decades. However, these benefits have not been evenly distributed. Some of the changes brought about by globalization also led to some people sinking into extreme poverty. As you might recall from our first two chapters, there are some prima facie reasons for thinking that people living in the global north have moral health aid obligations toward people living in the global south.

13.5   Two influential lines of reasoning in support of such health aid obligations have emerged, they are Kantian and utilitarian or consequentialist inspired respectively. The first rationale was developed by renowned political philosopher Thomas Pogge. He argues, essentially, that health aid is owed, because most of the worst instances of extreme poverty in the world, and the **known health consequences that extreme poverty entails**[3], are directly or indirectly caused by a world economic system forced by the countries of the global north on countries of the global south. (Pogge 2008; Lowry and Schüklenk 2009) How does this claim square against the earlier mentioned improvements in average life expectancy and the declining number of people living in abject poverty globally? Pogge does *not* need to dispute that *on balance* globalization has done more good than harm as far as the issue of impoverished citizens of the global south is concerned, his argument would succeed if he could show that particular, identifiable people living there live in abject poverty *because* of the same economic system that might have benefited others like them. These individuals would have been harmed by that system.

13.6   This kind of analysis is arguably primarily directed at people who are opposed to giving health aid for any number of reasons, including 'my fellow citizens first' (that is, nationalism). Even **libertarians**[4] who might be opposed to the state-financed (that is, tax financed) provision of international health aid, because they do not believe it is the state's role to provide such aid, should be open to arguments showing that their country's wealth is partly a consequence of demonstrable harm inflicted unjustly on others. Libertarians typically accept that if we have attained our wealth by unjust means, compensation could be justifiable.

A number of criticisms have been mounted against Pogge's analysis. One 13.7
counter argument is of a consequentialist nature. The argument suggests
that if – in balance – globalization has done more good than harm, it is
unfortunate that a smaller number of people has lost out as a result of globalization, but given the much larger number of people who are demonstrably better off than they would have been had globalization not occurred,
globalization was the morally right thing to do under the circumstances.
Those who were the beneficiaries of this project should not be held responsible for its foreseeable harmful consequences, especially if the only way to
achieve the desirable outcomes was at the cost incurred by those who saw
their quality of life deteriorate (Risse 2005).

Another criticism maintains that there will be people in the global south 13.8
who might find themselves in dire need of health aid but who are unable to
demonstrate that they are directly victims of globalization. Who could find
themselves in that situation? Think, for instance, of victims of natural catas-
trophes like tsunamis or earthquakes. Wealthy people in the global north
with the capacity to assist would be under no moral obligation to render
assistance in the form of health aid, at least not those whose decisions,
about who to provide health aid to, base their actions on Pogge's analysis.
Christopher Lowry has suggested that Pogge's analysis could be rescued
from such a counter-intuitive conclusion (Lowry and Schüklenk 2009). He
argues that the reason why natural disasters (such as, for instance, the 2010
earthquake in Haiti[5]) cause enormous damage in many countries of the
global south, is because impoverished nations cannot afford to invest
(unlike, for instance **Japan**[6]) in the infrastructure necessary to prevent significant loss of human lives.

Finally, it has been suggested that even if Pogge's analysis was sound, it 13.9
would mean little, practically, because it would be next to impossible to
quantify the harm done and the compensation owed in individual cases.
Say, even if we acknowledged that the slave trade and colonialism did significant damage to West African nations and their citizens, what would that
mean for the question of whether we had a moral obligation to assist specifically Sierra Leonians during the 2014 Ebola virus outbreak?

Consequentialists have developed a different case in support of the view 13.10
that people with the capacity to assist owe health aid to those in dire need.
Fairly prominent among those arguing this case is the utilitarian Peter Singer
(Singer 1972, 2004). The key feature relevant to a being's moral standing is, as
we have seen in Chapter 2, the capacity to feel pain. Suffering is something we
try to avoid, if we can. The premature, preventable deaths of impoverished

people and the suffering that that usually entails, have negative moral value. This moral badness remains the same regardless of our geographical distance to their suffering. The premature preventable death of a person in the global south is just as bad as the premature preventable death of a comparable person in the global north. Our obligations to people in far-away places do not diminish as a result of their distance to us. If we are in a situation, either individually or as a community, to prevent the moral bad that these preventable deaths would be, we have an obligation to act, provided we do not incur unreasonably high cost ourselves. Among consequentialists as well as critics of consequentialism there has been intensive debate about what constitutes unreasonably high cost, but we cannot get into this discussion here. If we accept Singer's premises, it would follow, for the case under consideration, that we would have a moral obligation to provide health aid. What remains a contested issue is the extent of those obligations.

13.2.1 Allocation Priorities

13.11   Let us assume, for the sake of the argument, that we agreed that some health aid was owed to people living in countries of the global south, and that those in the global north, with the means to assist, agreed to provide it. The odds are that the amount of health aid made available would remain insufficient (Chatham House 2011). Given the relative scarcity of available health aid, how should we go about deciding who among those in need should be prioritized? We have discovered already that, all other things being equal, distance as such is not a morally defensible decision-making criterion. What guidance, if any, would the two approaches to global health obligations provide us with? It is worth noting, of course, that even if we were to consider one or another of these models persuasive, it would not follow that the same model would also have to be deployed to guide us in making resource allocation decisions. You have already read a fair bit about justice in the allocation of scarce resources in Chapter 12, so we will not rehash that content at this point. We are following closely an analysis presented by Lowry and Schüklenk (Lowry and Schüklenk 2009). They claim that Pogge's model is unable to guide our prioritization decision-making concerning the allocation of health aid. While it might provide us with good reasons for why health aid is owed, it has nothing to contribute when we are trying to figure out who to assist in particular.

13.12   Typically, when we are faced with the necessity to make and justify allocation decisions, we are looking at three criteria to help us in that process: *need, efficiency* and *responsibility*. It does not take a lot of imagination to appreciate why each of these criteria matters. If someone is in more urgent need than another, we should, all other things being equal, prioritize the neediest person. By taking into account need we are also less likely to waste scarce resource on someone who might not need assistance to begin with. Efficiency is another uncontroversial criterion. If I have limited health care resources, I should aim at deploying them as efficiently as is possible to ensure the greatest possible return on the resources utilized. Then there is the matter of responsibility. Who is responsible for the health need? Answers to the responsibility question could potentially assist us in determining who should contribute to addressing the problem at hand. Pogge's approach to global health aid obligations would, as we have already seen, ask us to focus exclusively on responsibility. Lowry and Schüklenk argue that responsibility is not a good decision-making criterion, because it would be fairly difficult, if not impossible, to determine precise causal responsibilities for particular health problems in the global south. Further complicating this matter is that it is also true that decisions by, say, the government of the United Kingdom, would have more uncontroversially demonstrable consequences for citizens of that country. A focus on degrees of responsibility would almost always lead us to focus first on what is happening at home, and rarely, if ever, on other parts of the world where people's health needs are often both greater as well as more urgent, and where greater amounts of positive health outcomes could be generated with the amount of health aid resources available to us.

Would the nature of someone's need offer us a more defensible decision-making criterion? Pogge's analysis does not address need. We have noted earlier that even great needs arising, for instance from natural disasters, would not result in a moral obligation to provide emergency health aid on Pogge's account, because they are not a result of the global economic order but of nature causing havoc. Accordingly, need does not feature as a relevant decision-making criterion. The same holds true for consequentialists. Being primarily concerned with generating the maximum amount of positive health outcomes that available health aid can reasonably produce, their focus would be on efficiency rather than need or responsibility. This could well mean that they would not assist those in most dire need if that required a highly resource intensive effort and if more people elsewhere could be assisted, promising an overall greater number of desirable health outcomes.

13.14   What is the problem with a singular focus on efficiency? It is conceivable that this could result in those most vulnerable, and those most in need, such as for instance people in war torn areas of the world, never receiving health aid, simply because the resource required to reach them would be disproportionately high and so efficacy would demand that the finite health aid resource available ought to be deployed elsewhere, to greater effect. That does seem unfair, doesn't it? The **victims of the Sudanese**[7] war were not exactly responsible for the predicament they found themselves in. The consequentialist charged with allocating scarce health aid donations could retort that if more lives worth living can be preserved with the means available, provided we give those in most need a lower priority ranking, then that's what we ought to do, otherwise we would practically ascribe greater value to the lives of those in most need. Apologetically the consequentialist might add that the state of the world is not of their making and that they merely aim to achieve the best outcomes with the limited resources they have available. All lives deserving of assistance could be preserved if we increased the amount of health aid made available, but until then, if allocation decisions have to be made at all, we should focus on efficiency as the decisive selection criterion.

13.15   We have seen that there are plausible accounts on why health aid is owed globally to others in far-away places. The same accounts, when put to the task of determining who should receive our aid, given that we are unlikely to be able to assist everyone who deserves assistance, lead to quite different responses. What is your view on the question of global health aid? Is it owed by those who have the capacity to assist, to others who could benefit from it? If not, why not? If you agree, how would you decide who should be prioritized as a recipient of health aid?

13.3 Population Health and Public Health

13.16 Population and public health ethics try to address the ethical implications of population or public health issues. Before we have a closer look at some of these issues, let us clear a bit of conceptual ground. What do we mean by 'population health', and how does it differ from 'public health'? Can there even be such a thing as 'public health' or 'population health'? Marcel Verweij and Angus Dawson are two experts in public health ethics. They are also the editors of a leading international journal called *Public Health Ethics*. They have tried to figure out what exactly 'public health' means. This is what they came up with (Verweij and Dawson 2013, 4221):

> Public health is a disputed concept. It refers to the health of the population as a group, as well as to organizations and practices that aim to promote health. In order to avoid confusion it is helpful to use the term 'population health' for the former and to define 'public health' as *collective interventions to promote or protect the health of the population.*

Verweij and Dawson's distinction is today widely used. Another writer, Adrian Viens comes up with a comparable definition for 'population ethics' (Viens 2014, 2415–6):   13.17

> Population ethics is an area of ethics concerned with questions and problems that arise about populations and how population-level issues present questions and problems that are distinct from traditional individual-level issues that have been the predominant focus of ethics.

John Duffy describes 'public health' as 'the collective action by community or society to protect and promote the health and welfare of its members' (Duffy 2014). Population health ethics then is concerned about the health of populations, public health ethics is concerned about the actions taken by society to protect the health of populations. If you were to extend that thinking to global matters, you would have global health. The health of populations is what public health policy makers want to protect. What could possibly be wrong with that, you ask? Well, at least one libertarian philosopher thinks that Verweij and Dawson and other population or public health ethics academics talk plain nonsense. Please note, when you read the following quote, that what the writer, Richard D. Mohr, criticizes in his 1980s article is what the above authors would refer today to as 'population health', except that in the 1980s he chose to refer to 'population health' as 'public health'. Let that not confuse you!   13.18

Here is Richard D. Mohr's* critique of mainstream views of what we would call public health today (Mohr 1987, 46–50):   13.19

---

* Mohr is not the only philosopher defending such a stance. Patricia Illingworth defended a similar line of reasoning in *AIDS and the Good Society* (1990). You might find the discussion between the public health focused Ronald Bayer (1989) and the individual liberties focused Patricia Illingworth (1990, 1991) in the journal *Bioethics* worth your time. We have referred to them in our Further Reading suggestions.

Doctors tend to hold the unrefined view that health policy is merely a matter of strategy because they, not surprisingly, tend to see health itself as a trumping good, second to none in importance. This is a dangerous view, especially when coupled with their idea that health is an undifferentiated good. They fail to distinguish between my harming my health and my harming your health. Behind this oversight lies the further presumption that you and I are both absorbed into and subordinated under something called the public health. ... No literal sense exists in which there could be such a thing as public health. To say the public has a health is like saying the number seven has a color: such a thing cannot have such a property. You have health or you lack it and I have health or lack it, because we each have a body with organs that function or do not function.

13.20   Let us halt for a moment and reflect on the significance of Mohr's point about the relative as opposed to the absolute value of health in our lives. Michael Allen, for instance, argues that health and individual liberty are of coequal value (Allen 2011). What is the value of health then? It is worthwhile perhaps to ask why health is important to us. Here is an attempt at an answer, provided by Christopher R. Lowry and Udo Schüklenk (2009). They write:

We can start by asking why health is important. Its importance is pervasive. Nearly every valuable human activity is ultimately supported by health and undermined by illness. There is a close connection between health and many prominent moral values. Health has a strong tendency to contribute to happiness or utility. Of course, a happy life is neither guaranteed by good health nor ruled out by illness, yet there is a clear enough correlation to ground a utilitarian commitment to pro-health policies. The same holds true for economic considerations. They give us sound utilitarian reasons to value health, since no society can prosper without a healthy workforce.

Furthermore, from a liberal egalitarian perspective, health greatly affects how well people can make use of their liberties; and it significantly shapes the range of valuable options a person is able to pursue. Illness is a barrier to education, employment and political engagement, and so health is also important for equality of opportunity.

13.21   Health clearly is very important to us, but it is also clear that its value is a function of its *instrumental nature*. It is always a means to achieve another end, namely to *enjoy* our existence, to *participate* in public life, to *have* a good time with friends and so on and so forth. It is conceivable then that there could be circumstances where other values are more important to us than the value we put on being healthy. This is the problem Mohr hints at in the quote we reproduced above. Public health understood as the aggregate form of the individual healths in a given population runs the risk of ignoring those individual valuations of particular states of health and competing other values. In fact, such an understanding of public health would align best with objectivist accounts of well-being. Proponents of **objectivist accounts of well-being**[8] insist that there are things that are objectively good for us, regardless of whether we value them. These kinds of lists of objectively good things could be hierarchically structured, but they could also offer us lists of things that are good without telling us which of these things trump other competing things. As Derek Parfit explains, 'according to this theory, certain things are good or bad for people, whether or not these people would want to have the good things, or to avoid bad things. ... The Objective List Theory appeals directly to facts about value' (Parfit 1994, 239). Aristotelian virtue ethics would also insist that there is an objective list of characteristics that is good to have in order to live a flourishing life.

Mohr, on the other hand, defends what is called a **subjectivist account of well-being**[9], whereby we as individuals decide what is best for us. Health turns out to remain an important value in this approach, but only an important value among other important values, and it is a value that individuals choose as important for themselves and that they weigh against other values that are also important to them. People could then well make rational choices that risk their health in the pursuit of the realization of other values. In fact, we make such choices more frequently than you might think. People risk their health in the pursuit of dangerous hobbies, ranging from **rock climbing**[10] to scuba diving in shark infested waters to engaging in **contact sports**[11]. Many of us also consume regularly food products that are known to contribute to a reduced life-expectancy and that are known to cause illnesses that reduce our quality of life, diabetes and alcoholism chief among these. Conflicts between individual lifestyle preferences and the maximization of individual health are a daily feature in our lives. In liberal societies the regulatory lines we draw in the sand are anything but consistent. For instance, we will be punished if we do not wear seatbelts in cars, but nobody stops us from smoking our way to lung cancer.

13.4 Communicable Disease Control Challenges

As this brief introduction shows, public health policies are quite likely to give rise to ethical conflict. We will now – in an extended section – review ethical issues in communicable disease control, with an initial focus on sexually transmitted illnesses, using HIV as an example.

13.24   To leave the discussion not entirely in the realm of theory, **consider the following real-world case**[12]. Michael Johnson, an African-American student at a United States college, who also happened to be a **local star athlete**[13], was incarcerated since October 2013. He had unprotected sex with a fair number of other gay men, mostly fellow white college students. Reportedly, he continued engaging in unsafe sex with his willing sex partners *after* he knew to be HIV infected. The athlete was charged under a Missouri law that made HIV transmission a class A felony, punishable by anywhere between 10 to 30 years, or even life imprisonment (State of Missouri). Compare that to other class A felonies such as murder and child abandonment. Johnson was eventually found guilty of transmitting the virus to one of his sex partners and subjecting various others to a transmission risk. The student was 23 years old at the time. He was found guilty during a jury trial and sentenced to 30.5 years in prison, by a jury consisting of 12 members, all identifying as heterosexual, eleven of the jurors were white. The prosecutor deliberately included among the jurors people who considered homosexuality a 'sin' (**Schreiber 2017**[14]). The legislation Johnson's conviction was based on came into force in 1988 when no medical treatment for an HIV infection existed, and when people died as a result of their infection. While an HIV infection remains a serious infection today, it can be brought under control with efficient drugs that permit infected people to live healthy and productive lives. In Missouri HIV infected people must prove that they have disclosed their infection, which, when you think about it, is close to impossible to do, given the intimate nature of most sexual encounters, involving typically two people and not a lot of witnesses.

13.25   As Michael Johnson discovered, States in the United States criminalize both subjecting someone knowingly to the risk of HIV infection as well as transmitting the virus while knowing that one is infected. The language that is used to describe what happened in this case is revealing of the views held by those who discuss the case. Many writers would hold the view that Johnson, and others like him, *infected* someone else with HIV or that he *transmitted* the virus to someone else. A smaller number of writers insist that his sex partners actually *acquired* the virus from him. In the former case they are portrayed as *passive* victims of a transmission, in the latter case they are seen to be participants in a sexual encounter during which they *actively* acquired the virus. We do not appear to have language sufficiently neutral as to acknowledge the role both parties played in their respective sexual encounters.

Are there ethical justifications for policies such as those in Missouri? 13.26
The argument that the Missouri legislation is based on contends that HIV
transmission always constitutes a case of harm to others. Is this view
ethically defensible? Consider the following three lines of reasoning in
this context.

13.4.1 Take One: Michael Johnson is Not Culpable

Proponents of this view argue that by *volunteering* to have unsafe sex with 13.27
someone whose HIV status is unknown to oneself one *consents to the risk* of
getting infected, even if not to an actual infection, especially if one belongs
to a population in which HIV is fairly prevalent. This logic relies heavily
on a well-established and quite uncontroversial legal principle that we
discussed on various occasions in this book, the *volenti non fit iniuria*
principle – to a willing person no injury is done. That is not to say that the
infection itself is not harmful, but, so goes the argument, no injustice
occurred to someone who consented to the infection risk. The transmission
then is interpreted as an act of harm to self as opposed to an act of harm to
others. This could be seen as agreeing with the point made by Richard
Mohr. People could have decided that they prefer unsafe sex over sex involving the use of protective condoms, despite the increased risk of acquiring an
infection.

13.4.2 Take Two: Michael Johnson is Culpable

It is possible that Johnson deceived some or perhaps all of his sex partners 13.28
into having unsafe sex with him. Their choice to have unsafe sex with him
could not be considered one that was truly based on voluntary informed
consent, because they did not have all relevant facts made available to them.
That would have required of Johnson to disclose his HIV status prior to
having sexual intercourse. This disclosure argument insists both that in this
case the uninformed students' autonomy was violated by Johnson's omission to disclose his status, and also that the student who eventually became
infected was actually harmed by the transmission of the virus itself. The
others were subjected to the risk of bodily harm without having consented
to that risk.

Are these arguments sound? It is difficult to argue against this conclusion 13.29
with regard to those of his sex partners who did ask him about his HIV
status and were lied to. It is less clear that that argument is persuasive in
circumstances where no questions were asked. It also is the case that

Johnson's sex partners could have insisted on the use of condoms. Perhaps we should be looking at a framework that permits for a sharing of responsibility.

13.4.3 Take Three: Shared Responsibility

13.30 The argument from shared responsibility suggests that the responsibility both for risk taking as well as a possible transmission of HIV should be shared by both parties. Johnson ought to accept responsibility for not disclosing his infection, and for subjecting his sex partners knowingly to the risk of an infection. However, equally, his sex partners knew how to protect themselves against acquiring HIV. They could have chosen to insist on the use of condoms during their sexual encounters. It is not a big secret that people lie about their HIV-status, many might not even be aware of it. Condoms are the obvious response to such vagaries. The point of the argument here is that the responsibility for the transmission/acquisition as well as its consequences should be shared, much as the transmission/acquisition was the result of a shared, voluntary, consensual activity.

13.31   Regardless of who is morally responsible when HIV transmission occurs or when someone is at risk of an infection during a sexual encounter, could a deterrence rationale justify the criminalization of non-disclosure of one's HIV status?

13.4.4 Deterrence

13.32 A different, consequentialist public health ethics rationale goes beyond merely wanting to *punish* Johnson for transmitting a life-threatening infection to others. It suggests that by threatening HIV infected people with jail if they refuse to disclose their HIV status societies would be able to create a strong *deterrent* effect. HIV infected people would think twice about not disclosing their infection to sex partners if there was the threat of a long prison term hanging over their heads. If the criminalization of HIV transmission or the criminalization of subjecting someone to the risk of an infection resulted in a measurable deterrence effect, public health campaigners would have a harm reduction rationale on their side. This argument relies on the truth of a particular empirical assumption, namely that we remain level-headed rational actors during sexual intercourse, and that we will be able to choose to disclose our HIV status or respond 'responsibly' to such a disclosure, as the case might be. There are various practical as well as conceptual problems with such disclosure requirements, not least the question of what constitutes disclosure. Empirical research has shown that 'the majority of communication in sex is non-verbal,' so, a duty to disclose understood as requiring of the HIV-positive person to *say* explicitly that they are infected could violate oftentimes the basic 'rule of conduct' in many situations involving sexual encounters (Davies 1993, 49). It is surprising that to date no reliable empirical evidence exists that shows that this deterrence effect actually operates in the minds of people who have sex. For that an infected person would, at a minimum, have to be worried that they might realistically be prosecuted if they get caught. In light of millions of such encounters and – at best – a few hundred successful prosecutions worldwide, it is arguable that the deterrence rationale rests on shaky empirical assumptions (Lazzarini et al. 2002, 250).

Patricia Illingworth argues that even if the deterrence effect worked to some extent, public health policy makers ought to be worried that such policies could be counterproductive. She writes: 'If Sam believes that it is Bob's moral responsibility to inform him of his antibody status, he may construe Bob's silence as an invitation not to practice safe sex' (Illingworth 1990, 42). The effect Illingworth describes here could well translate into mistaken assumptions about the HIV status of people who do not disclose their infection to their sex partners. Placing the responsibility for avoiding HIV transmission exclusively on the infected person risks offering a false sense of security to uninfected people who might wrongly conclude that (HIV-focused) safe sex is unnecessary if their sex partner did not disclose an infection. Even today, **many infected people are ignorant of their infection**[15], hence the false sense of security that disclosure policies could produce might be counterproductive from a public health perspective. 13.33

What we have encountered so far are arguments discussing the ethics of the transmission of a sexually transmitted illness between two arguably volunteering adults during unsafe sexual encounters. If these were truly acts affecting only individuals, this matter should be of no concern to public health professionals. That, however, would not quite do justice to this issue, given the global spread of diseases like HIV/AIDS. There are societal-level consequences. 13.34

13.4.5 *Private Acts and Social Consequences*

Public health ethics rationales challenge the idea that HIV transmission is merely a problem between two individuals. Ronald Bayer, a public health ethicist, points out that private (sexual) acts between consenting adults can have 13.35

public consequences that go beyond merely the two individuals involved (Bayer 1989). When you reflect on Johnson engaging in unprotected sexual intercourse, his actions made it more likely that others who willingly had unsafe sex with him would pick up the virus and subject – possibly unwittingly – others to the same risk during their next sexual encounter, some of whom would get infected and unwittingly subject others to the same risk, etc. It is true that for many of those transmissions there are no culpable actors, because those infected were oblivious of their infection, and their sex partners volunteered to have unsafe sex. Still, so goes Bayer's argument, eventually a critical mass of such infected people would be reached and society would have to face an out-of-control epidemic with concomitant cost implications for economic productivity, national expenditure on life preserving medication, and so on and so forth. In many societies this cost would eventually have to be borne by the community, hence Bayer is correct when he claims that private acts can have societal-level consequences.

13.36   Bayer's argument is a version of the kind of analysis that was attacked by Richard Mohr. He is concerned that the spread of an expensive (or at the time impossible-to-treat) infectious disease is likely to cause sufficient havoc in society that there is a societal interest in reducing the number of transmissions, if not in putting a stop to them altogether. While things, on this occasion, with this disease, did not turn out to reach such dramatic proportions in countries of the global north, the same isn't true for other parts of the world, like for instance sub-Saharan Africa (Selgelid 2005).

13.37   Let us return briefly to Michael Johnson's story. **His verdict was overturned in 2017**[16] due to prosecutorial misconduct that rendered his trial, in the words of a superior court, 'fundamentally unfair'. He was released from prison in 2019.

13.38   To some extent these issues will be less pressing in the future, due to developments in the availability of new classes of drugs that **render HIV infected people who take them non-infectious**[17] for all intents and purposes. As a result of this **governments in some countries have begun to remove disclosure obligations**[18] on HIV infected people vis a vis their sex partners, provided they have demonstrably an undetectable viral load. The same kinds of drugs also permit HIV negative people to protect themselves against an infection.

13.4.6 Novel Coronavirus Pandemic

13.39   While HIV is not that easy to transmit or acquire, corona viruses are much easier to transmit or acquire. They are somewhat comparable to flu viruses.

On November 17, 2019 Chinese medical doctors encountered a 55-year old patient from Hubei province who became patient zero in what turned into a global novel coronavirus outbreak (Davidson 2020). Since then countries like Italy, Spain and the UK in Europe, and the United States have faced up to waves of infections and deaths the likes of which countries in the global north have not seen in many years. Most patients infected with the virus experience no or mild flu-like symptoms, but a significant percentage requires hospitalization, and of those some need access to intensive care unit beds and ventilators in particular. Those most at risk are older people and others with significant co-morbidities. None of the countries we mentioned, wealthy as they are, had initially sufficient quantities of these facilities and medical devices available where and when they were needed. One of the ethical challenges that all of these societies faced was that of triage decision-making, that is the effort to develop a just decision-algorithm aimed at placing patients into categories based on their needs and their prospective benefits from particular interventions, and then ranking them to establish an order of priority, if there are not enough resources to go around for everyone who could benefit from them. You might want to re-read Chapter 12 to refresh your memory of the ways in which societies could go about doing this. Utilitarians would want to maximise lives, or quality- or disability adjusted life years. On that account it might be ethically required, for instance, to remove a patient from a life-preserving ventilator and move them to palliative care only, if a higher amount of such life-years could be created by allocating that scarce resource to a different patient. Other approaches could entail a lottery among those in need, regardless of age and future prospects, or there could be a first-come-first-served approach, where access to a resource like an intensive care unit bed is granted based on when a patient arrived in the hospital. It all depends on what a society values.

Surprisingly, given that outbreaks like the COVID19 pandemic were predicted by global health experts for many years (Garrett 1994), in most societies no ethical decision-making frameworks were in place to provide those at the frontlines of health care delivery with the necessary decision-making tools (Schüklenk 2020). 13.40

Given that this particular coronavirus was novel, no successful therapies existed to treat those whose bodies had trouble fighting the virus off on their own. In fact, many health care workers lost their lives trying to provide professional care to patients fighting for their own survival. How did that happen? These health care workers did not have what is known as 13.41

personal protective equipment (PPE), or they were provided with suboptimal equipment unable to protect them from acquiring infections themselves (Keshavan 2020). Very much in line with what their predecessors did during pandemics gone by (Schwartz 2007), health care workers responded in quite idiosyncratic manners: in Hungary's capital Budapest, reportedly many resigned, in Zimbabwe health care workers went on strike, in other countries they merely complained about the lack of equipment. What are health care professionals' obligations during public health emergencies, when protective equipment is unavailable in the required quantities? Interestingly, we cannot take here recourse to health care workers traditional conduct in such situations, because their responses have been idiosyncratic at best. We also cannot take recourse to their professed values, because crucial guidance documents such as the World Medical Association's Declaration of Geneva are silent on this. Some have argued that if the lack of such equipment in an otherwise well-resourced, wealthy country is merely a function of government cost-cutting decisions, they are under no ethical obligation to provide care (Schüklenk 2020a). Others have gone so far as to claim that unless there was certainty of significant harm, health care workers were under a professional obligation to offer their services, given that society relied on them, and given that they had a monopoly on the provision of these kinds of services. Patients couldn't go anywhere else if their health care workers declined to work (British Columbia 2020).

13.42   Let us briefly look at one further issue among many other ethical challenges that arose during this particular outbreak, namely that of the justifiability of the public health policies governments across the globe instituted. The consensus among public health professionals was that it was necessary to 'flatten the curve', that is to reduce the rate at which an infection spreads in a community. The idea here was to slow the spread of the virus to such an extent that there would be a sufficient number of intensive care beds and ventilators to care for every patient, or even most patients. This seems on the face of it, like a good idea, even though it wasn't quite clear for how long such responses needed to be instituted, and also how the cost of these measures could be balanced against the cost of a controlled faster spread of the virus, with a view to establishing what is called 'herd immunity'. Herd immunity exists when a sufficiently large number of people got infected and became eventually immune to the virus so that individuals who are not immune also were protected. The obvious problem with the latter approach is that the spread of the virus might run out of control and too many people eventually die preventable deaths.

On the other side were arguments noting that actions to slow or halt the   13.43
spread of the virus would lead to large numbers of people falling back into
abject poverty across the globe. The charity Oxfam America predicted that
up to half a billion people could have to face such a fate (Oxfam 2020).
Poverty, of course, is the cause of many avoidable deaths, so the question of
whether public health interventions that led to a shutting down of most of
the world's countries' economies is not merely a question of money and
wealth, it is fundamentally also about human well-being. The South African
philosopher Alex Broadbent brings this point home quite vividly, he wrote,

> 'At the bottom of the global pile, recession isn't just a matter of falling
> property prices and disappointing pensions, it's a matter of life and death.
> When we lock down, we are making a choice. We are saving the lives of some
> older people [who are disproportionately likely to succumb to the virus], and
> causing the deaths of some younger people, especially children, who are most
> at risk of malnutrition and diseases of poverty. … Lower respiratory tract
> infection, caused by a prior bacterial or viral disease, is the largest cause of
> death on the continent. Covid-19 might increase that risk, but it's hardly
> something to write home about, and not preferable to the hunger caused by
> recession' (Broadbent 2020).

Assuming that Broadbent's factual claims are correct, governments in the
global south face truly difficult ethical questions.

Let us move on to a different question that has gained a high profile   13.44
both in public health ethics, but also in society generally, namely that of
ethically defensible vaccination policies. Vaccines are typically – but not
always – means to protect those vaccinated from either getting infected by
diseases or, if they get infected, prevent them from getting sick.

13.4.7 Vaccines

In recent years there has been much societal controversy, typically stoked   13.45
by so-called anti-vaxxers; they are essentially activists who claim that societal policies should not force, for instance, parents to vaccinate their children against the flu virus each flu season, before they send them to school.
Why would parents object to protecting their children against potentially
life-threatening diseases? Much of this is related to long-debunked claims
about a link between vaccines and autism in children (Hotez 2019). Others
have religious reasons. Some parents are also concerned about rare reported
cases of allergic reactions to vaccines. They tend to object to compulsory flu
and measles vaccinations policies. Arguably as a result of their activities

measles outbreaks have increased in countries like, for instance the United States of America (Olive et al. 2018). Measles is highly contagious, and was eliminated in that country in 2000. In 2019 various measles outbreaks were reported in the United States, with the majority of patients being unvaccinated. About 1 in 10 of them needed to be hospitalized (Patel et al. 2019). The island nation of Samoa, meanwhile, to choose one other example, had to **declare a state of emergency in late 2019**[19] over its deadly measles epidemic, with 5667 cases and 81 measles related deaths by December 28, 2019, mostly among children, in a population of only about 200,000.

13.46   While it is true that some people have a higher risk than others to experience an allergic reaction to a vaccine, it is also the case that an informed assessment of that risk requires specialist expertise, for instance in vaccine immunology. It is an expertise that lay people do not have, no matter how much time they spend on the internet investigating the matter. However, not everything in this context is about scientific illiteracy. What is also often on display are conflicting values. To public health experts the science should dictate our actions. Many vaccine refusers, on the other hand, think that measles, for instance, is a natural part of growing up, and that there is nothing wrong with their children developing immunity during a naturally occurring infection. As the evidence suggests, however, such a stance also means that a fair number of children will die preventable deaths as a result of measles related complications. Some children who get infected because their parents refused them to get vaccinated, will infect other children who will die as a result of that parental decision. For this reason, in many countries, children are only permitted to attend school after they have been vaccinated against a range of diseases, often including measles as well as the flu virus. Here, as an example, **is an overview**[20] of United States state school and childcare vaccination laws. In other countries there is an ongoing lively debate about the rights and wrongs of mandatory vaccine for school-aged children (e.g. Weeks 2019).

13.47   Other vaccine refusers decline to participate for more individualistic reasons. They hope that a sufficient number of their fellow citizens will get vaccinated, which, in turn, should ensure herd immunity. Under such circumstances they would have little reason to get vaccinated themselves. This phenomenon is also known as the free-rider phenomenon, because these people benefit from others behaving more responsibly than they themselves do. Alberto Giubilini has argued that:

> There is a principle of fairness in the distribution of the burdens of collective obligations, and that such principle entails that each of us has the individual

moral responsibility to make their fair contribution to herd immunity through vaccination. These individual moral obligations, in turn, entail a further individual obligation to support policies aimed at realizing herd immunity. (Giubilini 2019)

Moral justifications for coercive state policies mandating vaccination 13.48 against communicable illnesses that pose significant health risks, except for people for whom vaccination is medically contraindicated, can be both utilitarian as well as contractualist in nature. The utilitarian rationale rests on the premise that health is a public good. Each citizen ought to contribute to the maximization of that good. In the case of vaccination each of us has a moral obligation to contribute toward enabling society to achieve a desirable outcome, in this case herd immunity. Contractualists would look for a rule that 'no one could reasonably reject as a basis for informed, unforced general agreement' (Scanlon 1998). It seems that requiring everyone for whom vaccination isn't medically contra-indicated to be vaccinated in order to achieve herd immunity is a reasonable proposition. As Giubilini and colleagues point out (2018):

It is rational for each person who is at risk of infection to demand that others contribute to keeping this risk of infection to a minimum. When keeping the risk of infection to a minimum comes at a small cost to others, as is the case with vaccination, this demand by persons at risk is not only rational, but also reasonable. We are here defining 'reasonable' in such a way that the objective costs one has to bear, such as the risks of side-effects the vaccinated takes on herself, make the option in question reasonable or an unreasonable to reject; thus, the small risks involved make a principle that prescribe (sic) to be vaccinated, in this sense, unreasonable to reject.

Another aspect of the vaccination ethics debates surrounds the question 13.49 of whether health care professionals should be vaccinated against influenza, measles, pertussis and hepatitis B. The same kind of analysis is applicable here, too (Galanakis et al. 2013).

13.5 Public Health Promotion

Health promotion campaigns exist in many different contexts. Earlier in 13.50 this chapter we have familiarized ourselves with some of the HIV-related public health issues. HIV prevention campaigns typically do not focus on infected people's legal obligations to disclose their status, rather they focus on motivating people to use condoms during sexual intercourse. Other health promotion campaigns aim to persuade us to reduce our sugar intake, stop smoking, exercise more and so on and so forth. There is nothing inherently problematic about persuading us with sound reasons to live a healthier life. After all, as we have seen, health is an important means to live a good life. What is controversial among bioethicists are some of the means that are deployed by public health campaigners to achieve those otherwise laudable objectives. Let us look at health promotion campaigns that have brought upon them the ire not just of bioethicists, but also the ire of some of the people these campaigns were targeting. The fundamental objection to certain campaign techniques is that they are not focused on *persuading through reason* but on bringing about behavioral change through the use of manipulative techniques that have the potential to subvert autonomy and, that some argue, are coercive in nature.

13.5.1 Communicable Disease: HIV

13.51   Patricia Illingworth analyzed health promotion campaigns conducted by the Canadian Public Health Association during the early days of the Canadian HIV epidemic, that is prior to the existence of life-preserving anti-HIV drugs (Illingworth 1991, 143–147). She argues that health promotion campaigns that are manipulative are a threat to our autonomy because they are designed to trigger choices that are not truly our authentic choices. An autonomous choice, argues Gerald Dworkin, is a choice that is authentically our own informed choice (Dworkin 1988, 20). What makes one's desires truly one's desires is that one, on reflection, accepts them to be one's desires.

13.52   Illingworth describes how a particular health promotion model has been used in those HIV campaigns, the so-called **Health-Belief Model**[21]. The objective, not surprisingly in the context of public health promotion campaigns, is to motivate people to adopt healthy behaviors and avoid unhealthy ones. Illingworth explains (2011):

> According to this model, people are more likely to change their behavior if they believe that (1) they are particularly vulnerable to a disease that will have (2) severe and harmful consequences for them; and if they also believe that (3) a particular health action will be efficacious and (4) will not carry with it higher costs than the benefits it promises.

How could such a model be a threat to our autonomy? It could be a threat   13.53
to our autonomy, because nothing in this model suggests that it is necessary
that what people believe about the threat they are facing is based on fact and
reason. If one's primary concern is to achieve behavioral changes, exagger-
ating the individual risk or the severity of a given illness could be more
efficient than a neutral presentation of pertinent facts and figures. A public
health promotion campaigner might also be tempted to exaggerate the
likely success of one's favored behavioral change, and, might consider
downplaying the cost of behavioral changes to individual lives. As an example of the latter concern, a health promoter could claim that the use of condoms is only a minor inconvenience given their obvious health benefits,
when for some people that cost might be anything but minor. Richard Mohr
noted in his article the centrality of sex in most of our lives (Mohr 1987).
For some people the use of condoms could seriously impact their ability to
enjoy a sex life they consider worth having. Using public health promotion
campaigns that rely on the health-belief model would be considered
ethically indefensible by libertarians like Mohr, but also by others, whenever
these campaigns use manipulative means to achieve otherwise desirable
behavioral change.

Consequentialist approaches to public health – and they arguably are the   13.54
normative engine driving public health policy – would have an easier task
defending manipulative campaign techniques. They could point to the
number of life years preserved as a result of bringing about protective
behavioral changes in the sexual conduct of many people who otherwise
would be at risk of acquiring HIV and other sexually transmitted illnesses.
Consequentialists might well consider violations of individual autonomy by
means of manipulative health promotion campaign techniques as a kind of
ethical cost, but unlike libertarians they could be persuaded that desirable
health outcomes can outweigh such costs.

Let us briefly turn to another prominent target of public health promo-   13.55
tion campaigners, obesity. Obesity is of interest, because it is one of a
number of *non-communicable* diseases that are responsible for a very significant disease burden not only in high-income, but increasingly also in
low- and middle-income countries. A high-level United Nations conference on sustainable development describes non-communicable diseases
as 'one of the major challenges for sustainable development in the twenty-
first century' (Clark 2013). To give just one example, smoking causes
about 6 million deaths globally, and reduces global GDP by anywhere
between 1–2 percent (ibid.).

13.5.2 Non-Communicable Disease: Obesity

13.56   Overweight and obesity are responsible for millions of preventable deaths globally every year (Ng et al. 2014). The obesity related cost to the United States economy alone was estimated to be around 215 billion US$ in 2010. Obesity is caused by surplus energy, simply put, energy consumed but not expended, that is stored in our bodies where it then causes disease. Obesity is closely correlated with a range of morbidities, including hypertension, diabetes, cardiovascular disease, as well as various cancers. It is today typically measured using a standard called the **Body Mass Index**[22] (BMI). The BMI, ranging from I to III is calculated by dividing one's weight by one's height squared. This use of the BMI is anything but unproblematic. For instance, BMI I actually correlates with an increased life expectancy in certain age groups, while BMI III is unquestionably linked to excess mortality, with the mortality risk increasing the higher the individual's BMI is. There have been some arguments about the BMI's method, given that it doesn't take into account factors such as gender, age, one's bone structure, muscle mass and fat distribution, and yet, despite all this, it is a reasonably reliable predictor of mortality risk (Schüklenk et al. 2014). What is uncontroversial is that severe obesity is associated with a significant reduction in life expectancy. A Caucasian male between the ages of 20–30 is likely to die on average more than a decade earlier than he would have had he not been severely obese (Fontaine et al. 2003).

13.57   Unsurprisingly, public health promotion campaigns and policies aim to reduce the incidence of obesity in a given population in order to reduce the obesity-related disease burden. Let us briefly investigate a public health ethics decision-making framework that utilizes principle-based bioethics (consider re-reading the relevant section on the *Georgetown Mantra* in Chapter 2 to familiarize yourself with this kind of approach). Our primary interest is in finding out whether this influential conceptual framework delivers action guidance and action justification in the context of public health promotion, or whether it falters for the reasons we discussed in Chapter 2.

13.58   A number of public health ethics frameworks have been developed that are variations of the *Georgetown Mantra* (Kass 2001; Childress et al. 2002; ten Have et al. 2012). We cannot discuss each of them in great detail here, however, given that only the work by ten Have and colleagues is explicitly focused on obesity and overweight, we shall have a closer look at that particular framework. A comprehensive critique of each mentioned framework, including those that we are not discussing in this chapter, can be found in an overview article by Schüklenk and Zhang (2014). ten Have and colleagues have produced a type of principlist public health ethics framework, consisting essentially of a list of eight questions that correspond to particular ethical principles or values. Here they are:

1. How does the program affect physical health?
2. How does the program affect psychosocial well-being?
3. How does the program affect equality?
4. How does the program affect informed choice?
5. How does the program affect social and cultural values?
6. How does the program affect privacy?
7. How does the program affect the attribution of responsibility?
8. How does the program affect liberty?

The claim here is, basically, that answers to these questions will serve as useful markers of a prospective health promotion program's ethical strengths and weaknesses. When you look at these questions, it is not difficult to appreciate that they are indeed useful. It's a good thing if a program does not impact negatively on equality or privacy or liberty, and ethical justifications for each of these questions can be created without great difficulty. However, keeping in mind that the twin goals of ethics are action guidance and action justification, it becomes apparent that the concerns critics expressed about the viability of principlism affects ten Have's model. The absence of an overarching ethical theory that would permit us to rank the values expressed in the eight questions, results eventually in a failure to offer uncontroversial action guidance. Uncertainty about the relative importance of the principles between each other is just one problem. Another challenge is uncertainty when we try to apply even one principle. Let us test principle 8: Whose liberty should policy makers be concerned about? The liberty of manufacturers of soft drinks to market their product to children? The liberty of parents to feed soft drinks to their underage offspring? The liberty of teenagers to spend their pocket money on soft drinks? Should it really be held against a policy proposal that certain liberties might be curtailed with rules and regulations? One public health ethics expert seems to think that that is a questionable guidance criterion. Ross Upshur argues:

13.59

> With respect to liberty impacts, it is considered a positive factor when pro-
> motion of autonomy and freedom of choice is preserved and a negative one
> if there is interference with autonomy and freedom of choice. This latter
> category includes interference with commercial factors, without any consid-
> eration of whether these commercial factors have public health within their
> purview of concern. (Upshur 2013)

13.60   This seems to confirm then what we said in Chapter 2. The absence of
a foundational ethical theory that would permit the creation of a hierarchy of ethical principles appears to be a recurring problem for the
Georgetown Mantra. However, a different view on this can also be taken:
given that we live in pluralistic societies, perhaps checklists like Ten
Have's are all that is actually needed to provide policy advice to politi-
cians and law makers. They are a reflection of the diverse values held in
our societies. Some of us will value equality (question 3) over liberty
(question 8), while others will hold exactly the opposite point of view.
Let ethicists lay out what the ethical issues are, and let society decide how
to respond to them.

13.61   Among bioethicists who argue that obesity constitutes a serious public, and indeed, global health problem, various recommendations have
been defended on consequentialist grounds. Daniel Callahan, for
instance, argued that overweight people should be stigmatized by society
in order to encourage them to lose weight (Callahan 2013). He notes that
similar strategies worked with regard to discouraging people from pick-
ing up smoking, or with regard to encouraging people to stop smoking.
Empirical evidence that consequentialist arguments like Callahan's must
rely on, do not support such approaches. 'Stigmatization is more likely to
contribute to weight gain than it is to contribute to weight loss. Many of
us resort almost by default to comfort food when we are downtrodden'
(Schüklenk and Zhang 2014). Bogart notes that government health promotion campaigns aimed at weight reduction have largely failed to
reduce the prevalence of obesity, and they have led to the harmful stigmatization of overweight people. He argues that public health promotion
campaigns ought to focus on better health and food products as well as
on lifestyles that are detrimental to our well-being. What should not be
the primary focus of public health promotion are our weight and the
BMI (Bogart 2013).

13.62   This chapter on global and public health ethics is, such is the nature of
these fields, wide-ranging. What are your considered ethical views on the
following questions, and what are your ethical the reasons for them?

Questions

Do well-off people in the global north have global health obligations to assist those in dire poverty in other parts of the world?

What is the ethics of Michael Johnson's past conduct that led to his prison sentence? Do you think he had a moral obligation to disclose his HIV status to his sex partners?

What is the ethics of compulsory vaccination policies?

Website Links

1   https://www.un.org/millenniumgoals/
2   https://www.un.org/millenniumgoals/poverty.shtml
3   https://www.children.org/global-poverty/global-poverty-facts/facts-about-world-poverty-and-health/
4   http://plato.stanford.edu/entries/libertarianism/
5   http://time.com/3662225/haiti-earthquake-five-year-after/
6   https://edition.cnn.com/2016/04/15/asia/japan-earthquake/
7   https://www.hrw.org/world-report/2015/country-chapters/south-sudan/
8   http://plato.stanford.edu/entries/well-being/#ObjLisThe/
9   http://spot.colorado.edu/~heathwoo/STWB.pdf/
10 http://www.sciencedirect.com/science/article/pii/S0196064489804639/
11 http://ajs.sagepub.com/content/40/4/747.short/
12 http://www.buzzfeed.com/steventhrasher/how-college-wrestling-star-tiger-mandingo-became-an-hiv-scap#.juwew8032/
13 http://mic.com/articles/115558/the-disturbing-way-america-s-legal-system-turns-people-s-bodies-into-weapons/
14 http://www.apa.org/pi/aids/resources/exchange/2017/03/michael-johnson.aspx/
15 http://america.aljazeera.com/articles/2015/12/30/Atlanta-alarming-rates-HIV-AIDS.html
16 http://www.apa.org/pi/aids/resources/exchange/2017/03/michael-johnson.aspx
17 https://www.cdc.gov/nchhstp/dear_colleague/2017/dcl-092717-National-Gay-Mens-HIV-AIDS-Awareness-Day.html/
18 http://www.cbc.ca/news/politics/liberals-hiv-criminalization-1.4428395/
19 https://samoaglobalnews.com/samoa-measles-outbreak-records-two-more-deaths-parents-urged-to-present-babies-in-early/
20 https://www.cdc.gov/phlp/publications/topic/vaccinations.html/
21 https://www.utwente.nl/cw/theorieenoverzicht/Theory%20Clusters/Health%20Communication/Health_Belief_Model/
22 https://www.cdc.gov/healthyweight/assessing/bmi/

BIBLIOGRAPHY

Chapter 1: Introduction to Ethics

Baker, Robert. (2013). *Before Bioethics: A History of American Medical Ethics From the Colonial Period to the Bioethics Revolution*. New York: Oxford University Press.

Feinberg, Joel. (1990). *The Moral Limits of the Criminal Law: Harmless Wrongdoing*. Oxford: Oxford University Press.

Graham, Gordon. (2004). *Eight Theories of Ethics*. London: Routledge.

Katchadourian, Herant. (2010). *Guilt: The Bite of Conscience*. Stanford: Stanford University Press.

Locke, John. 1689 (1983). *A letter Concerning Toleration*. Indianapolis: Hackett.

McMillan, John. (2018). *The Methods of Bioethics: An Essay in Meta-Bioethics*. Oxford: Oxford University Press.

Proctor, Robert. (1988). *Racial Hygiene: Medicine Under the Nazis*. Cambridge, MA: Harvard University Press.

Quong, Jonathan. (2013). Public Reason. In: *The Stanford Encyclopedia of Philosophy* (ed. Edward N. Zalta). (Summer 2013 Edition). http://plato. stanford.edu/archives/sum2013/entries/public-reason/

Schwitzgebel, Eric. (2015). Are professional ethicists good people? According to our research, not especially. So what is the point of learning ethics? *Aeon*July14http://aeon.co/magazine/philosophy/how-often-do-ethics-professors-call-their-mothers/

Singer, Peter. (ed.) (1991). *A Companion to Ethics. Part 6. The Nature of Ethics*. Oxford: Blackwell.

Singer, Peter. (1995). *Rethinking Life and Death: The Collapse of Our Traditional Ethics*. New York: St Martin's Press.

Singer, Peter. (2011). *Practical Ethics*. Cambridge: Cambridge University Press.

Sowle Cahill, Lisa. (1990). Can Theology Have a Role in 'Public' Bioethical Discourse? *Hastings Center Report* 20(4): 10–14.

Stanford Encyclopedia of Philosophy. Online resource produced by Stanford University.

Syndicat Northcrest v. Amselem (2004). 2 S.C.R. 551, 2004 SCC 47.

Valles, Sean A. (2015). Bioethics and the framing of climate change's health risks. *Bioethics* 29(5): 334–341.

Veatch, Robert M. (2012a). *Hippocratic, Religious, and Secular Medical Ethics: The Points of Conflict*. Washington DC: Georgetown University Press.

Veatch, Robert M. (2012b). Hippocratic, religious and secular ethics: The points of conflict. *Theoretical Medicine and Bioethics* 33: 33–43.

Williams, Bernard. 1972. *Morality: An Introduction to Ethics*. New York: Harper Torchbooks.

Williams, Bernard. (1974–1975). The Truth in Relativism. *Proceedings of the Aristotelian Society* 75(1): 215–228.

Chapter 2: Ethical Theory

Baron, Jonathan. (2006). *Against Bioethics*. Cambridge MA: MIT Press.

Beauchamp, Tom L. and James F Childress. (2019). *Principles of Biomedical Ethics*, 8th edition. New York: Oxford University Press.

Clement, Grace. (2013). Feminist ethics. In: *The International Encyclopedia of Ethics*. Vol 4. (ed. Hugh LaFollette), 1925–1938. Oxford: Wiley Blackwell.

Dawson, Angus. (2005). The determination of 'best interests' in relation to childhood vaccinations. *Bioethics* 19: 187–205.

Foot, Philippa. (1977). Euthanasia. *Philosophy and Public Affairs* 6: 85–112.

Gilligan, Carol. (1972). *In a Different Voice: Psychological Theory and Women's Development*. Cambridge, MA: Harvard University Press.

Goodin, Robert. (1989). The ethics of smoking. *Ethics* 99: 574–624.

Graham, Gordon. (2004). *Eight Theories of Ethics*. London: Routledge.

Gruen, Lori. (2011). *Ethics and Animals: An Introduction*. Cambridge: Cambridge University Press.

Hardwig, John. (2000). *Is There a Duty to Die and Other Essays in Medical Ethics*. New York: Routledge.

Harsanyi, John. (1977). Morality and the theory of rational behavior. *Social Research: An International Quarterly* 44: 623–656.

Hursthouse, Rosalind. (1991). Virtue ethics and abortion. *Philosophy and Public Affairs* 20: 223–246.

Kamm, Frances M. (1992). *Creation and Abortion: A Study in Moral and Legal Philosophy.* New York: Oxford University Press.

Kamm, Frances M. (1994). *Morality, Mortality: Vol. 1 – Death and Whom to Save From It.* New York: Oxford University Press.

Kamm, Frances M. (1996). *Morality, Mortality: Vol. 2 – Rights, Duties and Status.* New York: Oxford University Press.

Kant, Immanuel. (1785). [1998]. *Grundlegung zur Metaphysik der Sitten (Groundwork to the Metaphysics of Morals – translated by Mary J Gregor).* Cambridge: Cambridge University Press.

Kass, Leon R. (1997). The wisdom of repugnance. *The New Republic June* 2: 17–26.

Kuhse, Helga. (1987). *The Sanctity-of-Life Doctrine in Medicine: A Critique.* Oxford: Clarendon Press.

Kuhse, Helga. 1997. *Caring: Nurses, Women and Ethics.* Oxford: Blackwell.

Kumar, Rahul. (2013). Contractualism. In: *The International Encyclopedia of Ethics.* Vol 2. (ed. LaFollette, Hugh), 1095–1105. Oxford: Wiley-Blackwell

Little, Margaret. (1996). Why a feminist approach to bioethics. *Kennedy Institute of Ethics Journal* 6(1): 1–18.

Lowry, Christopher and Udo Schüklenk. (2009). Two models in global health ethics. *Public Health Ethics* 2: 276–284.

Mackenzie, Catriona. (1992). Abortion and embodiment. *Australasian Journal of Philosophy* 70: 136–155.

Mill, John Stuart. (1871). [1910] *Utilitarianism, Liberty, Representative Government.* London: J. M. Dent & Sons, New York: E. P. Dutton & Co.

O'Neill, Onora. (2002). *Autonomy and Trust in Bioethics.* Cambridge: Cambridge University Press.

Oakley, Justin. (1998). A virtue ethics approach. In: *A Companion to Bioethics.* (eds Helga Kuhse and Peter Singer), 86–97. Oxford: Blackwell.

Savulescu, Julian. (2001). Procreative beneficence: why we should select the best children. *Bioethics* 15: 413–426.

Scully, Jackie L. (2008). *Disability Bioethics: Moral Bodies, Moral Difference.* Totowa, NJ: Rowman and Littlefield.

Sherwin, Susan. (1992). *No Longer Patient: Feminist Ethics and Health Care.* Philadelphia: Temple University Press.

Singer, Peter. (1995). *Rethinking Life and Death: The Collapse of Our Traditional Ethics.* New York: St Martin's Press.

Smart, J.J.C. and Bernard Williams. (1973). *Utilitarianism: For and Against.* Cambridge: Cambridge University Press.

Takala, Tuija. (2001). What is wrong with global bioethics? On the limitations of the four principles approach. *Cambridge Quarterly of Healthcare Ethics* 10: 72–77.

Veatch, Robert M. (2003). Is there a common morality? *Kennedy Institute of Ethics Journal* 13: 189–192.

Chapter 3: Basics of Bioethics

Baker, Robert. (2013). *Before bioethics: a history of American medical ethics from the colonial period to the bioethics revolution*. New York: Oxford University Press.

Ballantyne, Nathan. (2013). Knockdown arguments. doi: 10.1007/s10670-013-9506-8.

Bayer, Ronald. (1987). *Homosexuality and American Psychiatry*. Princeton: Princeton University Press.

Bullock, Allan and Stephen Trombley. (1999). *The New Fontana Dictionary of Modern Thought*. London: Harper-Collins.

CIOMS, the Council for International Organizations of Medical Sciences. (2016). *International Ethical Guidelines for Health- related Research Involving Humans*.

Cox Macpherson, Cheryl. (2013). Climate change is a bioethics question. *Bioethics* 27: 305–308.

Beecher, Henry. (1966). *Ethics and clinical research. New England Journal of Medicine* 274: 1354–1360. (Reprint starting p. 357 of hyperlinked document.)

Benatar, David. (2005). The trouble with universal declarations. *Developing World Bioethics* 5: 220–224.

Burgess, John A. (1993). The great slippery-slope argument. *Journal of Medical Ethics* 19: 169–174.

Caplan, Arthur and Kenneth Moch. (2014). Rescue me: the challenge of compassionate use in the era of social media. *Health Affairs blog* August 27. http://healthaffairs.org/blog/2014/08/27/rescue-me-the-challenge-of-compassionate-use-in-the-social-media-era/

Crooks, Robert and Baur, Karla. (2014). *Our Sexuality*, 14th edition. Belmont, CA: Wadsworth.

Evans, John. (2012). *The History and Future of Bioethics: A Sociological View*. New York: Oxford University Press.

Gillon, Ranaan. (1999). Human reproductive cloning – a look at the arguments against it and a rejection of most of them. *Journal of the Royal Society of Medicine* 92(1): 3–12.

Goodin, Robert. (1981). The political theories of choice and dignity. *American Philosophical Quarterly* 18 (2): 79.

Harkness, Jon, Lederer, Susan E. and Daniel Wikler. (2001). Laying ethical foundations for clinical research. *Bulletin of the WHO* 79(4): 366.

Hoche, Alfred and Binding, Karl. (1920). *Die Freigabe der Vernichtung lebensunwerten Lebens.* Felix Meiner Verlag: Leipzig.

Hume, David. (2000). *A Treatise of Human Nature.* (eds David Fate Norton and Mary J. Norton). Oxford: Clarendon Press.

Hunter, David A. (2009). *A Practical Guide to Critical Thinking: Deciding What to Do and Believe.* Hoboken, NJ: Wiley.

Hyman DA. (2003). Does technology spell trouble with a capital 'I'?: Human Dignity and Public Policy. *Harvard Journal of Law and Policy* 27: 3–18.

Jonsen, Albert. (1998). *The Birth of Bioethics.* New York: Oxford University Press.

Jonsen, Albert. (2014). History of bioethics. In: *Encyclopedia of Bioethics*, 4th edition. (ed. Bruce Jennings), 331–336. Farmington Hills, MI: Gale.

Kuhse, Helga and Peter Singer. (1987). Bioethics: What? and Why? *Bioethics* 1(1): iii–v.

Macklin, Ruth. (2003). Dignity is a useless concept. *BMJ* 327: 1419.

Michalczyk, John J. (1994). *Medicine and Ethics in the Third Reich: Historical and Contemporary Issues.* New York: Sheed and Ward, 8.

O'Neill, O. (1991). Kantian ethics. In: *A Companion to Ethics.* (ed. P. Singer), 175–185. Oxford: Blackwell.

Pence, Gregory. (1998). *Who is Afraid of Human Cloning?* Lanham: Rowman & Littlefield.

Potter, Van Rensselaer. (1971). *Bioethics: Bridge to the Future.* Englewood-Cliffs, NJ: Prentice-Hall.

Rothman, David. (1991). *Strangers at the Bedside: A History of How Law and Bioethics Transformed Medical Decision Making.* New York: Basic Books.

Sartin, Jeffrey S. (2004). J. Marion Sims, the father of gynecology: hero or villain. *Southern Medical Journal* 97(5): 500–505.

Sass, Hans-Martin. (2007). Fritz Jahr's 1927 concept of bioethics. *Kennedy Institute of Ethics Journal* 17: 279–295.

Schaler, Jeffrey A. (ed.) (2004). *Szasz Under Fire: The Psychiatric Abolitionist Faces His Critics.* Chicago: Open Court.

Schöne-Seifert, Bettina and Rippe, Klaus-Peter. (1991). Silencing the Singer: Antibioethics in Germany. *Hastings Center Report* 21(6): 20–27.

Schüklenk, Udo, Stein, Edgar, Kerin, Jacintha and Willam Byne. (1997). The ethics of genetic research on sexual orientation. *Hastings Center Report* 27(4): 6–13.

Schulman, Adam. (2008). Bioethics and the question of human dignity. In: *Human Dignity and Bioethics: Essays commissioned by the President's Council on Bioethics* (ed. President's Council on Bioethics), 3–18. Washington, DC: US Independent Agencies and Commissions.

Sensen, Oliver. (2011). Human dignity in historical perspective: the contemporary and traditional paradigms. *European Journal of Political Theory* 10: 71–91.

Sidgwick, Henry. (1907). *Methods of Ethics*, 7th edition. London: Macmillan.

Singer, Peter. (2011). *Practical Ethics*. Cambridge: Cambridge University Press.

Somerville, Margaret. (2014). Euthanasia's slippery slope can't be prevented. *Calgary Herald* March 03. (Available at www.catholiceducation.org/en/controversy/euthanasia-and-assisted-suicide/euthanasia-s-slippery-slope-can-t-be-prevented.html)

Soble, Alan. (2003). Kant and Sexual Perversion. *The Monist* 86(1): 55–89.

Sommer, Volker and Vasey, Paul L. (eds.) (2006). *Homosexual Behaviour in Animals – An Evolutionary Perspective*. Cambridge: Cambridge University Press.

Vaughn, Lewis and Chris MacDonald. (2010). *The Power of Critical Thinking: Second Canadian Edition*. Toronto: Oxford University Press.

Wright, Walter. (2000). Historical Analogues, Slippery Slopes, and the Question of Euthanasia. *Journal of Law, Medicine and Ethics* 28:176–186.

Chapter 4: Moral Standing: What Matters

Bentham, Jeremy (1789). *Introduction to the Principles of Morals and Legislation*. Oxford: Clarendon Press.

Buchanan, Allen. (2009). Moral status and human enhancement. *Philosophy and Public Affairs* 37(4): 346–381.

DeGrazia, David. (2008). Moral status as a matter of degree? *Southern Journal of Philosophy* 46(2): 181–198.

Frankena, William K. (1979). Ethics and the environment. In: *Ethics and Problems of the 21st Century*. (eds K.E. Goodpaster and K.M. Sayre) 3–20. Notre Dame: Notre Dame University Press.

Marquis, Don. (1989). Why abortion is immoral. *The Journal of Philosophy* 86(4): 183–202.

Nussbaum, Martha. (2006. 1). The moral status of animals. *Chronicle of Higher Education* 52(22): B6–8.

Nussbaum, Martha. (2006. 2). *Frontiers of Justice: Disability, Nationality, Species Membership*, Cambridge, MA: Harvard University Press.

Pimentel, David and Marcia Pimentel. (2003). Sustainability of meat-based and plant-based diets and the environment. *American Journal of Clinical Nutrition* 78(3): s660–s663.

Regan, Tom. (1988). *The Case for Animal Rights*. London: Routledge.

Singer, Peter. (1975). *Animal Liberation: A New Ethics for Our Treatment of Animals*. New York: HarperCollins.

Sparrow, Robert. (2004). The Turing Triage Test. *Ethics and Information Technology* 6(4): 203–213.

Stone, Christopher D. (1972). Should trees have standing: toward legal rights for natural objects. *Southern California Law Review* 45: 450–487.

Stone, Christopher D. (2010). *Should Trees Have Standing: Law, Morality, and the Environment*, 3rd edition. Oxford: Oxford University Press.

Streiffer, Robert. (2005). At the edge of humanity: Moral status, human stem cells, and chimeras. *Kennedy Institute of Ethics Journal* 5(4): 347–370.

Tooley, Michael. (1972). Abortion and Infanticide. *Philosophy and Public Affairs* 2: 37–65.

Vines, Timothy, Bruce, Alex, and Faunce, Thomas. (2013). Planetary medicine and the Waitangi Tribunal Whanganui River Report: Global health law embracing ecosystems as patients. *Journal of Law and Medicine* 20: 528–541.

Wetlesen, Jon. (1999). The moral status of beings who are not persons: A casuistic argument. *Environmental Values* 8: 287–323.

Chapter 5: Beginning of Life

Abortion Act 1967.

ACB v. Thomson Medical Pte Ltd, 2017.

American Medical Association. (1996). Opinion 2.161 Medical Applications of Fetal Tissue Transplantation AMA/

Blackshaw, Bruce P. (2019). The impairment argument for the immorality of abortion: A reply. *Bioethics* 33(6): 723–724.

Brake, E. 2005. Fatherhood and child support: do men have a right to choose? *Journal of Applied Philosophy*. 22 (1): 55–73.

Capps, Ben et al. (2013). An ethical analysis of human elective egg freezing. In: *Reproductive Issues in Singapore on Elective Freezing: a BELRIS Report*. Singapore: Centre for Biomedical Ethics.

Carter-Walshaw, Sarah. (2019). In vitro gametogenesis: the end of egg donation? *Bioethics* 33(1): 60–67.

Chadwick, Ruth and Childs, Richardo. (2012). Ethical issues in the diagnosis and management of fetal disorders. *Best Practice Research in Clinical Obstetrics and Gynaecology* 26 (5): 541–550.

Chadwick, Ruth and Levitt, Mairi. (2016). Genetic technology: a threat to deafness? In: *Bioethics: An Anthology*, 3rd edition. (eds Kuhse, Helga, Schüklenk, Udo and Peter Singer), 127–135. Chichester/Oxford: Wiley Blackwell.

Clarke, L. (1989). Abortion: a rights issue? In: *Birthrights: Law and Ethics at the Beginning of Life* (eds R. Lee and D. Morgan), 155–171. London: Routledge.

Crummett, Dustin (2020). Violinists, demandingness and the impairment argument against abortion. *Bioethics* 34(2): 145–220.

Dimond, Rebecca. (2015). Social and ethical issues in mitochondrial donation. *British Medical Bulletin* 115: 173–182. doi.org/10.1093/bmb/ldv037.

Foley, J. (2012). Uterine transplantation: a step too far? *Clinical Ethics* 7(4): 193–198.

Hamzelou, Jessica. (2015). The fertility calculator. *New Scientist* 227(3032): 6–7.

Hendricks, Perry. (2019). Even if the fetus is not a person, abortion is immoral. The impairment argument. *Bioethics* 33(2): 245–253.

Holm, Søren. (2008). The expressivist objection to prenatal diagnosis: can it be laid to rest? *Journal of Medical Ethics* 34: 24–25.

Human Fertilization and Embryology Act, 1990.

Hursthouse, Rosalind. (1991). Virtue theory and abortion. *Philosophy and Public Affairs* 20: 223–246.

Johnson, B.R., Kismödi, E., Dragoman, M.V. and Temmerman, M. (2013). Conscientious objection to provision of legal abortion care. *International Journal of Gynecology and Obstetrics* 123(3): S60–62.

Johnston, J. and Zacharias, R.L. (2017). The future of reproductive autonomy. *Hastings Center Report* 47(6): S6–S11.

Jotkowitz, A.B. and Glick, S. (2006). The Groningen Protocol: another perspective. *Journal of Medical Ethics* 32: 157–158.

Kuhse, Helga and Peter Singer. (1986). Severely handicapped newborns: For sometimes letting and helping die. *Journal of Law, Medicine and Ethics* 14(3/4): 149–154.

Kuhse, H. and Singer, P. (1985). *Should the Baby Live?: The Problem of Handicapped Infants*. Oxford: Oxford University Press.

Marquis, Don. (1989). Why abortion is immoral. *Journal of Philosophy* 86: 183–202.

McMahan, Jeff. (2013). Infanticide and moral consistency. *Journal of Medical Ethics* 39: 273–280.

Medical Research Council. (2014). *Human Tissue and Biological Samples for Use in Research: Operational and Ethical Guidelines* London: MRC.

Meilander, Gilbert. (2014). No to infant euthanasia. *Journal of Thoracic and Cardiovascular Surgery* 149(2): 533–534.

National Institute for Clinical Excellence (NICE). (2010). *Specialist Neonatal Care Quality Standard*. London: NICE.

O'Donovan, L., Williams, N.J., and Wilkinson, S. (2019). Ethical and policy issues raised by uterus transplants. *British Medical Bulletin* 131(1): 19–28. https://academic.oup.com/bmb/article/131/1/19/5554327

Parfit, Derek. (1984). *Reasons and Persons Oxford:* University Press.

Parit, Derek. (2017). Future people, the non-identity problem, and person-affecting principles. *Philosophy and Public Affairs* 45(2): 118–57.

Parker, Michael. (2007). The best possible child. *Journal of Medical Ethics.* 33(3): 279–283.

Polkinghorne, J. (Chairman) (1989a). *Code of Practice on the Use of Fetuses and Fetal Material in Research and Treatment.* London: HMSO.

Polkinghorne, J. (Chairman) (1989b). *Review of the Guidance on the Research Use of Fetuses and Fetal Material* London: HMSO.

Robertson, John. (1983). Procreative liberty and the control of conception, pregnancy and childbirth. *Virginia Law Review* 69(3): 405–464.

Savulescu, Julian. (2001). Procreative beneficence: why we should select the best children. *Bioethics* 15(5/6): 413–426.

Schüklenk, Udo. (2014). Physicians can justifiably euthanize severely handi-capped neonates. *Journal of Thoracic and Cardiovascular Surgery* 149(2): 535–537.

Shakespeare, Tom. (2006). *Disability Rights and Wrongs*. London: Routledge.

Sheldon S, and S Wilkinson. (2004). Should selecting saviour siblings be banned? *Journal of Medical Ethics* 30: 533–537.

Singer, Peter. (2011). *Practical Ethics*. Cambridge: Cambridge University Press.

Sparrow, Robert. (2008). Is it 'Every man's right to have babies if he wants them'? Male pregnancy and the limits of reproductive liberty. *Kennedy Institute of Ethics Journal* 18(3): 275–299.

Strange, Heather. (2010). Non-medical sex selection: ethical issues. *British Medical Bulletin* 94(1): 7–20.

Strange, Heather and Chadwick, Ruth. (2010). The ethics of nonmedical sex selection. *Health Care Analysis* 18(3): 252–266.

Strathern, Marilyn. (1994). *The Relation: Issues in Complexity and Scale.* Inaugural lecture before the University of Cambridge.

Taylor-Sands M. (2013). *Saviour Siblings*. Oxford: Routledge.

Thomson, J.J. (1971). A defense of abortion. *Philosophy & Public Affairs* 1(1): 47–66.

Tooley, Michael. (1972). Abortion and infanticide. *Philosophy and Public Affairs* 2(1): 37–65.

Transeuro. (2015). Innovative Approach for the Treatment of Parkinson's Disease. www.transeuro.org.uk/

Vawter, D.E., Kearnery, W., Gervais, K.G., Caplan, A.L., Garry, D., and C. Taue. (1990). *The Use of Human Fetal Tissue: Scientific, Ethical, and Policy Concerns*. Minneapolis: University of Minnesota.

Verhagen, E. (2005). The Groningen Protocol – euthanasia in severely ill newborns. *New England Journal of Medicine* 352: 959–962.

Warnock, Mary. (1985). *A Question of Life: The Warnock Report on Human Fertilisation and Embryology*. Oxford: Blackwell.

Wilkinson, S. (2008). Saviour siblings and organ transplantation. *Clinical Ethics* 3(3): 107–108.

Wilkinson, S. (2015). Do we need an alternative 'relational approach' to saviour siblings? *Journal of Medical Ethics* 41: 927–928.

Chapter 6: Health Care Professional Patient Relationship

Buchanan, Allen E. (1988). Advance Directives and the Non-Identity Problem. *Philosophy and Public Affairs* 17(4): 277–302.

Buchanan, Allen E and Dan W Brock. (1990). *Deciding for Others: The Ethics of Surrogate Decision Making*. New York: Oxford University Press.

Charo, Alta R. (2005). The celestial fire of conscience – refusing to deliver medical care. *New England Journal of Medicine* 352: 2471–2473.

Collins, Joseph. (1927). Should Doctors Tell the Truth? *Harper's Monthly* 155 (August): 320–326.

Cowley, Christopher. (2016). A defence of conscientious objection in medicine: A reply to Schüklenk and Savulescu. *Bioethics* 30: 358–364.

Daniels, Norman. (1991). Duty to treat or right to refuse? *Hastings Center Report* 21(2): 36–46.

Dilling, Daniel. (2007). Diagnostic criteria for persistent vegetative state. *AMA Journal of Medical Ethics* 9: 359–361.

Dresser, Rebecca. (1986). Life, death, and incompetent patients: conceptual infirmities and hidden values in the law. *Arizona Law Review* 28(6): 373–405. https://www.researchgate.net/publication/11698488_Life_Death_and_Incompetent_Patients_Conceptual_Infirmities_and_Hidden_Values_in_the_Law

Evans, Kenneth G. (2016). *Informed consent*. Canadian Medical Protective Association. https://www.cmpa-acpm.ca/en/advice-publications/handbooks/consent-a-guide-for-canadian-physicians

Faden, Ruth R and Tom L Beauchamp. (1986). *A History and Theory of Informed Consent*. New York: Oxford University Press.

Feinberg, Joel. (1986). *The Moral Limits of the Criminal Law: Harm to Self*. New York: Oxford University Press.

Hebert, Phillip C, Hoffmaster, Barry, Glass, Kathleen C, and Peter A Singer. (1997). Bioethics for clinicians: truth telling. *CMAJ* 156: 225–228. www.cmaj.ca/content/156/2/225.full.pdf+html/

Higgs, Roger. (1985). On telling patients the truth. In: *Moral Dilemmas in Modern Medicine*. (ed. Lockwood, Michael), 186–202, 232–233. Oxford: Oxford University Press.

Kant, Immanuel. (1909).*Critique of Practical Reason and Other Works on the Theory of Ethics* 6th edition, trans. T.K. Abbott. 361–363. London.

Kuhse, Helga and Peter Singer. (1985). *Should the Baby Live? The Problem of Handicapped Infants*. Oxford: Oxford University Press.

Kuhse, Helga. (1987). *The Sanctity of Life Doctrine in Medicine: A Critique*. Oxford: Clarendon Press.

Minerva, Francesca. (2015). Conscientious objection in Italy. *Journal of Medical Ethics* 41: 170–173.

Multi-Society Task Force on PVS 1. (1994a). Medical aspects of the persistent vegetative state – first of two parts. *New England Journal of Medicine* 330:1499–1508.

Multi-Society Task Force on PVS 2. (1994b). Medical aspects of the persistent vegetative state – second of two parts. *New England Journal of Medicine* 330: 1572–1579.

Petrini, Carlo. (2014). Ethical and legal aspects of refusal of blood transfusions by Jehovah's Witnesses, with particular reference to Italy. *Blood Transfusion* 12(suppl 1): s395–401. www.ncbi.nlm.nih.gov/pmc/articles/PMC3934270/

Reid, Lynette. (2005). Diminishing returns? Risks and the duty to care in the SARS epidemic. *Bioethics* 19: 348–361.

Ries, NM. (2004). Public health law and ethics: lessons from SARS and quarantine. *Health Law Review* 13(1): 3–6.

Savulescu, Julian and Udo Schüklenk. (2017). Doctors have no right to refuse medical assistance in dying, abortion or contraception. *Bioethics* 31(3): 162–170.

Schachter, Madeleine and Joseph J. Fins. (2008). Informed Consent Revisited: A Doctrine in the Service of Cancer Care. *The Oncologist* 13(10): 1109–1113.

Schüklenk, Udo. (2015). Physicians can justifiably euthanize certain severely impaired neonates. *Journal for Thoracic and Cardiovascular Surgery* 149: 535–537.

Schüklenk, Udo and Ricardo Smalling. (2017). Why medical professionals have no moral claim to conscientious objection accommodation in liberal democracies. *Journal of medical ethics* 43: 234–240. doi: 10.1136/medethics-2016-103560 http://jme.bmj.com/content/early/2016/04/27/medethics-2016-103560.abstract.

Schüklenk, Udo. (2019). Non-informed consent can be ethically defensible. *Annals of Thoracic Surgery* 106: 1612–1613.

Schüklenk, Udo. (2020). What health care professionals owe us: why their duty to treat during a pandemic is contingent on personal protective equipment (PPE). *Journal of medical ethics* 46: doi: 10.1136/medethics-2020-106278.

Siegler, Mark. (1982). Confidentiality in medicine – a decrepit concept. *New England Journal of Medicine* 307: 1518–1521.

Smolkin, D. (1997). HIV infection, risk taking, and the duty to treat. *Journal of Medicine and Philosophy* 22: 55–74.

Sulmasy, Daniel P. (2008). What is conscience, and why is respect for it so important? *Theoretical Medicine and Bioethics* 29: 135–149.

West-Oram Peter and Alena Buyx. (2016). Conscientious objection in health care provision: a new dimension. *Bioethics* 30: 336–343.

Wicclair, Mark R. (1991). Patient decision-making capacity and risk. *Bioethics* 5(2): 91–104.

Wicclair Mark R. (2000). Conscientious objection in medicine. *Bioethics* 14: 205–27.

WMA (World Medical Association). (2017). Declaration of Geneva https://www.wma.net/policies-post/wma-declaration-of-geneva/

Chapter 7: Research Ethics

Adebamowo, Clement, Bah-Sow, Oumou, Binka, Fred, Bruzzone, et al. (2014). Randomised controlled trials for Ebola: Practical and ethical issues. *The Lancet* 384: 1423–1424.

Angelski, Calra, Fernandez, Conrad V., Weijer, Charles and Jun Gao. (2011). The publication of ethically uncertain research: attitudes and practices of journal editors. *BMC Medical Ethics* 2012; 13(4) doi: 10.1186/1472-6939-13-4.

Annas George J. (1990). (Healing), Hope, and Charity at the FDA: The Politics of AIDS Drug Trials. In: *AIDS and the Healthcare System*. (ed. Lawrence O. Gostin), 183–194. New Haven (CT): Yale University Press.

Arras, John. (1990). Non-compliance in AIDS Research. *Hastings Center Report* 20(5): 24–32.

Ballantyne Angela J. (2010). How to do research fairly in an unjust world. *American Journal of Bioethics* 10(6): 26–35.

CIOMS (2016). *International Ethical Guidelines for Health-Related Research Involving Humans*. Geneva: CIOMS.

Cohen, Baruch. (1990). The ethics of using medical data from Nazi experiments. *Journal of Halacha and Contemporary Society* 19: 103–126.

Delaney, Martin. (1989). The case for patient access to experimental therapy. *Journal of Infectious Diseases* 159: 416–419.

Dixon, John. (1991). Catastrophic rights: vital public interests and civil liberties in conflict. In: *Perspectives on AIDS: Ethical and Social Issues*. (eds Christine Overall and William P. Zion). Toronto: Oxford University Press.

Donaldson, Sue, and Will Kymlicka. (2011). *Zoopolis: A Political Theory of Animal Rights*. Oxford: Oxford University Press.

Emanuel, Ezekiel, Wendler, David, Grady, Christine. (2000). What makes clinical research ethical? *JAMA* 283: 2701–2711.

Freedman, Benjamin. (1987). Equipoise and the ethics of clinical research. *New England of Medicine* 317: 141–145.

Hellman, S. and D. Hellman. (1991). Of mice but not men: problems of the randomized clinical trial. *New England Journal of Medicine.* 324: 1585–1589.

ICMJE International Council of Medical Journal Editors (2010). Uniform Requirements for Manuscripts Submitted to Biomedical Journals. www. icmje.org/urm_main.html/

Levine, Robert J. (1998). The 'best proven therapeutic method' standard in clinical trials in technologically developing countries. *IRB – A Review of Human Subjects Research* 20(1): 5–9.

Lie, Reidar K. (2010). The fair benefit approach revisited. *Hastings Center Report* 40(4): 3.

Lo, Bernard, Padian, Nancy, and Barnes, Mark. (2007). The obligation to provide antiretroviral treatment in HIV prevention trials. *AIDS* 21(10): 1229–1231.

London, Alex John and Kevin J.S. Zollman. (2010). Research at the auction block: problems for the fair benefits approach to international research. *Hastings Center Report* 40(4): 34–45.

Lowry, Christopher and Udo Schüklenk. (2009). Two models in global health ethics. *Public Health Ethics* 2: 276–284.

Macklin, Ruth. (2006). Changing the presumption: providing ART to vaccine research participants. *American Journal of Bioethics* 6(1): W1–W5.

Macklin, Ruth and Gerald Friedland. (1986). AIDS research: the ethics of clinical trials. *Law, Medicine and Health Care* 14: 273–280.

Miller, Seumas and Michael Selgelid. (2008). *Ethical and Philosophical Consideration of the Dual-Use Dilemma in the Biological Sciences*. Dordrecht: Springer.

Moe, Kristine. (1984). Should the Nazi research data be cited? *Hastings Center Report* 14(6): 5–7.

National Commission for the Protection of Human Subjects of Biomedical and Behavioral Research (1979). The Belmont Report: Ethical Principles and Guidelines for the Protection of Human Subjects of Research. https://www.hhs.gov/ohrp/regulations-and-policy/belmont-report/index.html/

Novick, Alvin. (1993). Reflections on a term of public service with the FDA Anti-Virals Advisory Committee. *AIDS and Public Policy Journal* 8(2): 55–61.

Orford, C. (2019). *N-of-1 trials take on challenges in health care. The Scientist.* July/Augusthttps://www.the-scientist.com/features/n-of-1-trials-take-on-challenges-in-health-car-66071

Participants in the 2001 Conference on Ethical Aspects of Research in Developing Countries. (2004). Moral standards for research in developing countries: from 'reasonable availability' to 'fair benefits'. *Hastings Center Report* 34(3): 17–27.

Proctor, Robert N. (1999). *The Nazi War on Cancer*. Princeton: Princeton University Press.

Regan, Tom. (1988). *The Case for Animal Rights*. London: Routledge.

Reiss, Michael. (2000). The ethics of genetic research on intelligence. *Bioethics* 14: 1–15.

Schüklenk, Udo. (1990). *Access to Experimental Drugs in Terminal Illness: Ethical Issues*. Binghamton: Pharmaceutical Products Press.

Schüklenk, Udo, Stein, Edward, Kerin, Jacintha, and William Byne. (1997). The ethics of genetic research on sexual orientation. *Hastings Center Report* 27(4): 6–13.

Schüklenk, Udo and Richard E. Ashcroft. (2000). International Research Ethics. *Bioethics* 14: 158–172.

Schüklenk, Udo and Anita Kleinsmidt. (2006). North-south benefit sharing arrangements in bioprospecting and genetic research: An ethical and legal analysis. *Developing World Bioethics* 6: 122–134.

Schüklenk, Udo, and Jim Gallagher. (2007). Obligations of the pharmaceutical industry. In: *Principles of Health Care Ethics*. (eds Ashcroft, Richard, Dawson, Angus, Draper, Heather, and John R. McMillan. West Sussex, UK: John Wiley & Sons, Ltd: 734–751.

Schüklenk, Udo and Ricardo Smalling. (2017). The moral case for granting catastrophically ill patients the right to access unregistered medical interventions. *Journal of Law, Medicine & Ethics* 45(3): 382–391.

Simon, Alan E., Wu, Albert W., Lavori, Philip W., and Jeremy Sugarman. (2007). Preventive misconception: its nature, presence, and ethical implications for research. *American Journal of Preventive Medicine* 32: 370–374.

Singer, Peter. 2011. *Practical Ethics*, 3rd edition. New York: Cambridge University Press.

Trials of War Criminals before the Nuremberg Military Tribunals under Control Council Law. (1994). [1949]. *Nuremberg Code* 2(10): 181–182. Washington, D.C.: U.S. Government Printing Office.

Weijer, Charles, and Guy J. LeBlanc. (2006). The Balm of Gilead. Is the provision of treatment to those who seroconvert in HIV prevention trials a matter of moral obligation or moral negotiation? *Journal of Law, Medicine & Ethics* 34: 793–808.

Wertheimer, Alan. (2008). Exploitation in clinical research. In:. *Exploitation and Developing Countries: The Ethics of Clinical Research.* (eds Hawkins, Jennifer and Ezekiel Emanuel), 63–104. Princeton: Princeton University Press.

World Medical Association (1964–2013). "Declaration of Helsinki", https://www.wma.net/policies-post/wma-declaration-of-helsinki-ethical-principles-for-medical-research-involving-human-subjects/

Chapter 8: Genetics

Arney, Kat. (2018). Change the genes to fix the skin: The largest organ in the body is a prime target for gene therapy. *Nature* S64: 14–15.

Bergmann, Mary Todd. (2019). Perspectives in gene editing: Harvard researchers, others share their views on key issues in the field. *The Harvard Gazette,* 9 January.

British Society for Human Genetics (BSHG). (2010). *Report on the Genetic Testing of Children.* Birmingham:BSHG.

Bush, George W. (President). (2001). President George W. Bush's announcement on stem cells. August 09. https://embryo.asu.edu/pages/president-george-w-bushs-announcement-stem-cells-9-august-2001

Chadwick, Ruth and O'Connor, Alan. (2013). Epigenetics and personalised medicine. *Personalised Medicine* 10(5): 463–471.

Chadwick, Ruth, Levitt, Mairi. and Darren Shickle. (eds). (2014). *The Right to Know and the Right not to Know.* Cambridge: Cambridge University Press.

Daar, Abdallah, S. and Peter A. Singer. (2005). 'Pharmacogenomics and geographical ancestry: implications for drug development and global health' *Nature Reviews Genetics* 6: 241–6.

Dimond, Rebecca. (2015). Social and ethical issues in mitochondrial donation. *British Medical Bulletin* 115(1): 173–182.

Elsner, Markus. (2018). Epigenome editing to the rescue. *Nature Biotechnology* 36(4): 315.

Elwyn, G., Gray, J and Clarke, Angus. (2000). Shared decision making and non-directiveness in genetic counseling. *Journal of Medical Genetics* 37(2): 135–138.

European Science Foundation (ESF). (2012). *Personalised Medicine for the European Citizen – towards more precise medicine for the diagnosis, treatment and prevention of disease.* Strasbourg: ESF.

Gottweis, Herbert, Petersen, Alan. (eds). (2008). *Biobanks: Governance in Comparative Perspective.* London: Routledge.

Green, M.J. and Botkin, J.R. (2003). "Genetic exceptionalism" in medicine: clarifying the differences between genetic and nongenetic tests. *Annals of Internal Medicine* 138(7): 571–575.

Holm, Søren. (2002). Going to the roots of the stem cell controversy. *Bioethics* 16(6): 496–497.

Human Genome Organisation. (2000). *Statement on Benefit-Sharing.* London: HUGO.

Husted, Jørgen. (2014). Autonomy and a right not to know. In: *The Right to Know and the Right not to Know.* (eds R. Chadwick et al.) Cambridge: University Press.

Kass, Leon R. (1997). The wisdom of repugnance. *The New Republic* June 2: 17–26.

Knoppers, Bartha Maria, Chadwick, Ruth. (2005). Human genetic research: emerging trends in ethics. *Nature Reviews Genetics* 6(1): 75-9.

Schüklenk, Udo and Smalling, Ricardo (2017). The moral case for granting catastrophically ill patients the right to access unregistered medical interventions. *The Journal of Law, Medicine and Ethics*, 45(3), 382–391: 75–79.

Knoppers, Bartha Maria and Chadwick, Ruth. (2015). The ethics weathervane. *BMC Medical Ethics* 16: 58. https://link.springer.com/content/pdf/10.1186%2Fs12910-015-0054-4.pdf/

Levitt, Mairi. (2013). Perceptions of nature, nurture and behaviour. *Life Sciences Society and Policy* 9: 13. doi: 10.1186/2195-7819-9-13.

Lunshof, Jeantine E., Chadwick, Ruth, Church, George, Vorhaus, Dan. (2008). From genetic privacy to open consent. *Nature Reviews Genetics* 9: 406–411.

Lunshof, Jeantine E. and Chadwick, Ruth. (2011). Editorial: genetic and genomic research – changing patterns of accountability. *Accountability in Research* 18(3): 121–131.

Mackley, Michael P. and Capps, Ben. (2017). Expect the unexpected: screening for secondary findings in clinical genomics research. *British Medical Bulletin* 122(1): 109–122.

[US]National Academy of Sciences (NAS). (2011). *Toward Precision Medicine: Building a Knowledge Network for Biomedical Research and a New Taxonomy of Disease.* Washington, DC: NAS.

Nelkin, D. and Lindee, M. Susan. (1995). *The DNA Mystique: The Gene as Cultural Icon.* New York: W.H. Freeman.

Nuffield Council on Bioethics. (1993). *Genetic Screening: Ethical Issues.* London: Nuffield Council on Bioethics.

Nuffield Council on Bioethics. (2003). *Pharmacogenomics: Ethical Issues.* London: Nuffield Council on Bioethics.

Nuffield Council on Bioethics. (2018). *Genome Editing and Human Reproduction.* London: Nuffield Council on Bioethics.

Pence, Gregory E. (1998). *Who's Afraid of Human Cloning?* Lanham: Rowman and Littlefield.

Savulescu, Julian and Singer, Peter (2019). An ethical pathway for gene editing. *Bioethics* 33: 2.

Scholl, H.P.N. and Sahel, J.A. (2014). Gene therapy arrives at the macula. *Lancet* 383 (9923): 1105–1107.

Stolberg, Sheryl Gay. (1999). The biotech death of Jesse Gelsinger. *New York Times* 28 November.

UNESCO. (1997). *Universal Declaration on the Human Genome and Human Rights.* Paris: UNESCO.

U.S. (1927). *Buck v Bell 274 U.S. 200.*

Zezulin, A. and Musunuru, K. (2017). Turning up the heat with therapeutic epigenome editing. *Cell Stem Cell* 22 (4 Jan): 10–11.

Chapter 9: Enhancement

Agar, Nicholas. (2010). *Humanity's End: Why We Should Reject Radical Enhancement.* Cambridge MA: MIT Press.

Agar, Nicholas. (2013). *Truly Human Enhancement: A Philosophical Defense of its Limits.* Cambridge, MA: MIT Press.

Aristotle. (1908). *Nicomachean Ethics.* D. Ross. (trans.) Clarendon: Oxford.

Baylis, Francoise and Robert, Jason Scott. (2004). The inevitability of genetic enhancement techniques. *Bioethics* 18(1): 1–26.

Carter, Sarah. (2015). Putting a price on empathy: against incentivising moral enhancement. *Journal of Medical Ethics* 41: 825–829.

Chadwick, Ruth. (2008). Enhancement, therapy and improvement. In: *Medical Enhancement and Posthumanity.* (eds B. Gordijn and R. Chadwick). Dordrecht: Springer.

Daniels, Norman. (2000). Normal functioning and the treatment-enhancement distinction. *Cambridge Quarterly of Healthcare Ethics* 9: 309–322.

Eisinger, François. (2007). Prophylactic mastectomy: ethical issues. *British Medical Bulletin* 81-2: 719.

Fukuyama, Francis. (2003). *Our Posthuman Future: Consequences of the Biotechnology Revolution.* New York: Picador.

Habermas, Jürgen. (2003). *The Future of Human Nature.* Beister, H., Rehg, W. (trans). Cambridge: Polity.

Hamzelou, Jessica. (2017). Brain implant boosts memory by mimicking how we learn. *New Scientist,* 13 November.

Harris, John. (2007). *Enhancing Evolution: The Ethical Case for Making Better People.* Columbia and Princeton University Presses.

Harris, John. (2012). Moral progress and moral enhancement. *Bioethics* 27(5): 285–290.

Harris, John. (2016). Germline modification and the burden of human existence. *Cambridge Quarterly of Healthcare Ethics* 25(1): 6–18.

Henrich, Daniel. (2011). Human nature and autonomy: Jurgen Habermas' critique of liberal eugenics. *Ethical Perspectives* 18: 249–268.

Holm, Søren. (1994). Genetic engineering and the North-South divide. In: *Bioethics and Biotechnology.* (eds Anthony Dyson and John Harris). London: Routledge.

Hume, David. (2000). [1739–40]. A Treatise of Human Nature. Oxford University Press.

Innes, Michael. (1951). *Operation Pax.* Harmondsworth: Penguin.

Kant, I. (2012). [1785]. *Groundwork of the Metaphysics of Morals. Translated by Mary Gregor, Jens Timmerman.* Cambridge: University Press.

Krutzinna, Jenny. (2016). Can a welfarist approach justify a moral duty to cognitively enhance children? *Bioethics* 30(7): 528–535.

Miah, Andy. (2004). *Genetically Modified Athletes: Biomedical Ethics, Gene Doping and Sport.* London: Routledge.

Ministry of Defence. (2010). *Global Strategic Trends, 4th edition – Out to 2040.* London: Ministry of Defence.

Persson, Ingmar and, Savulescu, Julian. (2008). The perils of cognitive enhancement and the urgent imperative to enhance the moral character of humanity. *Journal of Applied Philosophy* 25(3): 162–177.

Rakić, Vojin. (2014). Voluntary moral enhancement and survival-at-any-cost bias. *Journal of Medical Ethics* 40(4): 246–250.

Sparrow, Robert. (2007). Revolutionary and familiar, inevitable and precarious: rhetorical contradistinctions in enthusiasm for nanotechnology. *Nanoethics* 1: 57–68.

Sparrow, Robert. (2015). Enhancement and obsolescence: avoiding an "enhanced rat race". *Kennedy Institute of Ethics* 25 (3): 231–260.

Sparrow, Robert. (2019). Yesterday's child: how gene editing for enhancement will produce obsolescence – and why it matters. *American Journal of Bioethics* 19(7): 6–15.

Sparrow, Rob and Cohen, Glenn. (2015). Genetically engineering humans: a step too far? *Pharmaceutical Journal* 295(7881).

Stapledon, Olaf. (1930). *Last and First Men.* York: Methuen.

Strathern, Marilyn. (1995). *The Relation: Inaugural Lecture.* Cambridge: Prickly Pear Press.

Sulekova, Maria and Fitzgerald, Kevin. (2019). Can the thought of Teilhard de Chardin carry us past current contentious discussions of gene editing technologies? *Cambridge Quarterly of Healthcare Ethics* 28(1): 62–75.

US President's Council on Bioethics Report. 2003. *Beyond Therapy: Biotechnology and the Pursuit of Happiness.* https://repository.library. georgetown.edu/bitstream/handle/10822/559341/beyond_therapy_final_ webcorrected.pdf.

Warnock, Geoffrey. (1971). *The Object of Morality.* London: Methuen.

Warwick, Kevin. (2010). Future issues with robots and cyborgs. *Studies in Ethics, Law and Technology.* 4 (3) Article 6.

Wellcome Collection. (2012). *Superhuman: Exploring Human Enhancement From 600 BCE to 2050.* London: Wellcome Trust.

Young, Emma. (2016). How sharing other people's feelings can make you sick. *New Scientist* 14 May: 33–35.

Chapter 10: Mental Health

Aleman, André and Denys, Damiaan. (2014). A road map for suicide prevention and research. *Nature* 509: 421–423.

American Psychiatric Association. (2013). *The Diagnostic and Statistical Manual of Mental Disorders (DSM) 5.* American Psychiatric Association.

Bayer, Ronald. (1987). *Homosexuality and American Psychiatry: The Politics of Diagnosis.* Princeton: Princeton University Press.

Brendel, David (2006). *Healing Psychiatry.* Cambridge: MIT Press.

Buchanan, Alec. (2014). Psychiatric detention and treatment: a suggested criterion. *Journal of Mental Health Law* 35: 35–41.

Chadwick, Ruth. (1994). Kant, thought insertion and mental unity. *Philosophy, Psychiatry and Psychology* 1(2): 105–113.

Chadwick, Ruth. (2016). Normality as convention and as scientific fact. In: T. Schramme and S. Edwards (eds) *Handbook of the Philosophy of Medicine*. Dordrecht: Springer.

De Hert, Marc. (2011). Physical illness in patients with severe mental disorders. I. Prevalence, impact of medications and disparities in health care. *World Psychiatry* 10(1): 52–77.

Eastman, Nick. (1994). Mental health law: civil liberties and the principle of reciprocity. *British Medical Journal* 308: 43.

Edwards, Steven D. and Hewitt, Jeanette. (2011). Can supervising self-harm be part of ethical nursing practice? *Nursing Ethics* 18(1): 79–87.

Fulford, K.W.M. (1987). *Moral Theory and Medical Practice*. Cambridge: Cambridge University Press.

Lindley, R. (1978). Social philosophy. In: R. Lindley et al. *What Philosophy Does*. London: Open Books.

Megone, Chris. (2000). Mental illness, human function, and values. *Philosophy, Psychology, Psychiatry*. 7(1): 45–56.

Mill, John Stuart. (1859). *Essay On Liberty*. London: J.W. Parker.

Mind. (2017). www.mind.org.uk/

New, Christopher. (1992). Time and punishment. *Analysis* 52 (1): 35–40.

Pies, R.W. (2014). The Bereavement Exclusion and DSM-5: an update and commentary. *Innovation in Clinical Neurosciences* 11(7–8): 19–22.

Radden, Jennifer and Sadler, John Z. (2013). Character virtues in psychiatric practice. In: D.A Susti, A.C. Caplan and H. Rimon-Greenspan (eds) *Applied Ethics in Mental Health Care: An Interdisciplinary Reader*. Cambridge: MIT Press.

Scholten, Matthé and Gather, Jakov. (2018). Adverse consequences of Article 12 of the UN Convention on the Rights of Persons with Disabilities and an Alternative Way Forward. *Journal of Medical Ethics* 44: 226–233.

Smilansky, S. (2007). Determinism and prepunishment: the radical nature of compatibilism. *Analysis* 67 (4): 347–349.

Szasz, Thomas S. (1962). *The Myth of Mental Illness*. London: Harper & Row.

Thaler, Richard H. and Sunstein, Cass R. (2008). *Nudge: Improving Decisions About Health*, Wealth and Happiness. New Haven: Yale University Press.

United Nations. (1991). *Principles for the Protection of Persons with Mental Illness and the Improvement of Mental Health Care*. Adopted by General Assembly Resolution 46/119 of 17 December 1991.

UN Convention on the Rights of Persons with Disabilities (2006).

van Voren, R. (2012). Political abuse of psychiatry. In M. Dudley (ed.), *Oxford Textbook on Mental Health and Human Rights*. Oxford: Oxford University Press.

Wilkes, K.V. (1988). *Real People: Personal Identity Without Thought Experiments.* Oxford: Clarendon Press.

World Health Organization (2014). Mental Health. www.who.int/mental_health/en/

Young, Robert. (1986). *Personal Autonomy: Beyond Negative and Positive Liberty.* Croome-Helm.

Chapter 11: End-of-Life Issues

Burgess, John A. (1993). The great slippery-slope argument. *Journal of Medical Ethics* 19: 169–174.

Downie, Jocelyn, Chambaere, Kenneth, and Jan L. Bernheim. (2012). Pereira's attack on legalizing euthanasia and assisted suicide: smoke and mirrors. *Current Oncology* 19(3). www.current-oncology.com/index.php/oncology/article/view/1063/913/

EIU. (2016). *The Quality of Death: Ranking End-of-Life Care Across the World.* https://eiuperspectives.economist.com/healthcare/2015-quality-death-index

Emanuel, Ezekiel J. (2014). Why I hope to die at 75. *The Atlantic* www.theatlantic.com/magazine/archive/2014/10/why-i-hope-to-die-at-75/379329/

Hardwig, John. (2000). *Is There a Duty to Die? And Other Essays in Medical Ethics.* New York: Routledge.

Harris, John. (1970). *The Value of Life, an Introduction to Medical Ethics.* London: Routledge and Keegan Paul.

Kamm, Frances M. (1997). A right to choose death? *Boston Review* 22. https://bostonreview.net/books-ideas/fm-kamm-right-choose-death

Kant, Immanuel. 1785 *(1993)*. *(J.W. Ellington trans.) Grounding for the Metaphysics of Morals*, 3rd edition. Indianapolis: Hackett.

Pereira, Jose. (2011). Legalizing euthanasia or assisted suicide: the illusion of safeguards. *Current Oncology* 18(2). www.current-moncology.com/index.php/oncology/article/view/883/645/

Schüklenk, Udo, van Delden, Johannes J.M., Downie, Jocelyn, et al. (2011). End-of-Life Decision-Making in Canada: The Report by the Royal Society of Canada Expert Panel in End-of-Life Decision-Making. *Bioethics* 25(S1): 1–71. http://onlinelibrary.wiley.com/doi/10.1111/bioe.2011.25.issue-s1/issuetoc/

Von Staden, Heinrich. (2009). *The discourses of practitioners in ancient Europe.* New York: Cambridge University Press: 352–358.

Velleman, David. (1999). A right to self-termination? *Ethics* 109: 606–628.
WHO. N.d. Definition of palliative care. www.who.int/cancer/palliative/
definition/en/

Chapter 12: Justice

Daniels, Norman. (2008). *Just Health: Meeting Health Needs Fairly.* Cambridge:
Cambridge University Press.
Daniels, Norman. (2010). Capabilities, opportunity and health. In: *Measuring Justice: Primary Goods and Capabilities.* (eds H. Brighouse and I. Robeyns).
Cambridge: Cambridge University Press.
Evans, Don. (2013). Resource allocation. In: R. Chadwick (ed.) *Encyclopedia of Applied Ethics,* 2nd edition, 813–820. Elsevier.
Gallie, W.B. (1955). Essentially contested concepts. *Proceedings of the Aristotelian Society, New Series* 56: 167–198.
Harris, John. (1985). *The Value of Life* London: Routledge.
Margalit, Avisha (1996). *The Decent Society.* Cambridge, Mass: Harvard University Press.
Nussbaum, Martha. (2011). *Creating Capabilities: The Human Development Approach.* Cambridge, Mass: Belknap.
Rawls, John. (1971). *A Theory of Justice Cambridge,* Mass: Harvard University Press.
Rogers, Wendy (2004a). Evidence-based medicine and women: do the principles and practice of EBM further women's health? *Bioethics* 18 (1): 50–71.
Rogers, Wendy (2004b). Evidence-based medicine and justice: a framework for looking at the impact of EBM upon vulnerable or disadvantaged groups. *Journal of Medical Ethics* 30(2): 141–145.
Segall, S. (2009). *Health,* Luck and Justice Princeton, NJ: University Press.
Sen, Amartya. (1996). On the status of equality. *Political Theory* 24(3): 394–400.
Ventakapuram, S. (2011). *Health Justice.* Cambridge: Polity Press.
World Health Organization https://www.who.int/about/who-we-are/constituion
Vergel, Y.B. and Schulpher, M. (2008). Quality-adjusted life years. *Practical Neurology* 8(3): 175–182.
Walzer, Michael. (1983). *Spheres of Justice: A Defense of Pluralism and Equality.* New York: Basic Books.
Williams, Alan. (1995). Economics, QALYs and medical ethics—A health economist's perspective. *Health Care Analysis* 3: 221–226. https://doi.org/10.1007/BF02197671

Williams, Bernard. (1973). The idea of equality. In: *Problems of the Self.* (ed. B. Williams). Cambridge: University Press.

Chapter 13: Population Health

Allen, Michael. (2011). Is liberty bad for your health? Towards a moderate view of the robust coequality of liberty and health. *Public Health Ethics* 4: 260–268.

Armstrong, Russell. (2008). Mandatory HIV testing in pregnancy – is there ever a time? *Developing World Bioethics* 8: 1–10.

Bayer, Ronald. (1989). *Private Acts and Social Consequences: AIDS and the Politics of Public Health.* New York: Free Press.

Bogart, W.A. (2013). *Regulating Obesity: Government, Society, and Questions of Health.* New York: Oxford University Press.

British Columbia Ministry of Health Provincial COVID-19 Task Force. (2020) COVID-19 Ethics Analysis: What is the Ethical Duty of Health Care Workers to Provide Care During COVID-19 Pandemic? March 28, 2020 https://www2.gov.bc.ca/assets/gov/health/about-bc-s-health-care-system/office-of-the-provincial-health-officer/covid-19/duty_to_care_during_covid_march_28_2020.pdf

Broadbent, Alex. (2020). Lockdown is wrong for Africa. *Mail&Guardian* April 08. https://mg.co.za/analysis/2020-04-08-lockdown-is-wrong-for-africa/

Callahan, Daniel. (2013). Obesity: chasing an elusive threat. *Hastings Center Report* 43: 34–40.

Chatham House. (2011). *Background Note: Commission on Macroeconomics and Health (2001) – Ten Years On.* London: Chatham House.

Childress, J.F., Faden, R.R., Gaare, R. (2002). Public health ethics: mapping the terrain. *Journal of Medicine, Law and Ethics* 30: 169–177.

Clark, Hellen. (2013). NCD: a challenge to sustainable human development. *Lancet* 381: 510–511.

Davidson, Helen. (2020). First Covid-19 case happened in November, China government reports show. *The Guardian* March 13. https://www.theguardian.com/world/2020/mar/13/first-covid-19-case-happened-in-november-china-government-records-show-report

Davies, P.M., Hickson, F.C.I., Weatherburn, P., and Hunt, A.J. (1993). *Sex, Gay Men and AIDS.* London: Falmer Press.

Duffy, John. (2014). *Public Health: History.* In: Jennings, Bruce (ed.). *Bioethics (4th ed.)* MacMillan: Farmington Hills, Mich., 2592–2597.

Dworkin, Gerald. (1988). *The Theory and Practice of Autonomy.* Cambridge, MA: Cambridge University Press.

Fontaine, K., Redden, D., Wang, C., et al. (2003). Years of life lost due to obesity. *JAMA* 289: 187–193.

Galanakis, E., Jansen, A., Lopalco, P.L., and J. Giesecke. (2013). Ethics of mandatory vaccination of health care workers. *Eurosurveillance* 18(45): pii=20627.

Garrett, Laurie. (1994). *The Coming Plague: Newly Emerging Diseases in the World*. New York: Farrar Straus & Giraux.

Giubilini, Alberto, Douglas, Thomas, and Julian Savulescu. (2018). The moral obligation to be vaccinated: utilitarianism, contractualism, and collective easy rescue. *Medicine, Health Care and Philosophy* 21: 547–560.

Giubilini, Alberto. (2019). *The Ethics of Vaccination*. Cham: Palgrave.

Haines, Andy and Krietie Ebie. (2019). The imperative for climate action to protect health. *New England Journal of Medicine* 380: 263–273.

Hotez, Peter. (2019). *Vaccines Did Not Cause Rachel's Autism*. Baltimore: Johns Hopkins University Press.

Illingworth, Patricia. (1990). *AIDS and the Good Society*. London: Routledge.

Illingworth, Patricia. (1991). Warning: AIDS Health Promotion Programs may be hazardous to your autonomy. In: *Perspective on AIDS: Ethical and Social Issues*. (eds Overall, Christine and William P. Zion), 138–154. Toronto: Oxford University Press.

Kass, N. (2001). An ethics framework for public health. *American Journal of Public Health* 91: 1776–1782.

Keshavan, Meghana. (2020). 'We're being put at risk unnecessarily': Doctors fume at government response to coronavirus pandemic. *STAT* April 09. https://www.statnews.com/2020/04/09/doctors-fume-at-government-response-to-coronavirus-pandemic/

Lazzarini, Zita, Bray, Sarah, and Scott Burris. (2002). Evaluating the Impact of Criminal Law on HIV Risk Behaviour. *Journal of Law, Medicine and Ethics* 30: 239–253.

Lowry, Christopher R and Udo Schüklenk. (2009). Two Models in Global Health Ethics. *Public Health Ethics* 2: 276–284.

Mohr, Richard D. (1987). AIDS, Gays and State Coercion. *Bioethics* 1: 35–50.

Ng, M., Fleming, T., Robinson, M., Thomson, B., Graetz, N. et al. (2014). Global, regional and national prevalence of overweight and obesity in children and adults during 1980–2013: a systematic analysis for the Global Burdens of Disease Study. *Lancet* 384: 766–781.

Olive, Jacqueline K., Hotez, Peter J., Damania, Ashish, and Melissa S. Nolan. (2018). The state of the antivaccine movement in the United States: A focused examination of nonmedical excemtions in states and counties. *PLOS Medicine* 15(7): e1002616.

Oxfam America. (2020). Dignity not Destitution. April 09. https://assets. oxfamamerica.org/media/documents/mb-dignity_not_destitution-an-economic-rescue-plan-for-all-090420-en.pdf

Patel, Manisha, Lee, Adria D., Clemmons, Nakia S., Redd, Susan B., et al. (2019). National update on measles cases and outbreaks – United States January 1–October 1, 2019. *Morbidity and Mortality Weekly Report* 68(40): 893–896.

Parfit, Derek. (1994). What makes someone's life go best? In: Peter Singer (ed). *Ethics*. Oxford: Oxford University Press: 235–242.

Pogge, Thomas. (2008). *World Poverty and Human Rights*, 2nd edition. Cambridge: Polity.

Risse, Matthias. (2005). Does the global order harm the poor? *Philosophy and Public Affairs* 33: 35–45.

Scanlon, Tim. (1998). *What We Owe to Each Other*. Cambridge, MA: Harvard University Press.

Schreiber, Mayo Jr. (2017). An update on the prosecution, conviction and appeal of Michael Johnson. *American Psychological Association Psychology and AIDS Exchange Newsletter* March.

Schüklenk, Udo and Erik Yuan Zhang. (2014). Public health ethics and obesity prevention: the trouble with data and ethics. *Monash Bioethics Review* 32(1–2): 121–140.

Schüklenk, Udo. (2020). COVID19: Why justice and transparency in hospital triage policies are paramount. *Bioethics* 34: https://doi.org/10.1111/bioe.12744.

Schüklenk, Udo. (2020a). What health care professionals owe us: why their duty to treat during a pandemic is contingent on personal protective equipment (PPE). *Journal of medical ethics* 46: doi: 10.1136/medethics-2020-106278.

Schwartz AR. Doubtful Duty: Physicians' Legal Obligation to Treat during an Epidemic. *60 Stan. L. Rev. 657 2007*, 660.

Selgelid, Michael. (2005). Ethics and infectious disease. *Bioethics* 19: 272–289.

Singer, Peter. (1972). Famine, affluence, and morality. *Philosophy and Public Affairs* 1: 229–241.

Singer, Peter. (2004). Outsiders: our obligations to those beyond our borders. In: Chatterjee, D.K., (ed.)*The Ethics of Assistance: Morality and the Distant Needy.*, 11–32. Cambridge: Cambridge University Press.

Singh, Jerome A., Upshur, Ross, and Nesri Padayatchi. (2007). XDR-TB in South AfricA: No Time for Denial or Complacency. *PLoS Medicine* 4:1: e50.

State of Missouri v. Michael L. Johnson, Case No. 1311-CR05915-01

Ten Have, M.A., van der Heide, A., Mackenbach, J., et al. (2012). An ethical framework for the prevention of overweight and obesity: a tool for thinking through a programme's ethical aspects. *European Journal of Public Health* 23: 299–305.

Verweij, Marcel and Angus Dawson. (2013). Public Health Ethics. In: *The International Encyclopedia of Ethics*. Vol. 7. (ed. LaFollette, Hugh), 4220–4230. Chichester: Wiley

Upshur, Ross. (2013). What does public health ethics tell (or not tell) us about intervening in non-communicable diseases? *Journal of Bioethical Inquiry* 10: 19–28.

Viens A.M. (2014). Population Ethics: History of Population Theories. In: Jennings, Bruce (ed). *Bioethics 4th edition*. 2409–2415. Farmington Hills, Mich: MacMillan.

Weeks, Carly. (2019). Should vaccines be mandatory for school-aged children? *Globe and Mail* August 29.

FURTHER READING

Chapter 1: Introduction to Ethics

Aristotle. (1980). *Nicomachean Ethics. (transl. by W.D. Ross)*. Oxford: Oxford University Press.

Barry, Vincent. (2012). *Bioethics in a Cultural Context: Philosophy, Religion, History, Politics*. Boston: Wadsworth.

Blackford, Russell, and Udo Schüklenk. (2021). Religion at work in bioethics and biopolicy: Christian bioethicists, secular language, suspicious orthodoxy. *Journal of Medicine and Philosophy* 46: (in press).

LaFollette, Hugh. (ed. 2013). *The International Encyclopedia of Ethics. Vol. 1–9*. Oxford: Wiley-Blackwell.

Louden, Robert B. (1998). Virtue Ethics. In: Ruth Chadwick (Ed.). *Encyclopedia of Applied Ethics. Vol. 4*. San Diego: Academic Press: 491–498.

Rawls, John. (1997). The idea of public reason revisited. *The University of Chicago Law Review* 64: 765–807.

Sidgwick, Henry. (1907). [1981]. *The Methods of Ethics* – 7th edition. Indianapolis: Hackett.

Singer, Peter. ed. (1990. *A Companion to Ethics*. Oxford: Blackwell.

Singer, Peter. ed. (1994). *Ethics*. Oxford: Oxford University Press.

Singer, Peter. (1995). *Rethinking Life and Death: The Collapse of Our Traditional Ethics*. New York: St Martin's Press.

Stanford Encyclopedia of Philosophy. Check, for instance its entry on Theory and Bioethics. https://plato.stanford.edu/entries/theory-bioethics/ (*or* Singer 1991, Part VI: *The Nature of Ethics*).

Valles, Sean A. (2015). Bioethics and the framing of climate change's health risks. *Bioethics* 29(5): 334–341.

Chapter 2: Ethical Theory

Johnson, Robert and Cureton, Adam (2016). Kant's moral philosophy. In: *The Stanford Encyclopedia of Philosophy* (Fall 2016 Edition). (ed. Edward N. Zalta) http://plato.stanford.edu/archives/fall2016/entries/kant-moral/.

LaFollette, Hugh. (ed. 2013). *The International Encyclopedia of Ethics. Vol 1–9.* Oxford: Wiley-Blackwell.

McMillan, John. (2018). *The Methods of Bioethics: An Essay in Meta-Bioethics.* Oxford: Oxford University Press.

Smart, J.J.C. and Bernard Williams. (1973). *Utilitarianism: For and Against.* Cambridge: Cambridge University Press.

Chapter 3: Basics of Bioethics

History and Scope

Baker, Robert B. and Laurence B. McCullough (eds). (2009). *The Cambridge World History of Medical Ethics.* Cambridge: Cambridge University Press.

Benatar, David. (2005). The trouble with universal declarations. *Developing World Bioethics* 5: 220–224.

CIHR, NSERC, SSHRC. 2010. *Tri-Council Policy Statement: Ethical Conduct for Research Involving Humans.* Ottawa. https://ethics.gc.ca/eng/policy-politique_tcps2-eptc2_2018.html

Jennings, Bruce. (ed.) (2014). *Encyclopedia of Bioethics,* 4th edition. Farmington Hills, MI: Gale.

Singer, Peter. (1975). *Animal Liberation,* 2nd edition. New York: New York Review of Books.

Singer, Peter and Bernard Unti. (2014). Animal Research – Philosophical Issues. In: *Policy Advice* Bayertz, Kurt. (ed.). (1994). *The Concept of Moral Consensus.* Springer-Kluwer: Dordrecht.

Fallacious Arguments

Damer, Edward T. (2013). *Attacking Faulty Reasoning: A Practical Guide to Fallacy-Free Arguments.* Boston: Wadsworth.

DelaPlante, Kevin. (2010). Fallacies: Slippery Slope. ww.youtube.com/watch?v=DtmAw9Ia7LA/

Perelman, Chaim. (1990). *The Realm of Rhetoric.* Notre Dame: Notre Dame University Press.

Vaughn, Lewis and Jillian Scott McIntosh. (2013). *Writing Philosophy – A Guide for Canadian Students.* New York: Oxford University Press.

Chapter 4: Moral Standing: What Matters

Barad, Judith and Ed Robertson. (2001). *The Ethics of Star Trek*. New York: Harper Perennial.

Decker, Kevin S and Jason T. Eberl. (eds). 2008. *Star Trek and Philosophy: The Wrath of Kant*. Chicago: Open Court.

Levy, David. (2009). The ethical treatment of artificially conscious robots. *International Journal of Social Robotics* 1(3): 209–216.

Resnik, David. (2001). *Environmental Health Ethics*. New York: Cambridge University Press.

Rowland, Martin. (2009). *Animal Rights: Moral Theory and Practice*, 2nd edition. Palgrave/MacMillan: New York.

Chapter 5: Beginning of Life

Frith, L. and E. Blyth. (2013). They can't have my embryo: the ethics of conditional embryo donation. *Bioethics* 27(6): 317–324.

Frith, Lucy. (2013). Donor conception and mandatory paternity testing: the right to know and the right to be told. *American Journal of Bioethics* 13(5): 50–52.

Harris, John and Holm, Søren. (1998). *The Future of Human Reproduction: Ethics, Choice and Regulation*. Oxford: University Press.

Horsey, Kirsty. (2015). *Revisiting the Regulation of Human Fertilisation and Embryology*. London: Routledge.

Overall, Christine. (1987). *Ethics and Human Reproduction: a Feminist Analysis*. Boston: Allen & Unwin.

Chapter 6: Health Care Professional Patient Relationship

Buchanan, Allen E. and Dan W. Brock. (1989). *Deciding for Others: The Ethics of Surrogate Decision-Making*. Cambridge: Cambridge University Press.

Emanuel, Linda L., Barry, Michael J., Stoeckle, John D., Ettelson, Lucy M., et al. (1991). Advance directives for medical care: a case for greater use. *New England Journal of Medicine* 324: 889–895.

Pellegrino, Edmund. (2002). The physician's conscience, conscience clauses, and religious belief: a Catholic perspective. *Fordham Urban Law Journal* 30: 221–244.

Singer, Peter A., Benatar, Solomon R., Bernstein, Mark, Daar, Abdallah S., et al. (2003). Ethics and SARS: Lessons from Toronto. *BMJ (British Medical Journal)* 327: 1342.

Tarasoff v. Regents of University of California, 551 P.2d 334 (Cal. 1976).

Weinstock, Daniel. (2014). Conscientious refusal and healthcare professionals: does religion make a difference? *Bioethics* 28: 8–15.

Chapter 7: Research Ethics

Barsdorf, Nicola, Maman, Suzanne, Kass, Nancy, and Catherine Slack. (2010). Access to Treatment in Prevention Trials: Perspectives from a South African Community. *Developing World Bioethics* 10: 78–87.

Emanuel, Ezekiel J, Grady, Christine, Crouch, Robert A, Lie, Reidar K, Miller, Franklin G., and David Wendler (eds). (2008). *The Oxford Textbook of Clinical Research Ethics*. New York: Oxford University Press.

London, Alex J. (2005). Justice and the Human Development Approach to International Research. *Hastings Center Report* 35(1): 24–37.

Macklin, Ruth. (1999). *Against Relativism: Cultural Diversity and the Search for Ethical Universals in Medicine*. New York: Oxford University Press.

Presidential Commission for the Study of Bioethical Issues. (2011). *Moral Sciences: Protecting Participants in Human Subjects Research*. Washington, DC. https:// bioethicsarchive.georgetown.edu/pcsbi/sites/default/files/Moral%20 Science%20June%202012.pdf

Schüklenk, Udo. (2000). Protecting the vulnerable: testing times for clinical research ethics. *Social Science and Medicine* 51: 969–977.

Chapter 8: Genetics

Bunnik, E.M., de Jong, A., Nijsingh, N, and de Wert, G.M. (2013). The new genetics and informed consent: differentiating choice to preserve autonomy. *Bioethics* 27(6): 348–355.

Burley, Justine and Harris, John. (2002). *A Companion to Genethics*. Oxford: Wiley Blackwell.

Fiore, R.N. and Goodman, K.W. (2016). Precision medicine ethics: selected issues and developments in next-generation sequencing, clinical oncology, and ethics. *Current Opinion in Oncology* 28(2): 83–87.

Gibbon, Sahra, Prainsack, Barbara, Hilgartner, Stephen, and Lamoreaux, Janelle. (2018). *The Routledge Handbook of Genomics, Health and Society*. London: Routledge.

Kumar, Dhavendra and Chadwick, Ruth (eds). (2015). *Genomics and Society: Ethical, Legal, Cultural and Socioeconomic Implications*. Elsevier.

Sabatello, M. (2017). Precision medicine, health disparities, and ethics: the case for disability inclusion. *Genetics in Medicine* 20: 397–399.

Scully, Jackie Leach. (2008). Disability and genetics in the era of genomic medicine. *Nature Reviews Genetics* 9: 797–802.

Chapter 9: Enhancement

Agar, Nicholas. (2004). *Liberal Eugenics*: In *Defence of Human Enhancement*. Oxford: Wiley-Blackwell.

Blackford, Russell. (2014). *Humanity Enhanced: Genetic Choice and the Challenge for Liberal Democracies*. Cambridge, MA: MIT Press.

Bostrom, Nick. (2009). The Future of Humanity. *Geopolitics, History and International Relations* 1(2): 41–78.

Giubilini, Alberto., Sanyal, Sagar. (2015). The ethics of human enhancement. *Philosophy Compass* 10 (4): 233–243.

Savulescu, Julian., Bostrum, Nick (eds) (2009). *Human Enhancement*. Oxford: Oxford University Press.

Ter Meulen, Ruud., Mohamed, Ahmed Dahir, and Hall, Wayne. (2017). *Rethinking Cognitive Enhancement*. Oxford: Oxford University Press.

Chapter 10: Mental Health

Barker, Phil. (2010). *Mental Health Ethics: the Human Context*. Abingdon: Routledge.

Bloch, Sidney, and Stephen A. Green. (eds) (2009). *Psychiatric Ethics*, 4th edition. Oxford: University Press.

Callard, Felicity. (2014). Psychiatric diagnosis: the indispensability of ambivalence. *Journal of Medical Ethics* 40: 526–530.

Dupré, John. (1998). Normal people. *Social Research* 665 (2): 221–249.

Glover, J. (1977). *Causing Death and Saving Lives*. Harmondsworth: Penguin.

Lindley, Richard. (1986). *Autonomy*. Houndmills: Macmillan.

Radden, Jennifer (ed,) (2004).*The Philosophy of Psychiatry: a Companion*. Oxford: Oxford University Press.

Radden, Jennifer, and John Sadler. (2009). *The Virtuous Psychiatrist: Character Ethics in Psychiatric Practice*. Oxford: Oxford University Press.

Chapter 11: End-of-Life Issues

Benatar, David. 2010. Assisted suicide, voluntary euthanasia, and the right to life. In: Yorke, Jon (ed.). *The Right to Life and the Value of Life: Orientations in Law, Politics and Ethics*. Aldershot, UK: Ashgate: 291–310.

Butler, Martha and Nicol, Julia, Tiedeman, Marlisa and Dominique Valiquet. (2013). Library of Parliament Background Paper: Euthanasia and Assisted Suicide in Canada. February 15. http://publications.gc.ca/collections/collection_2013/bdp-lop/bp/2010-68-1-eng.pdf?/

Dworkin, Ronald, Nagel, Thomas, Nozick, Robert, Rawls, John, Scanlon, Thomas and Judith Jarvis Thomson. (1997). Assisted Suicide: The Philosophers' Brief. New York Review of Books March 27.

Foot, Philippa. (1977). Euthanasia. *Philosophy and Public Affairs* 6(2): 85–112. www.nybooks.com/articles/archives/1997/mar/27/assisted-suicide-the-philosophers-brief/?pagination=false/

Kelley, Amy S. and R. Sean Morrison. (2015). Palliative care for the seriously ill. *New England Journal of Medicine* 373: 747–755. doi: 10.1056/NEJMra1404684.

National Library of Medicine. (2002). Hippocratic Oath (translated by Michael North). https://www.nlm.nih.gov/hmd/greek/greek_oath.html

World Medical Association. (2019). WMA Declaration on Euthanasia and Physician-Assisted Suicide. https://www.wma.net/policies-post/declaration-on-euthanasia-and-physician-assisted-suicide/

Chapter 12: Justice

Chadwick, Ruth and O'Connor, Alan. (2015). Ethical theory and global challenges. In: *The Routledge Handbook of Global Ethics* (eds Darrel Moellendorf and Heather Widdows), 24–34. Abingdon: Routledge.

Dickenson, Donna. (2002). *Risk and Luck in Medical Ethics*. Cambridge: Polity Press.

Dworkin, Ronald. (2013). *Justice for Hedgehogs*. Cambridge, Mass: Belknap Press.

Miller, David. (2001). *Principles of Social Justice*. Harvard: University Press.

Nozick, Robert. (1974). *Anarchy, State and Utopia*. New York: Basic Books.

O'Neill, Onora. (2000). *Bounds of Justice*. Cambridge: University Press.

Pogge, Thomas. (2002). *World Poverty and Human Rights*. Cambridge: Polity Press.

Sandel, Michael. (2010). *Justice: What's the Right Thing to Do?* New York: Farrar, Strauss and Giroux.

Sen, Amartya. (2009). *The Idea of Justice*. Harvard: University Press.

ter Meulen, Ruud. (2015). Solidarity and justice in health care: a critical analysis of their relationship. *Diametros* 43: 1–20.

Walzer, Michael. (1983). *Spheres of Justice: A Defense of Pluralism and Equality*. New York: Basic Books.

Chapter 13: Population Health

Bayer, Ronald. (1992). AIDS and Liberalism: A Response to Patricia Illingworth. *Bioethics* 6: 23–27.

Bogart, W.A. (2014). *Regulating obesity? Government, Society and Questions of Health*. Toronto: Oxford University Press.

Illingworth, Patricia. (1990). Review Essay: *Private Acts and Social Consequences*. *Bioethics* 4: 340–350.

Illingworth, Patricia. (1992). Bayer revisited. *Bioethics* 6: 28–34.

Macklin, Ruth. (2012). *Ethics in Global Health: Research, Policy, and Practice*. Oxford: Oxford University Press.

Moellendorf, Darrel and Heather Widdows (eds). (2015). *The Routledge Handbook of Global Ethics*. London: Routledge.

Mosse, George L. (2003). *Nazi Culture: Intellectual, Cultural, and Social Life in the Third Reich*. Madison, WI: University of Wisconsin Press.

Rodger, Alison J., Cambiano, Valentina, Bruun, Tina, Vernazza, Pietro, Collins, Simon, et al. (2016). Sexual activity without condoms and risk of HIV transmission in serodifferent couples when the HIV-positive partner is using suppressive antiretroviral therapy. *JAMA* 316: 171–181.

Schüklenk, Udo and Anita Kleinschmidt. (2006). North-south benefit-sharing arrangements in bioprospecting and genetic research: a critical ethical and legal analysis. *Developing World Bioethics* 6: 122–134.

Schüklenk, Udo and Anita Kleinsmidt. (2007). Rethinking mandatory HIV testing during pregnancy in areas with high HIV prevalence rates: Ethical and policy issues. *American Journal of Public Health* 97: 1179–1183.

Selgelid, Michael J, Battin, Margaret P., and Charles B. Smith. (2006). *Ethics and Infectious Disease*. Oxford: Blackwell.

Wynberg, Rachel, Schroeder, Doris, and Roger Chennells. (eds.) (2009). *Indigenous Peoples, Consent and Benefit-Sharing*. Dordrecht: Springer.

INDEX

Abnormal, 47
Abortion, 12, 41, 69, 70, 79, 82, 83, 86
  and fetal transplants, 83, 84
  impairment argument, 82
  and virtue ethics, 82, 83
Acts and omissions, 87, 88
Advance directive, 97, 201
AI (Artificial Intelligence), 66
AMA (American Medical Association), 6
  on law and ethics, 10
Animals, 38, 61–64, 119, 120
APA (American Psychiatric Association), 40
  and homosexuality, 40
Aquinas, Thomas, 47
Aristotle, 21, 24, 32, 172, 175, 182, 243
ASBH (American Society for Bioethics and Humanities), 43, 91

Assisted Dying, 195, 202, 209
  burden on others, 198
  quality of life, 199, 200
Autonomy, 31, 80, 97, 149, 169, 174, 182, 186, 188–190, 203, 205, 206, 224
  dispositional, 190
  relational, 73
  reproductive, 70
  and responsibility, 224
  thick, 149

Baker, Robert, 6, 39
Bayer, Ronald, 247, 248
Beecher, Henry K., 40
Beneficence, 31, 96, 188
  procreative, 71
Bentham, Jeremy, 26, 62, 63
Biobanks, 147
Biocentrism, 64

This Is Bioethics: An Introduction, First Edition. Ruth F. Chadwick and Udo Schüklenk.
© 2021 John Wiley & Sons, Inc. Published 2021 by John Wiley & Sons, Inc.

Bioethics
  definition, 38
  Nazi arguments, 51
Brain death, 100
Buchanan, Allen, 98

Capabilities approach, 64, 231
Capacity (decisional), 186, 187
Categorical Imperative, 30, 55,
  121, 204, 208
Chadwick, Ruth R., 137, 146,
  149, 185
Clinical ethics, 39, 91
Cloning, 48, 151
  reproductive human,
    48, 153
  therapeutic human, 151
Communicable disease, 243, 253
Confidentiality, 22, 105–107
Conscientious objection, 107
Consequentialism, 71, 80, 84,
  85, 87, 92, 98, 100, 103–
  105, 112, 122, 155, 237, 238
Contractualism, 18, 34, 111,
  253–255
Coronavirus, 248–251
  ethical societal response,
    250, 251
CRISPR, 144

DALY (disability-adjusted life
  year), 181, 226
Daniels, Norman, 34, 35, 111,
  164–166, 229, 231
Declaration of Geneva, 49, 50,
  105, 112

Declaration of Helsinki, 116
Depression, 181, 185, 186
Developing country, 1, 123, 124,
  130, 237
Dignity, 48–51
Disability, 78, 140
  infant, 86
Dresser, Rebecca, 98
Duty-to-treat, 110, 111,
  249–250
  COVID, 249–250
  HIV, 111, 112
  SARS, 111

Embryo, 79, 153
  and personhood, 79
Emergency assistance, 1
End of Life, 195, 202
Enhancement, 159
  cognitive, 176
  and improvement, 161
  and justice, 184
  moral, 173
  quantitative account of, 164
  and species-normal
    functioning, 164
  and therapy, 163
  umbrella view of, 165
Environment, 38
Ethics, 1
  and animals, 38, 61–64,
    119, 120
  capabilities, 64
  care, 24
  feminist, 23–25
  and God, 7

impartialist, 25
and law, 9–13
and public health, 41
purpose of, 2, 4
and relativism, 13
and religion, 6–8
of research, 115
rule-based, 29, 30
utilitarian, 25–28
and virtues, 21–23
Euthanasia, 202
Euthyphro, 7

Fair innings (argument of),
    197
Fallacy, 48
naturalistic, 48
Feinberg, Joel, 11, 95, 96
Feminist ethics, 23, 73, 185
Fetus, 72, 79–82, 138
Fundraising, 1

Gene editing, 46, 73, 144
playing God, 46
Gene therapy, 135, 140–144
germline, 142–146, 160
Genetic relatedness, 75
children's right to know, 76
Genetics, 135
exceptionalism, 136
right not to know, 137
screening, 139, 140
testing and counseling,
    137, 138
Georgetown Mantra
    (Principlism), 31, 96

and public health ethics,
    256–258
Gilligan, Carol, 24
Global south, 237
God, 7, 46, 47
playing God, 46, 47, 77, 144
Groningen Protocol, 86, 87

Habermas, Jürgen, 169, 170
Hardwig, John, 23, 29, 198,
    199, 219
Harris, John, 166, 168, 197, 198
Health, 230, 235
aid obligations, 236, 237
definition of, 230
global, 235
value of, 242
Health care (right to), 228,
    229, 231
Hegel, Georg Wilhelm
    Friedrich, 24
Hendricks, Perry, 82
Heterotaxy syndrome, 87, 88
HGP (Human Genome Project),
    146, 147
Hippocratic Oath, 3, 21, 214
HIV, 106, 107, 111, 112, 119,
    122, 127–130, 145, 232,
    244, 253–255
deterrence, 246, 247
transmission, 244–246
Holism, 65
Homosexuality, 40, 47, 116,
    131, 183
Hume, David, 48, 174
Hursthouse, Rosalind, 23, 82

Illingworth, Patricia, 254, 255
Infanticide, 80, 85–88
    heterotaxy syndrome, 87, 88
Informed consent, 92–96, 116,
    117, 121, 128, 130, 143,
    148, 149, 186, 205
Interest, best, 182, 186, 188
Involuntary (definition of), 202
IVF (in-vitro fertilization),
    40, 74

Johnson, Michael, 244–246, 248
Justice, 32, 170, 171, 217
    and discrimination, 218
    distributive, 32, 219
    and equality, 222
    and exploitation, 220
    needs based, 225
    and personalized medicine,
        233
    procedural, 220

Kant, Immanuel, 24, 29, 30, 47,
    55, 64, 103, 121, 155, 174,
    190, 203, 207, 208, 228
Kass, Leon R., 30, 154
Kuhse, Helga, 37, 38, 86, 99

Law, 9–13
    and ethics, 9–11
Little, Margaret, 25
Lowry, Christopher, 238,
    239, 242

Marquis, Don, 61, 81
McMahan, Jeff, 86

McMath, Jahi, 100
Means, treating someone as a
    mere, 55, 121
Medical ethics, 39, 108
Meilander, Gilbert, 87
Mental health, 181
Metaethics, 4
Mill, John Stuart, 26, 189
Moral, 59, 60
    standing, 59, 60, 67
    status, 59, 60, 67

Nazis, 51–53, 115, 125, 126, 136
NCD (non-communicable
    disease), 256
Neuroethics, 41
NGO (non-governmental
    organization), 1, 2, 16, 28
Nicomachean Ethics, 21
Non-identity problem, 72, 73
Non-maleficence, 31
Non-voluntary (definition of),
    202
Nuremberg Code, 116, 117,
    121, 122
Nussbaum, Martha, 64, 231

Oakley, Justin, 23
Obesity, 256

Palliative care, 195, 196,
    209, 211
Pappworth, Maurice H., 40
Parfit, Derek, 72, 243
Paternalism, 31, 96, 103
Patient, 105

Pence, Gregory E., 153–155
Persistent vegetative state, 100
Personhood, 61, 67, 72, 79,
    80, 204
  and embryos, 79
Plato, 3, 6, 7, 174
Pogge, Thomas, 236, 239
Population health, 240
Principlism (Georgetown
    Mantra), 31
Privacy, 105, 149, 221
Procreative beneficence, 71,
    72, 78
  criticism of, 72
Professionalism, 39, 41, 42, 91,
    92, 108–110, 213
  and conscientious objection,
    107–110
  and duty to treat, 110
Public health, 240
  criticism of, 241, 242
  definition of, 241
  ethics, 247, 248, 253–258
  promotion, 253–258
Public reason, 8

QALY (quality-adjusted life
    year), 226–228

Rasouli, Hassan, 100, 101
Rawls, John, 34, 229
Regan, Tom, 61, 62, 120
Relativism (ethical), 13, 39
Religion, 4
  and ethics, 4
  and secular state, 8–9

Reproduction, 69–88
  assisted, 74–79
  procreative liberty, 70
Research ethics, 40, 115–133,
    145, 146, 218
  CIOMS guidelines, 44,
    45, 130
  elements of, 117
  standards of care, 131
Resource (health care), 1
  allocation, 219, 238, 239
  efficiency, 1
Rights, 12, 13
  legal and moral, 12, 13
  negative and positive, 12

Savior siblings, 84, 85
Savulescu, Julian, 71, 72, 78, 110,
    145, 146, 172
Schüklenk, Udo, 87, 92, 110,
    196, 213, 238, 242, 250
Sentientism, 62–65, 120
Sex selection, 77
Siegler, Mark, 107
Simpson, James, 39
Sims, J. Marion, 39
Singer, Peter, 16, 18, 37, 38,
    51–53, 62, 86, 99, 120, 145,
    146, 172, 237
Slippery-slope, 51, 53, 88, 154,
    202, 208–213
  causal arguments, 54
  conceptual arguments, 53
Socrates, 3, 7
Sophist, 3
Sparrow, Robert, 167, 171

Suicide, 189–191, 207
  assisted (definition of), 202
Sulmasy, Daniel, 107, 108
Surrogacy, 71, 220
Szasz, Thomas, 40, 182–184

Tarasoff, Tatiana, 105, 106
Thomson, Judith Jarvis, 81
Tooley, Michael, 61, 62, 80, 86
Tradition (arguments from),
  213–215
Transgender, 71, 218
Truth telling, 102–104

Ubuntu, 67
UNESCO, 50
  Declaration on Bioethics and
    Human Rights, 50
Unnatural, 47
Utilitarianism, 25, 62–64, 120,
  155, 203, 225, 237, 253
  act utilitarianism, 26
  preference utilitarianism,
    27, 198
  rule utilitarianism, 26

Vaccines, 251
  coercive policies, ethics of,
    253, 254
  free-rider phenomenon, 252
Veatch, Robert M., 3, 33
Ventakapuram, Sridhar,
  230, 232
Virtue ethics, 21–23, 73, 82,
  182, 243
Voluntary (definition of), 202

Warnock, Mary, 75, 79, 80
WHO (World Health
  Association), 3, 97,
  181, 230
Wicclair, Mark, 108
Williams, Bernard, 13,
  14, 225
WMA (World Medical
  Association), 3, 49, 50, 105,
  112, 214
  Declaration of Geneva, 49, 50,
    105, 112
  Declaration of Helsinki, 116,
    117